The Management of Head and Neck Cancer

Edited by
J.E. Hamner, III

With Contributions by
L.W. Brady S.K. Choksi L.W. Davis J.B. Drane
J.E. Hamner, III J.M. Lore, Jr. D.P. Shedd

With a Foreword by Th. E. Malone

With 248 Figures, Partly in Colour

Springer-Verlag
Berlin Heidelberg NewYork Tokyo 1984

James E. Hamner, III, Ph.D.
The University of Tennessee
Center for the Health Sciences
Hyman Building, Room 316
62 South Dunlap
Memphis, Tennessee 38163, USA

ISBN-13: 978-3-642-69651-0 e-ISBN-13: 978-3-642-69649-7
DOI: 10-1007/978-3-642-69649-7

Library of Congress Cataloging in Publication Data. Main entry under title: The Management of head and neck cancer. Includes bibliographical references and index. 1. Head – Cancer – Treatment. 2. Neck – Cancer – Treatment. I. Hamner, James E. II. Brady, Luther W., 1925–. [DNLM: 1. Head and Neck Neoplasms WE 707 M2664]
RC280.H4M27 1984 616.99′4 84-10530
ISBN-13: 978-3-642-69651-0

Softcover reprint of the hardcover 1st edition 1984

Typesetting, printing and bookbinding: Universitätsdruckerei H. Stürtz AG, Würzburg
2122/3130-543210

Dedicated to Joan

List of Contributors

BRADY, LUTHER W., M.D., Professor and Chairman, Department of Radiation Oncology & Nuclear Medicine, College of Medicine, Hahnemann University, Philadelphia, Pennsylvania, USA

CHOKSI, SOLI K., B.D.S., M.S., Assistant Professor, Department of Oral Diagnosis & Radiology, College of Dentistry, Howard University, Washington, D.C., USA

DAVIS, LAWRENCE W., M.D., Professor of Radiation Therapy, College of Medicine, Thomas Jefferson University, Philadelphia, Pennsylvania, USA

DRANE, JOE B., D.D.S., Professor of Dental Oncology, M.D. Anderson Hospital & Tumor Institute, University of Texas System Cancer Center, Houston, Texas, USA

HAMNER, III, JAMES E., D.D.S., M.S., Ph.D., M.B.A., Executive Assistant to the Chancellor, University of Tennessee Center for the Health Sciences, Professor of Pathology, College of Medicine, Professor of Oral Pathology, College of Dentistry, Memphis, Tennessee, USA

U.S. Public Health Service, National Cancer Institute (1973–1982), National Institutes of Health, Bethesda, Maryland, USA

LORE, JOHN M., JR., M.D., Professor and Chairman, Department of Otolaryngology, School of Medicine, State University of New York at Buffalo, Buffalo, New York, USA

SHEDD, DONALD P., M.D., Chief, Department of Head & Neck Surgery and Oncology Roswell Park Memorial Institute, Buffalo, New York, USA

Foreword

Statistically speaking, head and neck cancer per se (excluding melanoma and basal cell carcinoma) does not outwardly seem to pose a serious threat – 27,500/870,000 total cancer cases estimated for 1984 (or 3.2% of all cancers) and 9,350/450,000 total cancer deaths in 1984 (or 2.1%) for the United States. Yet in clinical practice, by the time that diagnosis is made, more than 60% of oral cancers have already spread to the nearby lymph node system. And while the overall five-year survival rate for localized oral cancer is 67%, this rate decreases drastically to only 25% when the original cancer has metastasized.

Scientific textbooks all too often are merely a compilation of discrete parts, rather than a correlated, integrated whole. Dr. Hamner and his colleagues have achieved such an integrated, succinct version in *The Management of Head and Neck Cancer*.

The outstanding group of contributors bring to the book a wealth of accumulated knowledge and expertise in their various cancer specialty disciplines. They are associated with some of the most distinguished cancer centers in the United States.

This concise book has been carefully arranged and logically organized with descriptive chapters on etiology/epidemiology, detection, diagnosis, pretreatment evaluation, treatment, follow-up, and rehabilitation. Each segment represents a vital component in comprehensive, multidisciplinary management of the head and neck cancer patient as a whole person. It concludes with five different, interesting, and unusual clinical cases that are well-documented and are of excellent teaching value.

The 248 illustrations are of surpassing quality, both microscopically and macroscopically, for use as teaching, educational examples, especially in the chapter on cancer diagnosis. These contribute immense strength and validity to the book. Also of tremendous value to the oncology clinician is the section on "Departure from Sound Management Practices" in the pretreatment evaluation chapter.

This book should have wide appeal to both the dental and medical specialties that relate to all phases of cancer management. It is both a pertinent, practical resource guide for clinicians and a clear, stimulating textbook for residents and students.

The authors are to be congratulated on this meaningful, scientific endeavor which has been compiled, organized, and edited with refined professional competence, combined with organizational skills of a high order.

Thomas E. Malone, Ph.D., Deputy Director
National Institutes of Health, Bethesda, Maryland USA

Preface

Even though an enormous amount of scientific endeavor and public attention has been rivoted on both basic cancer research and clinical investigations over the past four decades, it is still tremendously difficult to comprehend the broad topic of "cancer", because this area of science continues to expand and change rapidly.

Just as any doctor is the sum total of all knowledge imparted by his academic learning regimen, his exposure to clinical experiences, the influence of his professors and mentors, and the special repoire developed with his patients – this book represents the accumulation of knowledge and experience in head and neck cancer management, garnered over many years by its various contributors, who have labored to present it in as correlated, cohensive, and beneficial fashion as possible.

In 1903, Sir William Osler stated: "The practice of medicine is an art, not a trade; a calling, not a business; a calling in which your heart will be exercised equally with your head." His sound advice is even more appropriate today in our fast changing world of computerized technology. Patients are individuals, and each one must be cared for – not just treated as a number – accordingly. Often, the best treatment concensus will be a balanced application of several treatment modalities, specifically geared for each unique patient.

It is our hope that this particular book will convey that philosophy – that it will be both appealing and practically useful to many of the various specialties in dentistry, medicine, nursing, and the other health care professions who care for head and neck cancer patients.

I wish to express my personal sincere appreciation to the fine fellow-contributors: Doctors Luther W. Brady, Soli K. Choksi, Lawrence W. Davis, Joe B. Drane, John M. Lore, Jr., and Donald P. Shedd for bringing this extensive project to a fruitful conclusion. The arduous task of typing the manuscripts in final form with accuracy, outstanding quality, and dedication to high standards was performed in exemplary fashion by Mrs. Betty Swerda.

A special debt of gratitude is owed to those persons who have aided in the painstaking review of all manuscript segments, and also to our publisher, Mr. Bergstedt of Springer-Verlag, for his able assistance and useful advice on all aspects of publishing this volume.

Lastly, I wish to thank my family for their warm support and encouragement, understanding, and patience during the lengthy time of writing and editing this work.

James Edward Hamner, III, D.D.S., Ph.D.
Memphis, Tennessee

Table of Contents

Introduction

James E. Hamner, III

I. General Remarks

Oral cancer is one of the most mutilating, fatal diseases afflicting mankind. It is estimated that 27,500 new cases will be diagnosed in 1984, and 9,350 Americans will die from oral cancer in 1984 [1].

Cancer itself is actually a group of diseases, found in all races and ages of man and in all other animal species. Marked differences do exist in the occurrence of cancer by both anatomic site and histopathological type within human populations. In the past, cancer has often been thought of as a single disease, and in a broad manner of interpreation, one could describe it as a single disease, in the limited sense of definition that all cancers are characterized by uncontrolled growth of cells. Typically, these unrestrained, immature cells develop into tumors which in turn compress, invade, and destroy normal tissues, eventually leading to death, if untreated.

Malignant neoplasms share four common characteristics: (1) a higher rate of cell growth than the normal tissue from which the cancer was derived, (2) failure to maintain the boundaries of normal tissues and organs, (3) a microscopic appearance of immaturity, and (4) a tendency to metastasize to distant parts of the body (2). While not all of these features necessarily accompany every malignant tumor, they are eventually typical for most forms of cancer.

The term "oral cancer" is an extremely ambiguous one and therefore is subject to numerous interpretations in its definition. In 1973 the World Health Organization's International Classification of Diseases Related to Dentistry and Stomatology listed 57 malignant neoplasms and 88 benign neoplasms or tumor-like conditions of the oral cavity and pharynx [3].

"Head and neck cancer" is likewise a misnomer, since brain tumors and eye tumors are customarily not included in the usual clinical understanding of this term. Also, skin tumors, e.g. basal cell carcinoma and cutaneous malignant melanoma, are frequently excluded from this grouping of upper respiratory and alimentary passage tumors [4].

Squamous cell carcinoma is the most common malignant neoplasm occurring in the oral cavity, so therefore, it will receive greater emphasis in this book, since it is the most frequent "oral" malignancy that the dentist/physician will likely encounter in clinical practice. Basal cell carcinoma, melanoma, salivary gland tumors, odontogenic tumors, and fibro-osseous tumors will be covered in this work. Together, these tumors constitute the generic term, "oral cancer", in the broadest sense and in the most general fashion.

II. Anatomy

For purposes of clinical-stage classification, the oral cavity is considered as one anatomic region, extending from the vermillion borders of the lips to the junction of the hard and soft palate above and to the line of the circumvallate papillae below [5]. It is divided into the following specific sites:

1. Lips (Upper and Lower)

The lips form the upper and lower anterior walls of the oral cavity and are composed of the mucosa from the mucocutaneous junction to the line of contact of the opposing lips, including the commissures. They may be subdivided into upper and lower lips, and right and left commissures.

2. Buccal Mucosa

Buccal mucosa includes all the membranes lining the inner surface of the cheeks and lips, from the line of contact of the opposing lips to the line of attachment of mucosa of the alveolar ridge (upper and lower) and the pterygomandibular raphe.

3. Lower Alveolar Ridge

This ridge includes the alveolar process of the mandible and its covering mucosa, which extends from the line of attachment of mucosa in the buccal gutter to the line of free mucosa of the floor of the mouth. Posteriorly, it extends to the ascending ramus of the mandible.

4. Upper Alveolar Ridge

The upper ridge is the alveolar process of the maxilla and its covering mucosa, which extends from the line of attachment of mucosa in the upper gingival buccal gutter to the junction of the hard palate. Its posterior margin is the upper end of the pterygopalatine arch.

5. Retromolar Gingiva (Retromolar Trigone)

This area is the attached mucosa overlying the ascending ramus of the mandible from the level of the posterior surface of the last molar tooth to the apex superiorly adjacent to the tuberosity of the maxilla.

6. Floor of the Mouth

This is a semilunar space over the mylohyoid and hypoglossus muscles, extending from the inner surface of the lower alveolar ridge to the undersurface of the tongue. Its posterior boundary is the base of the anterior pillar of the tonsil. It is divided into two sides by the frenulum of the tongue and contains the ostia of the submaxillary and sublingual salivary glands.

7. Hard Palate

This is the semilunar area between the upper alveolar ridges and the mucous membrane, covering the palatine process of the maxillary palatine bones. It extends from the inner surface of the superior alveolar ridge to the posterior edge of the palatine bone.

8. Anterior Two-Thirds of the Tongue

This is a freely mobile portion of the tongue which extends anteriorly from the line of circumvallate papillae to the undersurface of the tongue at the junction of the floor of the mouth. It is composed of four areas: the tip, the lateral borders, the dorsum, and the non-villous undersurface [5].

The arrangement of the management of head and neck cancer per se will be divided into seven broad sections:

I. Etiology and Epidemiology
II. Detection
III. Diagnosis
IV. Pre-Treatment Evaluation
V. Treatment
VI. Follow-up
VII. Rehabilitation

To conclude, a series of five case examples are presented.

III. Purpose

The purpose of this book is to collate basic background information in these seven areas and to present management approaches of steps and procedures customarily taken, and considerations involved, in the management of head and neck cancer. In the portions related to treatment and rehabilitation, there is no intent to subvert the broad exercise of sound clinical judgement by each dentist/physician in relation to his individual patient care, which of course, must be tailored to the overall needs and condition of each patient.

References

1. Silverberg, E.: "Cancer Statistics, 1984", CA – A Cancer Journal for Clinicians 34:7–23, 1984
2. Lynch, M.A.: Oral Medicine, Ed. 7, (J.B. Lippincott Co.: Philadelphia, Pa.), 1977
3. W.H.O. International Classification of Diseases Related to Dentistry and Stomatology, (W.H.O.: Geneva, Switzerland), 1973
4. Holland, J.F. and Frei, E., III: Cancer Medicine, (Lea & Febiger: Philadelphia, Pa.), 1973
5. Hamner, J.E., III: Management Guidelines for Head & Neck Cancer, (N.I.H. Publication #80-2037), 1979

Chapter 1. Etiology and Epidemiology

JAMES E. HAMNER, III

I. Overview

It is neither the purpose nor the intention of this chapter to become involved in a lengthy discussion concerning the merits, pros, and cons, etc., of the various theories regarding cancer formation. However, it is felt that a few general remarks are in order prior to delving more deeply into the better known, suggested predisposing factors that have related, rightly or wrongly, with head and neck cancer.

Over many years of basic and clinical research, the concept of neoplasia has changed from that of a single disease entity, involving a single causative agent or a single common intracellular mechanism, to that concept of a general disease category that embraces a multiplicity of diseased states [1–3]. Thus, cancer can be caused by a wide variety of agents (carcinogens), which may be chemical physical, viral, and/or hormonal.

One theory that seems most applicable, when thinking in terms of these known carcinogenic agents, is the deletion biochemical theory, which hypothesizes an irreparable loss of intracellular factors related to histological structure and associated functional specialities [4]. Basically, this theory states that within the cell there is an immediate deletion of certain vital protein constituents through direct binding with carcinogenic chemicals, thereby removing these proteins from the intracellular interacting system. Therefore, they are not able to undergo normal replication in subsequent mitoses and are irretrievably lost to all future descendent cells. The absence of these components deprives the affected cells of the normal restraining and control mechanisms necessary for normal cell growth. Lacking this restraint, the affected cells can grow without host control and exhibit the classical behavior of malignant cells [4–7].

Cancer has been induced in laboratory animals and in man by many agents, including chemicals, viruses, and irradiation. It is thought that these carcinogenic agents may interact with one or more human host factors, including age, sex, hormone balance, immune status, and/or genetic structure, to cause cancer per se [8]. However, many cancers would not develop if certain substances were not present in the host's environment. Some investigators believe that environmental factors, such as: (A) work place or occupational exposure, (B) life-style habits, (C) iatrogenic exposures, and (D) general environmental exposures are implicated and may contribute to 80% of all cancers – others disagree with such a high estimate [8, 9].

Any discussion of this mix of internal and external factors that may induce cancer in various combinations, leads one to the concept of co-carcinogenesis.

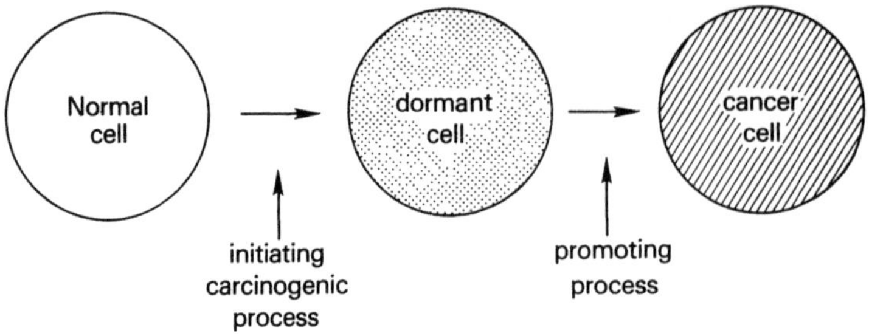

Fig. 1.1. Co-carcinogenesis

Co-carcinogenesis is the enhancement of the potency of a carcinogen by another substance, which may or may not, produce cancer when used alone [10, 11]. It implies that specific types of irritation, when added to a tumor-producing compound used in subminimal doses, will cause a malignant change to occur. This concept indicates that there are two steps in carcinogenesis, similar to a chemical chain reaction. First, a subtle intrinsic change within a cell due to a carcinogen, and second, gross manifestation of the tumor by some promoting irritant (see Fig. 1.1) [12]. This concept meshes well with the idea of external carcinogens and internal host factors, acting in an additive or synergistic fashion to induce cancer.

Many examples of co-carcinogenesis abound in the scientific cancer literature. Different solvents, having no independent carcinogenic effect, will variously accelerate the effect of a known carcinogen [13, 14]. Mottram found that a 800–2,500 R single dose of beta radiation from a radium source given 60 days after painting twice a week with a 0.5% 3,4 benzpyrene solution, (insufficient in itself to produce cancer in this time span), resulted in the increased formation of benign and malignant tumors in laboratory animals. Here, radiation acted as the promoting agent [15]. Shubik used beta rays from thallium-204 on mouse skin and observed that tumors were produced after subsequent painting with croton oil. In this case, raditation acted as a initiating process [16]. Such examples as these are but a few of co-carcinogenesis. For a more detailed review of co-carcinogenic examples in the literature, one is referred to Southam's article [10].

II. Possible Predisposing Factors

The following eight entities have been suggested as possible predisposing factors in the formation of head and neck cancer:

1. Tobacco

Tobacco is definitely a proven carcinogen for oral cancer. In the United States, cigarette, pipe, and/or cigar smoking multiplies the risk of lip, mouth, tongue, and pharyngeal cancer by a factor of about 3 to 10, depending on the type and amount of smoking [17]. Nine out of ten persons suffering from oral cancer in this country are smokers, indicating an extremely high risk for tobacco users [18].

Silverman studied 174 California patients with primary intraoral carcinoma, 159 (91%) of which habitually used tobacco for long periods of time. Eighty percent used cigarettes (more than double the estimate for an age-matched segment of the general population), and 41% of these cigarette smokers consumed over two packs per day. Thus, a sixfold relative risk for developing oral cancer existed for cigarette smokers, when compared to non-smokers in his study. Of the 174 treated oral cancer patients, 61 continued to smoke after treatment, and 22 of these 61 individuals afterwards developed second primary oral cancers [19, 20]. A similar magnitude of risk between continued smoking after cancer treatment, and secondary primary oral cancers developing in these same persons has also been reported by Moore [21].

Wynder found that cancer of the vocal cord was predominantly related to cigarette smoking [22]. He also noted that the risk for developing laryngeal carcinoma was much lower for ex-smokers and long-term (over 10 years) filter cigarette smokers in comparison with non-filter smokers [23]. The safest practice, however, was to not smoke any type of cigarette.

Numerous publications on the high incidence of oral cancer in India have emphasized the relationship between tobacco chewing and smoking habits and oral cancer in that country [24–30]. The longest reported survey and ten year follow-up of oral cancer and oral precancerous lesions in the world has been described by the Mehta group of researchers at the Tata Institute of Fundamental Research in Bombay, India. No case of oral cancer was detected by this study among individuals who had no tobacco habit. All of the new oral cancer cases developed among patients who had a prior diagnosis of a precancerous lesion, and all such patients used tobacco in some form of habit [31].

The betal quid, or "pan-chewing" habit, is one of the most widely practiced chewing habits in India. The basic "pan" consists of a combination of betel leaf (Piper betel), areca palm nut (Areca catechu), slaked lime (calcium hydroxide) and catechu, (Acacia catechu) – (see Fig. 1.2). Many other condiments, sweeteners, and flavoring agents are sometimes added to this basic chew to suit the user's individual taste. There are also differences in the variety of all the ingredients. Betel leaf varieties vary in different parts of India. The areca nuts may be used raw, baked, or boiled. Stone lime is perferred in most Indian localities except in Kerala, the southern-most state, where shell lime made from sea shells is more prevalent. The fifth ingredient most often added to the basic betel chew is tobacco. In normal use, a "pan" is folded into a quid, chewed and/or sucked, and is kept compressed against the buccal mucosa. It is normally chewed after meals. If it does not contain tobacco, the quid bolus may be swallowed. If it does contain tobacco, it may be spat out. "Pan" is frequently kept in the moth for long periods of time, and many "pans" may be consumed by a user in a single day [29].

Each of these ingredients in the betel quid have been studied for possible carcinogenic effect. Numerous clinical studies have indicated that tobacco ap-

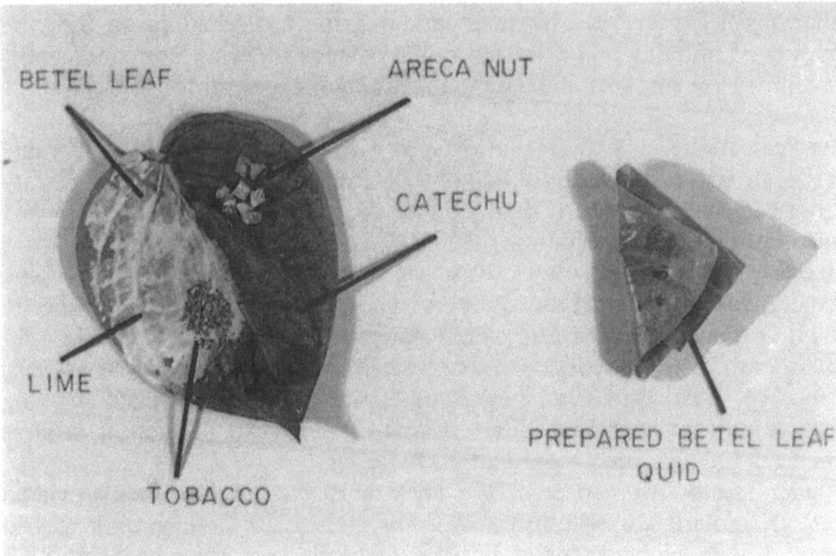

Fig. 1.2. Components of a "Pan-chew". (Courtesy of Drs. Mehta, Pindborg, and Hamner)

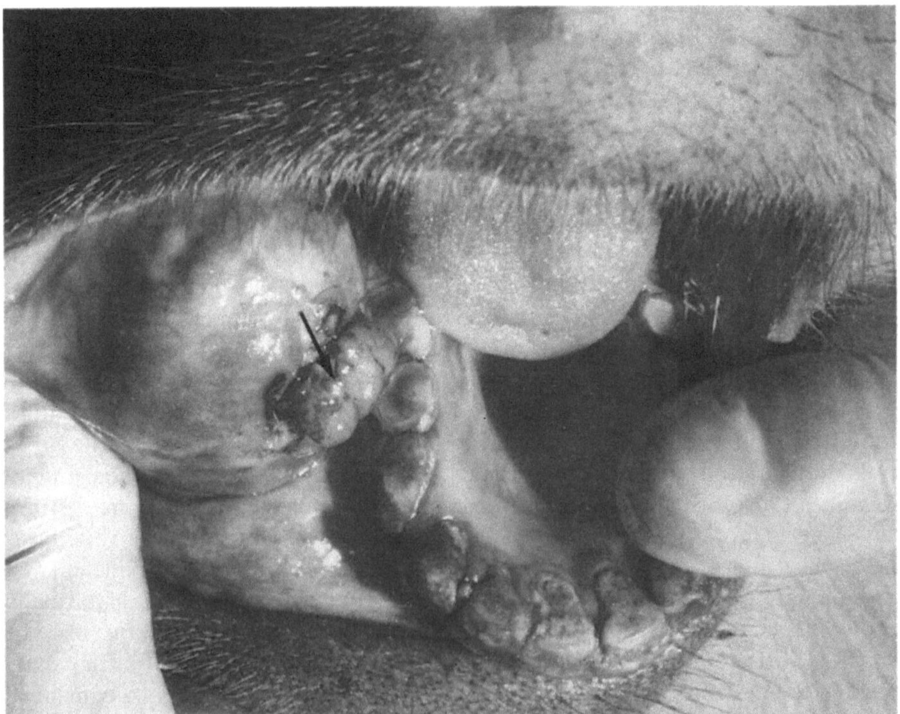

Fig. 1.3. Clinical lesion in a baboon's buccal mucosa (*arrow*) after 30 months of treatment with betel/tobacco quid

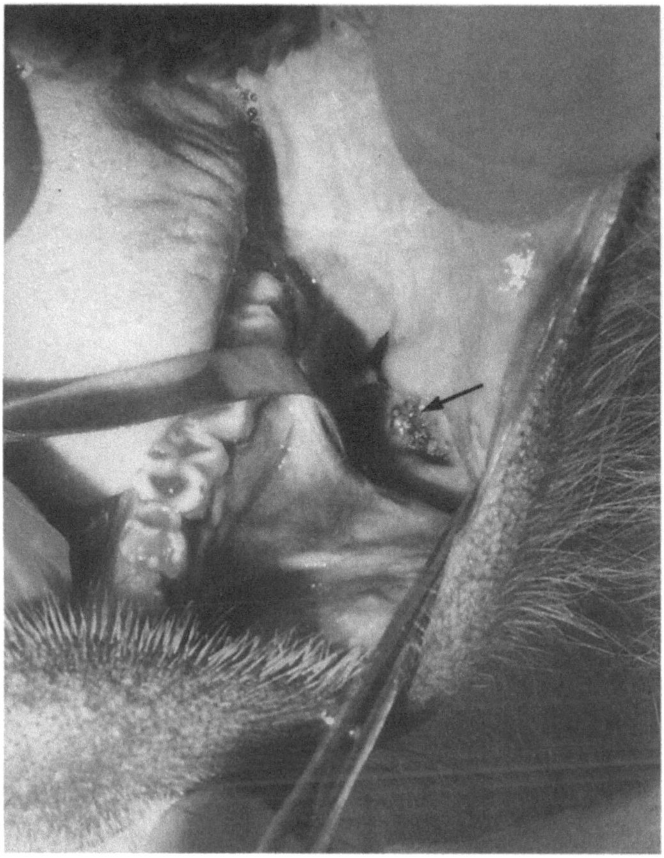

Fig. 1.4. Clinical lesion in a baboon's buccal mucosa (*arrow*) after 30 months of treatment with betel/tobacco quid

pears to be the carcinogenic agent [29–32]. Dunham and Herrold failed to produce tumors in the buccal mucosa of hamsters, using various combinations of betel leaf, areca nuts, tobacco, and gambier in a beeswax pellet [33]. Two deficiencies existed in their experimental design: first, not using lime as an ingredient (it is essential), and second, putting the ingredients in a beeswax pellet instead of using them directly against the hamster's buccal mucosa, as betel quid is used in the typical human habit. Later, Dunham and Hamner induced epithelial atypia by repeated applications of lime (calcium hydroxide) alone over an extended period of time in 3 out of 26 hamster cheek pouches [34]. Sirsat and Kandarkar produced similar epithelial atypia, following initial irritating inflammatory reactions due to the burning effect of lime, after 12 months of applying lime to the oral mucosa of Wistar rats. This result led them to agree that lime most likely acts as the co-carcinogen by the irritant reaction that it causes to oral mucosa [35].

Basic research investigations, involving tobacco as an oral carcinogenic agent, have confirmed the earlier clinical impressions as to its action as a weak

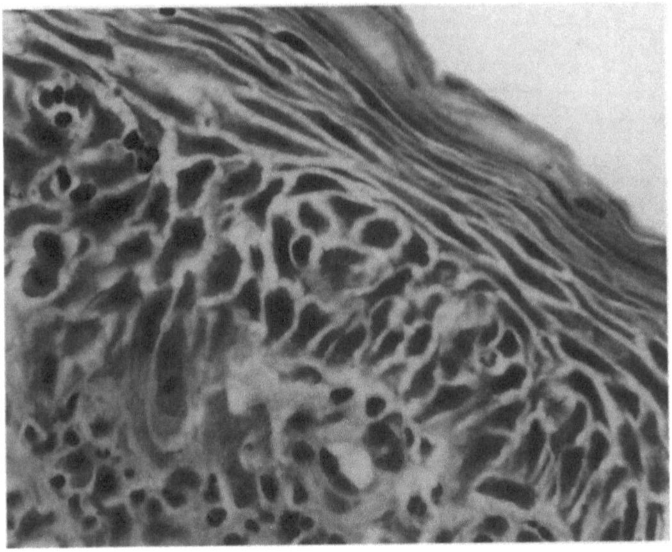

Fig. 1.5. Carcinoma-in-situ, buccal mucosa, 34 months treatment with betel/tobacco quid. H.&E. stain, ×450

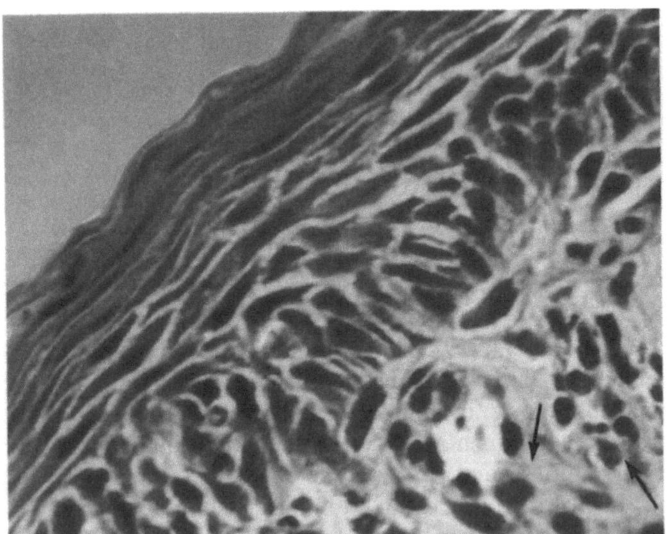

Fig. 1.6. Early localized cancer, buccal mucosa. Note malignant cells beginning invasion of lamina propria (*arrows*), 34 months treatment with betel/tobacco quid. H.&E. stain, ×450

carcinogen. In 1967, Cohen and Smith reported ballooning of epithelial cells in the buccal pouch mucosa of monkeys that had been exposed to a tobacco paste. This histopathologic atypia was similar to histologic changes seen in human snuff users [36–38]. Later, Cohen, Poswillo, and Woods produced premalignant lesions by sealing a Mainpuri tobacco quid into monkey's cheek pouches for periods of 1–42 months duration [39].

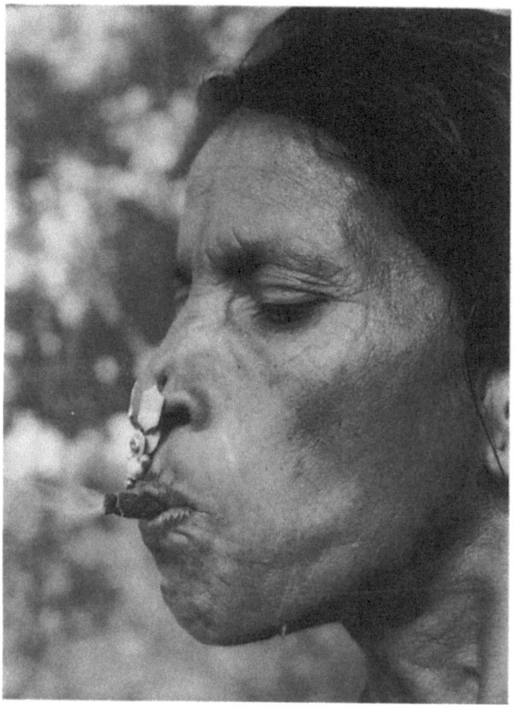

Fig. 1.7. "Chutta" reverse smoking habit in India. (Courtesy of Dr. Fali S. Mehta)

Using fresh betel leaves, areca nuts, lime, and Maharashtran sun-died tobacco to simulate the normal "pan" (betel quid) chewing habit in Indians, Hamner and Reed produced carcinoma-in-situ lesions in the cheek pouch mucosa of protein-deficient baboons after repeated exposure to a fresh tobacco-betel quid three times per week for 34 to 42 months duration (see Fig. 1.3, 1.4, 1.5, and 1.6). The control group, receiving the betel quid without tobacco, did not develop similar lesions [40, 41]. The two subhuman primate studies definitely demonstrate that tobacco acts as a weak carcinogen on the oral mucosa, while lime serves as the promoting co-carcinogenic agent in the betel quid/tobacco chewing habit.

Clinical studies in the Southeastern United States have demonstrated that a high percentage of oral cancer develops in women snuff dippers, usually at the bucco-gingival sites where the tobacco snuff was held [12, 20, 38].

A definite clinical relationship between the "chutta" habit (the reverse smoking of home-made cigars) and palatal cancer has been shown in India [29]. This habit is demonstrated in Fig. 1.7, and the resulting palatal carcinoma is revealed in Fig. 1.8.

The Surgeon-General's original Report on Smoking in 1964 concluded that a causal relationship existed between pipe smoking and lip cancer. The current 1982 Surgeon-General's Report on Smoking confirms the original report's findings and strongly indites tobacco as the carcinogen, whether by smoking cigarettes, pipes, or cigars, as the major cause of cancers of the oral cavity [42].

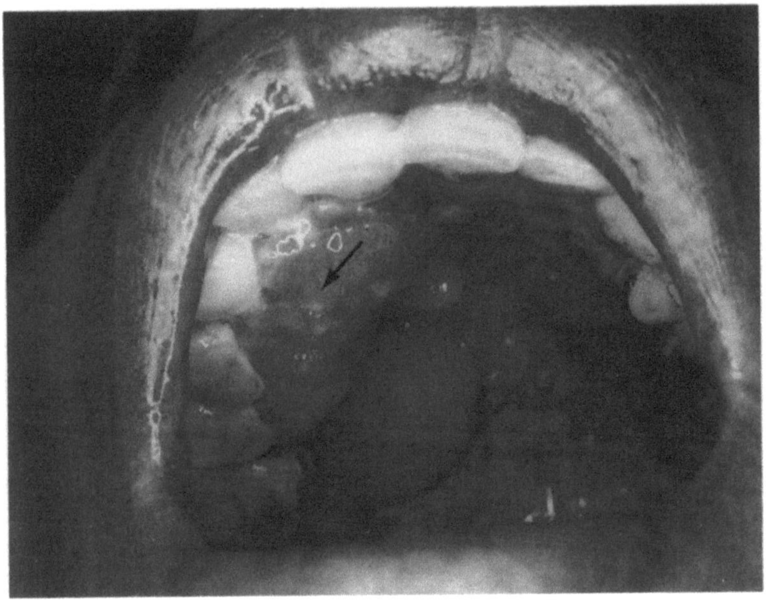

Fig. 1.8. Palatal carcinoma (*arrow*) resulting from the "chutta" habit. (Courtesy of Dr. Soli K. Choksi)

Clinical and basic science investigations have proven overwhelmingly that tobacco is a definite etiological cause of oral cancer.

2. Radiation

Human clinical studies and animal research investigations have verified that radiation, under certain conditions related to dosage and duration, can produce cancer [10, 12, 15, 43, 45, 46]. Upton has reported that an association between irradiation and neoplasia has been detected in human populations at lower levels of exposure than heretofore suspected. Data indicate that the relation may vary due to the type of tumor, age at irradiation, and other factors [47]. In experimental animals, complex factors such as constitutional, environmental, and radiobiological variables make it impossible to define the exact characterization and mechanism of radiation carcinogensis [47]. Again, similar to chemical carcinogenses, a succession of changes appears to be involved.

Various cancers (i.e. leukemias, malignant lymphoma, multiple myeloma, breast cancer, etc.) have been shown to evolve in the survivors of the atomic bomb casualities at Hiroshima and Nagasaki [48–50]. Breast cancer in women has been related to x-ray treatments for acute post-partum mastitis and multiple fluoroscopies during artificial pneumothorax treatment of pulminary tuberculosis [51, 52]. Childhood cancers have been shown to be related to obstetrical radiation dosage that the mother inadvertently received [53]. Also, iatrogenic inducement of cancer was unknowingly caused by irradiation for thymic enlargment and overzealous treatment of tinea capitis by irradiation [54, 55].

In regard to the head and neck region, we are mostly concerned with tumors of the thyroid and of the facial bones, both directly related to irradiation. In experimental animals, tumors have been produced in the thyroid gland by irradiation [56, 57].

In September 1975 the National Cancer Institute convened a workshop on the "Late Effects of Irradiation to the Head and Neck in Infancy and Childhood." Currently, it is recognized that one of the high-risk groups for developing cancer are those individuals who received therapeutic doses of x-radiation or radium applications to the head, neck, or upper thorax for various benign conditions (enlarged thymus, enlarged tonsils or adenoids, mastoiditis, sinisitis, keloids, tinea capitis, acne, etc) during infancy and childhood. This particular population has shown a statistically significant increase in cancer incidence of the thyroid gland and, to a leser extent, of the salivary glands and other tissues, developing latently 5–35 or more years after the initial radiation [46, 58–64].

The second iatrogenic radiation induced tumor of the head and neck area is osteosarcoma. Bone sarcomas have been produced experimentally by various types of irradiation in the bones of rats, rabbits, guinea pigs, and foul [65]. Cahan et al. emphasized in 1948 the role irradiation may play in producing malignant change in bone in his presentation of 11 patients in whom osteogenic sarcoma developed in irradiated bones 6 to 22 years after x- or gamma-ray therapy [65]. Osteosarcoma arising in irradiated bones was first described in 1922, and by 1936, 14 other cases were reported. In 17 postradiation bone sarcomas reported initially by the Mayo Clinic, 3 were in the head area (1 in the mandible, 2 in the maxillae) [66]. The second Mayo Clinic study on osteogenic sarcoma of the jaws and facial bones reported 19 cases in the mandible, 14 in the maxillae, and 11 in the antrum and ethmoid region [67]. Further clinical reports confirm the relationship between radiation and formation of bone sarcomas in certain cases [68, 69]. Again, radiation given unknowingly for treatment of benign conditions such as enlarged thymus, enlarged tonsils, acne, etc., was to cause production of osteogenic sarcoma years later.

There is no evidence to indicate that periodic exposure to routine dental diagnostic x-rays has any carcinogenic effect to cause head and neck cancer, especially in the modern era of using high-speed x-ray film and low dosage machines [20]. However, in the early years of x-ray usage, some dentists were guilty of careless, injudicious exposure to themselves by the erroneous habit of holding the film in place in the patient's mouth, while x-rays were taken. Such action over a period of years led to carcinomas of their fingers and subsequent loss of the fingers.

Another form of radiation known to produce cancer in both humans and experimental animals is ultraviolet radiation [18]. There is a striking inverse relationship of non-melanoma skin cancer incidence and latitude, due to repeated prolonged exposure of ultraviolet rays [70]. Persons, who carry dominant genetic traits for freckling and an incomplete melanin screen (chiefly Celts, such as the Irish, Scots, and Welsh) and who tan irregularly, have the highest incidence of skin cancer [70, 71]. Clinical studies also have implicated solar exposure of ultraviolet light as a factor affecting the incidence of cutaneous basal cell carcinoma and malignant melanoma since these lesions are more prevalent in the Southwestern United States and Australia than they are in Great Britain or Scandinavia [18, 72–74].

3. Nutritional Factors

Dietary or nutritional factors have recently entered on stage in the discussion of environmental carcinogens, however, there is a paucity of well-documented carcinoginic situations [9]. Aflatoxins, lactones produced by strains of Aspergillus florus growing on peanuts, grains, and other foods, produce liver cancer in fish and in rats [75]. Oettle emphasized the concentration of human liver cancer in African regions of high humidity where Aspergillus growth is favored [76].

Nitrosamines, known powerful carcinogens for animals, are frequently found in our foods, and are near the top of every food hazard list. However, in regard to human cancer in the United States, there is no conclusive incriminating link between them and any major amount of cancer [77]. A correlation between nitrosamine – containing foods and gastric cancer may exist in Japan, as their customary diet contains salted fish, a major source of nitrosamines [78]. A possible overlap in carcinogenic activity may exist due to the fact that a goodly portion of smoked fish is also consumed in the Japanese diet, so you have the high level of polycyclic hydrocarbons in smoked fish to complicate matters [77, 79].

Food additives (dyes, cyclamate, and saccharin), food contaminants (pesticides, antibiotics, etc.), and trace elements (metals) have been mentioned as possible carcinogens in man as well as laboratory animals [77].

Vitamin A is very essential to normal functioning of the epithelium, and therefore, has received more attention than the other vitamins in regard to its effects on carcinogenesis. Adding vitamin A has been shown to decrease the tumor-producing effect of polycyclic hydrocarbons in several rodent systems [80, 81]. In constrast, decreasing Vitamin A enhances salivary gland carcinogensis and increases bowel carcinogenesis in rats [82, 83]. Most importantly, vitamin A has been demonstrated to have direct and indirect therapeutic properties against human skin cancers [9, 84].

The best known example of oral carcinogenesis attributed to a dietary imbalance in humans is the Plummer-Vinson iron deficiency syndrome [18]. The Pulmmer-Vinson syndrome, first described by Plummer in 1914 and Vinson in 1922, is one manifestation of iron-deficiency anemia, most commonly seen in northern Scandinavian women [85]. Presenting symptoms usually include cracks or fissures at the corners of the mouth, a yellow-tinted skin, smooth, red, painful tongue, and dysphagia. In 1936, Ahlbom defined the relationship between atrophy of the mucous membranes of the upper alimentary tract and a predisposition to the development of carcinoma of the mouth, pharynx, and esophagus in these women [86]. He reported that 50% of the women patients with carcinoma of the hypopharynx and upper esophagus, treated at the Radiumhemmet in Stockholm, Sweden, also suffered from Plummer-Vinson syndrome [86]. Later studies reported similar results [87]. Improved nutrition, due to awareness of this problem, has caused a decrease in both Pulmmer-Vinson syndrome and cancer of the head and neck among women in northern Sweden [22].

4. Alcohol

Most studies indicate that alcohol is a cancer hazard, causing an increased cancer risk for carcinomia of the mouth, pharynx larynx, esophagus, liver, and lung, among excessive drinkers [8, 18, 20].

In 1958–1959, Tregier reported that 44% of 108 patients with carcinoma of the tongue and 59% of 68 patients with cancer of either the floor of the mouth, palate, or tonsillar fossa also exhibited proven cirrhosis of the liver [88]. Nearly 75% of both groups reportedly were excessive alcohol drinkers. In a separate study, Keller confirmed a definite association between hepatic cirrhosis, excessive alcohol consumption, excessive smoking, and carcinoma of the floor of the mouth and pharynx [89, 90]. Wynder observed that 33% of male patients suffering from oral cancer in his study series drank over 7 ounces of whiskey per day [91].

A recent study in Washington, D.C. among black men, who were heavy drinkers, correlated an increased risk for esophageal cancer [92]. Ninety-six percent of those men who died of esophageal cancer consumed large amounts of alcohol. Nearly half of those who died from this cancer drank the equivalent of 15 ounces or more of hard liquor per day [92].

Good has postulated that alcohol may act in an ambivalent fashion as a possible etiological agent, since depression of cellular immunological function is seen in alcoholics with head and neck cancer, but it is not evident in alcoholics without head and neck cancer [93]. It has been suggested that alcohol may aid in the absorbing of tobacco carcinogens, or perhaps nutritional deficiencies related to heavy alcohol intake cause squamous cells to be more susceptible to malignant conversion [22].

Because quite often excessive alcohol drinkers are also heavy smokers, it is difficult to separate the emphasis of alcohol from tobacco when studying possible modes of carcinogenesis. Studies have confirmed a synergistic relationship between oral cancer and the consumption of tobacco and alcohol [94–97].

We are left with the fact that there is no concrete evidence at this time that alcohol is carcinogenic per se. Yet the preponderance of clinical and basic research evidence does support the opinion that alcohol probably does act as a co-carcinogen, thus magnifying the carcinogenic potential of other cancer-inducing substances, such as tobacco [98].

5. Genetic Susceptibility

Because of their genetic make-up, certain people are at a higher risk for cancer. There are three types of genetic factors in cancer:

a) Chromosomal, with genetic imbalance because entire lengths of genetic material are absent or present in excess.

b) Single-gene locus, with disease arising from mutation either in one allele as in a dominant trait, or in paired alleles as in a recessive trait.

c) Polygenic, implying that many genes interact, perhaps with environmental factors, to cause disease, with no one factor or gene playing a major role [99].

Of the known single-gene traits in humans, 161 (9%) have neoplastic or preneoplastic manifestations or complications [9, 99]. If we eliminate the single-gene traits associated primarily with either skin, thyroid, or parathyroid cancer, we are left with three others that do definitely relate to head and neck cancer. The first is nevoid basal cell carcinoma syndrome, that is manifested with basal cell carcinoma, medulloblastoma, jaw cysts, and ovarian fibromas/carcinomas. The second is Garder's syndrome, which is associated with intestinal polyps, osteomas, fibromas, sebaceous cysts, and carcinomas of the colon, ampulla of vater, pancreas, thyroid, and adrenal. The third disorder is cherubism, which is manifested by multiple giant cell-type tumors of the jaws, that can cause life-threatening situations such as asphyxia [85, 100].

It has already been mentioned earlier that Celtic persons, such as the Scots, Irish, and Welsh, who possess the genetic trait for freckling and who do not tan regularly, exhibit a high incidence of skin cancer [70, 71]. Certain cancers appear to predominate among certain genetic pools. For example, narophyngeal cancer is common among Chinese, Malays, and Indonesians, yet is rarely seen in Caucasians. Yet even among the Chinese, nasopharyngeal cancer rates vary, being higher in South China. To complicate matters, American-born Chinese have a much lower rate of nasopharyngeal cancer. These facts suggest a possible genetic susceptability to some environmental carcinogen.

6. Viruses

Of all the possible microbial agents, only the viruses are of real importance in regard to carcinogenesis. If viruses do cause cancer in man, particular host factors, such as: time of infection, immune status, co-factors and other diseases, genetic susceptibility, and depression of cellular immunity, are involved.

Both RNA and DNA viruses have been incriminated as well-established causes of various cancers in experimental animals, including non-human primates. In 1908, Ellermann and Bang in Copenhagen discovered the first of the tumor viruses, transmitting leukemia in chickens by the innoculation of cell-free filtrates. In 1910, Rous transmitted his chicken sarcoma. Shope followed in 1932, producing papillomas in rabbits with the Shope virus. The next year he transmitted papillomas with cell-free tumor extracts, and some of these progressed to carcinomas – the first malignant mammalian tumors induced by a virus. Bittner next produced mammary tumors in mice via an oncogenic virus. Lucke induced tumors in the frog kidney in 1938, but the frog-kidney carcinoma was not proven conclusively to be caused by a filterable virus until 1956. The 1950's also saw numerous strains of mouse leukemia (lymphoid, myeloid, and histiocytic types) virus isolated. Later in 1958, Stewart discovered that the polyoma virus could give rise to a great variety of tumors in many animal species. In the 1960's investigators, using the SV40 simian virus, were able to induce tumors in mastomys and hamsters. Lastly, four types of human adenovirus have been shown to be tumor producing in animals [9, 101–103].

At this point in time, members of the herpesvirus family are highly suspected in relation to human carcinogenicity, although prima facie evidence of oncogenicity is lacking. The human viruses of particular interest are herpes simplex virus type 2 (HSV-2) and the Epstein-Barr virus (EBV).

Much evidence has accumulated to suggest that infection with HSV-2 (genetic virus) predisposes to cancer of the uterine cervix. The consistent association between the presence of anti-HSV-2 antibodies and cervical cancer holds true not only for frank invasive cervical carcinoma, but also for earlier stages of dysplasia and carcinoma-in-situ [104–106]. Nonviron antigen-antibody studies have suggested an association between HSV infection and head and neck cancers, but a review of the same studies failed to confirm them [107–109].

Considerable circumstantial evidence has been assembled to link the Epstein-Barr virus (EBV) to the Burkitt African lymphoma, since indentification of this virus in cell cultures of the lymphoma [110]. With almost no exceptions, African lymphoma cases exhibit serum antibodies against EBV with mean titers being markedly increased over control patients [111, 112]. Tissue from the nontropical Burkitt's tumor does not appear to contain EBV viral DNA [113].

In addition to Burkitt's African lymphoma, the only other neoplasm that exhibits consistent elevations of anti-EBV antibody is nasopharyngeal carcinoma. Here again, virtually every patient with this tumor demonstrates anti-EBV antibodies with mean titers much higher than control patients [114].

The etiological relationship of EBV and these tumors remains uncertain. Knowing that EBV is closely associated with lymphoid cells generally, observations have raised the possibility that increases in anti-EBV antibody among these cancer patients reflects a result rather than a cause of altered lymphoid function. Thus, the role of the virus may be one of secondary opportunist, rather than the primary etiological factor.

7. Syphilis

Early studies by Levin, Wynder, and Treiger reported a greater prevalence of syphilis in male patients with oral cancer, especially cancer of the lip and tongue [22, 91, 115, 116]. Later reports by Keller, Myer, and Silverman do not indicate that syphilis is a significant etiological factor in the causation of oral cancer [20, 89, 117]. In Heath's discussion of viruses and other microbes in their relationship as possible factors in persons who are at high risk for cancer, there is no mention of syphilis in conjunction to oral cancer [103].

Thus, the ralationship between syphilis and oral cancer is very equivocal because the case can easily be argued that in earlier times, the typical male case of syphilis tended to be elderly, used alcohol and tobacco to excess, and was frequently malnourished – all of which could play a contributing role in producing oral cancer [18].

8. Traumatic Irritation

The concept that traumatic irritations may be a predisposing factor in cancer formation originated with Berenblum's work in 1944. He compiled a review of the influence of non-carcinogenic irritants on carcinogenesis in which: (a) an irritant and a carcinogen were applied concurrently, (b) an irritant was applied prior to the carcinogen treatment, and (c) an irritant was applied after the carcinogen treatment. Intensity of irritation was not the deciding factor in carcinogenesis. The effect of applying an irritant concurrently with a carcinogen varied according to the irritant, from inhibition to acceleration of tumor formation. The application of irritants preceeding the carcinogen was unsuccessful in producing a preneoplastic skin lesion, but after carcinogen treatment, many precipitated a tumor response. These results indicated that carcinogenesis is not a singular process, but has several component phases, which may be dissociated. Preneoplastic hyperplasia is a highly specific type of hyperplasia, and once the preneoplastic state has been initiated by a true carcinogen, a tumor will be produced. Thus, it may be said that all carcinogens are irritants, but not all irritants are carcinogens [118].

For many years, chronic irritation from jagged teeth, rough dental restorations, and ill-fitting dentures has been postutated as a cause of oral cancer. However to date, none of these irritating factors has been proven to be a carcinogenic factor, per se [18].

Silverman has pointed out that with 20 million denture wearers in the United States, carcinoma of the palate and alveolar mucosa account for less than 11 per center of all oral cancers, and less than 0.5% of all cancers [20]. Wynder agreed that there is no solid evidence to link jagged teeth, rough dentures, or hot spicy foods to the pathogenesis of cancer [22, 91].

III. Oral Precancerous Conditions

The recognition of precancerous conditions and their accurate diagnosis forms an important segment of the cancer problem. Three conditions will be discussed – leukoplakia, erythroplakia, and submucous fibrosis – because in certain cases of each of these three conditions, the lesion will process on to frank carcinoma.

Histologically speaking, the individual cellular changes are referred to as epithelial atypia, while the general epithelial disturbance itself is termed epithelial dysplasia. The individual epithelial atypia changes may include: loss of polarity of the basal cells, the presence of more than one layer of cells having basaloid appearance, an increased nuclear-cytoplasmic ratio, drop-shaped rete pegs, irregular epithelial stratification, increased number of mitotic figures (a few abnormal mitoses may be present), the presence of mitotic figures in the superficial half of the epithelium, cellular pleomorphism, nuclear hyperchromatism, enlarged nucleoli, reduction of cellular cohesion, and keratinization of single cells or cell groups in the stratum spinosum [119]. Not all of these above changes are necessarily seen in any one case. Slight degrees of epithelial dysplasia do not indicate great danger for the patient. Moderate epithelial dysplasia is of more concern, and severe epithelial dyplasia places the patient in the high-risk category for cancer.

Carcinoma-in-situ is a separate histopathologic term, meaning that the entire thickness of a segment of epithelium shows through and through severe dysplastic change, but the basement membrane has not yet been penetrated by the cancerous-appearing cells [3, 85].

1. Leukoplakia

The World Health Organization's Collaborating Center for Oral Precancerous Lesions has advocated and recommended that the term "leukoplakia" should carry no histologic connotation and should be used in a clinical descriptive sense only. It may be defined as a white plaque or patch on the oral mucosa, that cannot be scraped off and cannot be delineated clinically or pathologically, as any other disease [119].

Three different clinical types of leukoplakia may exist:

a) Homogenous leukoplakia is characterized by raised white plaques, either solitary or multiple, which may vary in size and have irregular edges. Most such lesions are white (Fig. 1.9), but may have areas of greyish yellow.

b) Ulcerated leukoplakia is caused by trauma from chewing or burning of the oral mucosa. This form is more commonly seen in India because of the

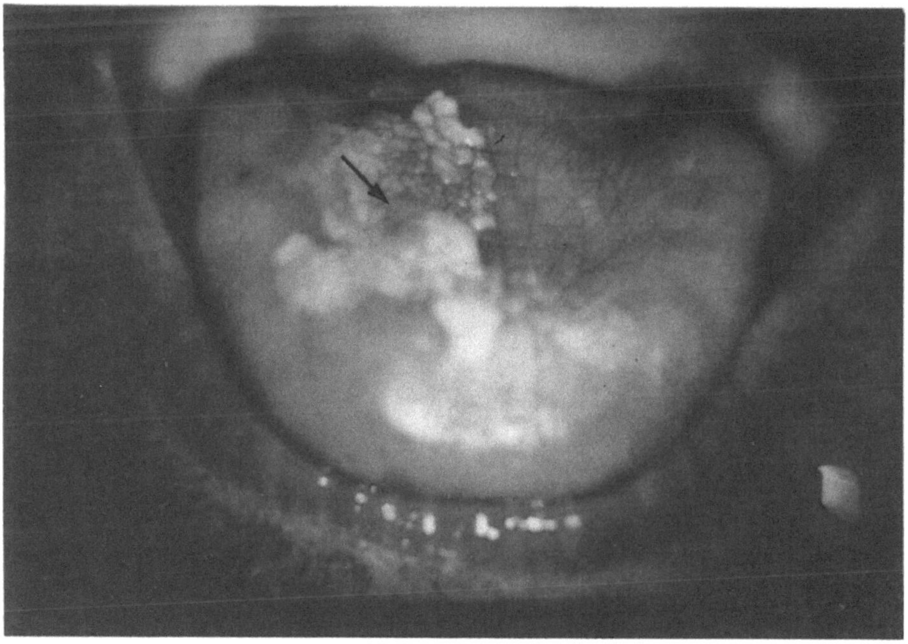

Fig. 1.9. Homogenous leukoplakia (*arrow*), tongue, Indian "bidi" smoker. (Courtesy of Dr. Soli K. Choksi)

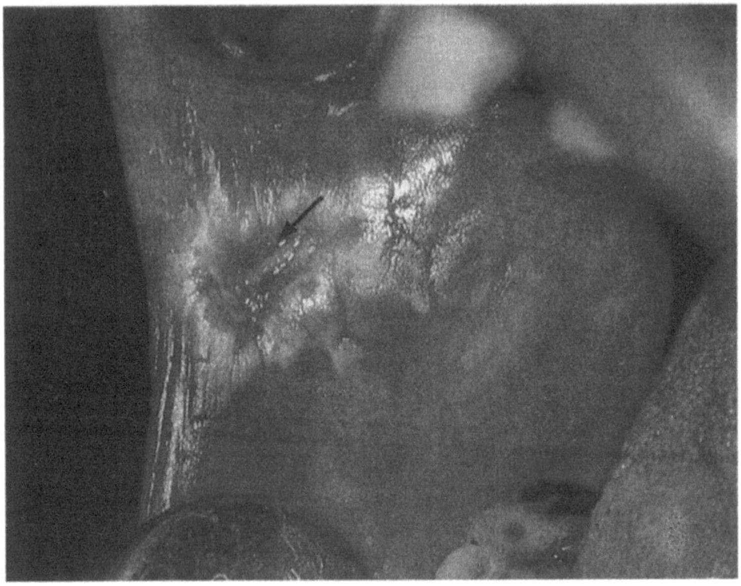

Fig. 1.10. Ulcerated leukoplakia (*arrow*) of commissure, Indian female reverse smoker. (Courtesy of Drs. Mehta, Pindborg, and Hamner)

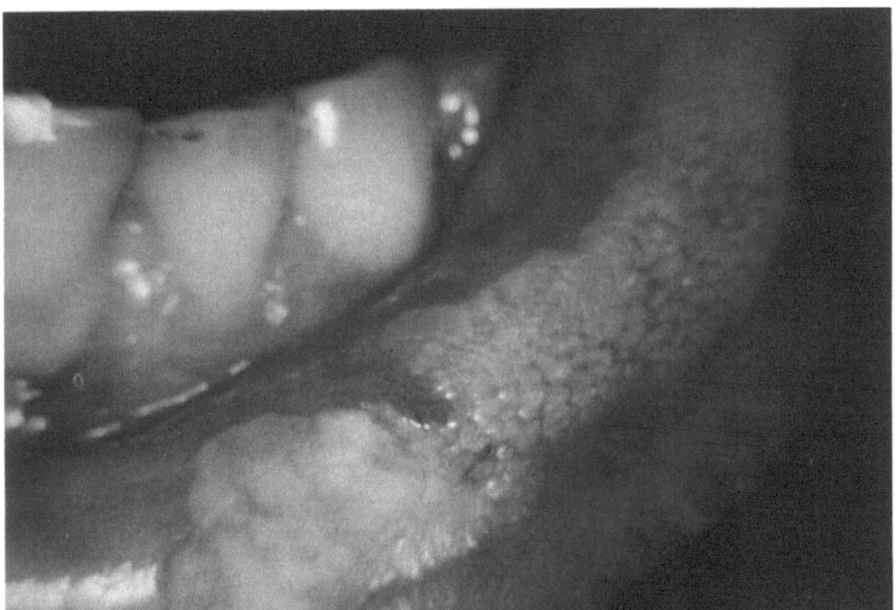

Fig. 1.11. Speckled leukoplakia, lower lip. (Courtesy of Dr. Soli K. Choksi)

many diverse smoking and chewing habits widely practiced there. The affected area is erythematous and ulcerated; usually wide white, radiating borders are seen as in Fig. 1.10.

c) Speckled leukoplakia is characterized as having white patches on an erythematous base, resulting clinically in a speckled appearance (Fig. 1.11). Speckled leukoplakia, also referred to as "nodular leukoplakia," is reported to have a higher potential for histopathological premalignant changes [29–31].

The histologic picture for leukoplakia can run the entire gamet from simple hyperkeratosis or hyperparakeratosis to epithelial dysplasia to actual carcinoma. Again, it should be emphasized that there is no close correlation between the clinical appearance of leukoplakia and the underlying histologic picture with the exception of speckled (nodular) leukoplakia, which often does present with epithelial atypia features.

2. Erythroplakia

The term "erythroplakia" is used to define oral mucosal lesions that appear as bright red, velvety patches or plaques, which cannot be established either clinically or pathologically as being caused by any other conditions [119]. A number of other conditions may appear as red areas within the mouth (e.g., inflammatory conditions, denture initiation, allergic reactions, fungal infections,

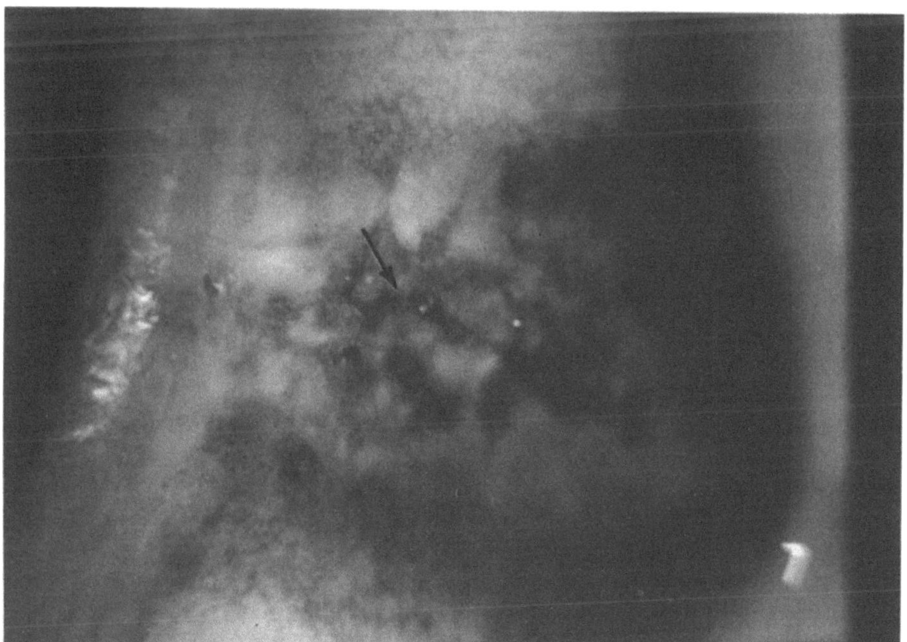

Fig. 1.12. Erythroplakia (*arrow*), buccal mucosa of an Indian male. (Courtesy of Dr. Fali S. Mehta)

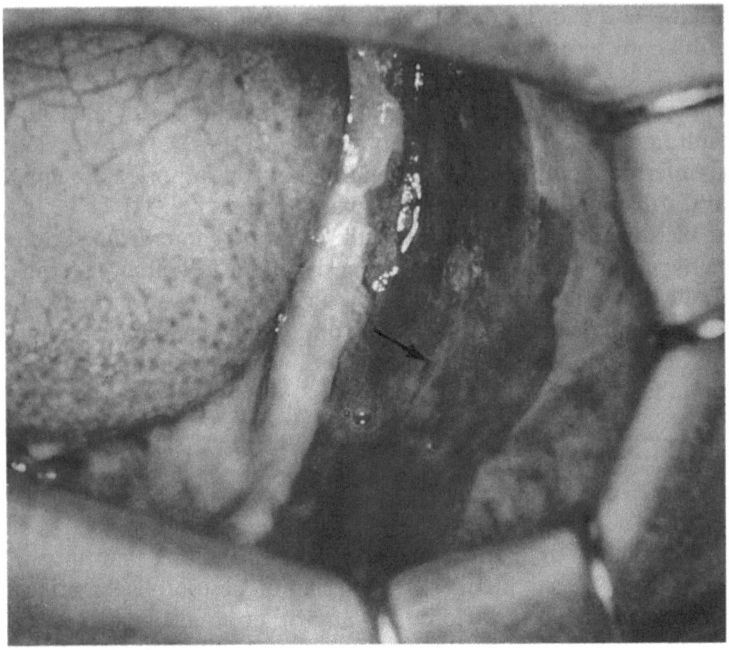

Fig. 1.13. Erythroplakia (*arrow*), buccal mucosa of a Danish male. (Courtesy of Dr. J.J. Pindborg)

some dermatoses, etc.), but these conditions can be differentiated from erythroplakia.

The relationship between red lesions in the mouth and oral cancer was initially pointed out by Pindborg [120]. Similar observations by other investigators have confirmed this opinion [18, 20, 121–123]. Mashberg found that most of his cases of erythroplakia were detected in high-risk patients, persons over 40, who were heavy drinkers and heavy smokers [122].

Clinically, the erythroplakia plaques are often irregular in outline, yet well-defined, and have a vivid red, velvety appearance (Fig. 1.12 and 1.13).

Fortunately, it is a rare lesion, and the most frequent site of occurence is the buccal mucosa [124]. Histopathological features of erythroplakia include marked epithelial atrophy, a variable degree of epithelial dysplasia, and usually a heavy chronic inflammatory infiltrate of the lamina propria.

3. Submucous Fibrosis

In 1952, submucous fibrosis was first described by Schwartz [125] in five Indian female patients from Kenya, East Africa, and a year later it was named as a distinct disease entity by Joshi in India [126]. While this malady is most often found in Indians [127–131], it has also been recorded in several Europeans living in Hyderabad, India [132], three Taiwanese males reported by Su [133], and an English woman married to a Pakistani living in England [134, 135]. Other isolated cases among Indians and Pakistanis dwelling in Great Britain, South Africa, Malaysia, Fiji Islands, and the United States have also been described in the literature [136–143].

Pindborg has defined submucous fibrosis best as: "an insidious, chronic disease affecting any part of the oral cavity and sometimes the pharynx, occasionally preceeded by vesicle formation, always associated with fibrous bands and a juxta-epithelial inflammatory reaction, followed by a fibro-elastic change of the lamina propria, with epithelial atrophy leading to a stiffness of the oral mucosa, trismus, and inability to eat" [135].

The prevalence rate of oral submucous fibrosis varies from 0.2 to 1.2% in India, with the higher percentage being found in the southern areas of that country [29, 144, 145, 147, 148]. Although reports of sex ratio vary in the literature, the majority demonstrate a female predominance [29, 31, 125, 128, 145, 146]. Most cases occur between the ages of 20 and 40 years, and no religious or caste group in India appears to be exempt from this disease [29, 145–147].

The most frequent initial symptom and presenting clinical complaint is a burning sensation in the mouth, most often experienced when the person is eating spicy food. This fact led many investigators to suspect chillies in the Indian diet as the responsible ingredient, especially capsaicin, the active irritant substance in chili peppers, which are universally used throughout India to season food [29, 135, 146, 149].

Sirsat and Khanolkar demonstrated changes similar to human submucous fibrosis after painting rat palates for 8 to 28 weeks with a 2% concentrated capsaicin [150]. Their results could not be duplicated in the hamster cheek pouch by using either 2% U.S.P. capsaicin or freshly ground chili peppers from the Indian states of Kerala and Gujarat three times per week for 2 years [143].

Other early clinical symptoms include: vesicle formation, ulceration, or recurrent stomatitis. As the disease progresses, rigidity of the oral tissues ensues, caused by dense bands of palpable fibrous tissue. The oral mucosa appears blanched, slightly opaque and white in areas, producing a marble-like effect, as demonstrated in Fig. 1.14. Scarlike fibrous bands can bind down the soft palate, shorten the uvula and faucial pillars, reduce the flexibility of the buccal mucosa, reduce the mouth opening (see Fig. 1.15), and impair normal chewing and swallowing. Figure 1.15 also demonstrates the peculiar bilateral dark brown hyperpigmentations at the corners of the mouth, first noted by Hamner, et al.. The patient's tongue usually exhibits a fibrous thickening, reduced mobility, and baldness due to atropy of the filiform papillae (see Fig. 1.16).

Histopathologically, the early stage of submucous fibrosis is characterized by atrophy of the oral epithelium with the loss of normal rete peg architecture, reduction of the stratum spinosum, vesicle formation, and a chronic inflammatory infiltrate (Fig. 1.17). The most distinctive histopathological feature of submucous fibrosis is the band of juxta-epithelial collagen [151], which is amorphous, non-bundular, and stains an abnormal greyish pink rather than the typical deep red for collagen, as demonstrated by the Rinehart stain (Fig. 1.18). This altered collagen appears atypically non-birefringent under polarized light.

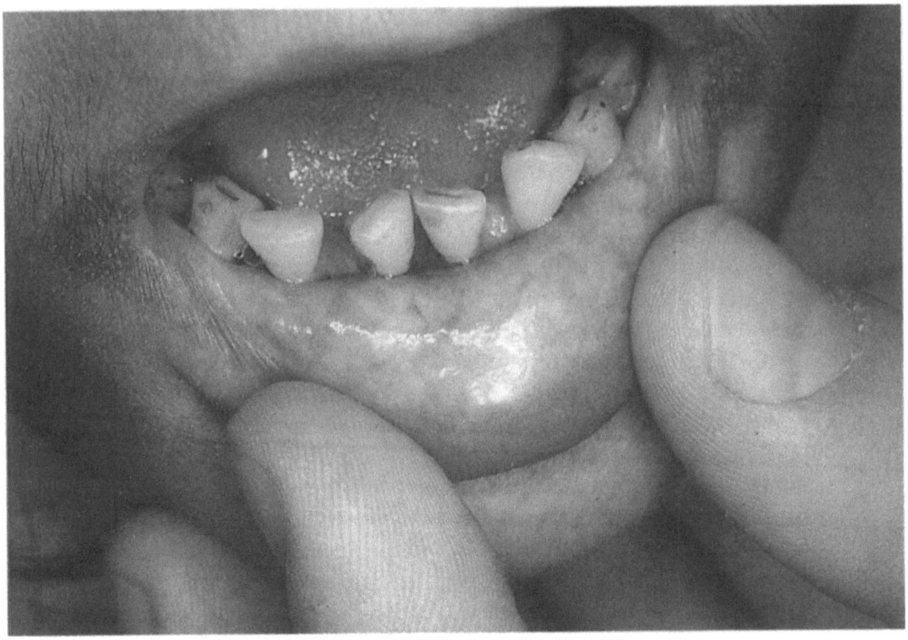

Fig. 1.14. Submucous fibrosis, 33 year old Pakistani female; note the marblelike appearance of the inner labial mucosa

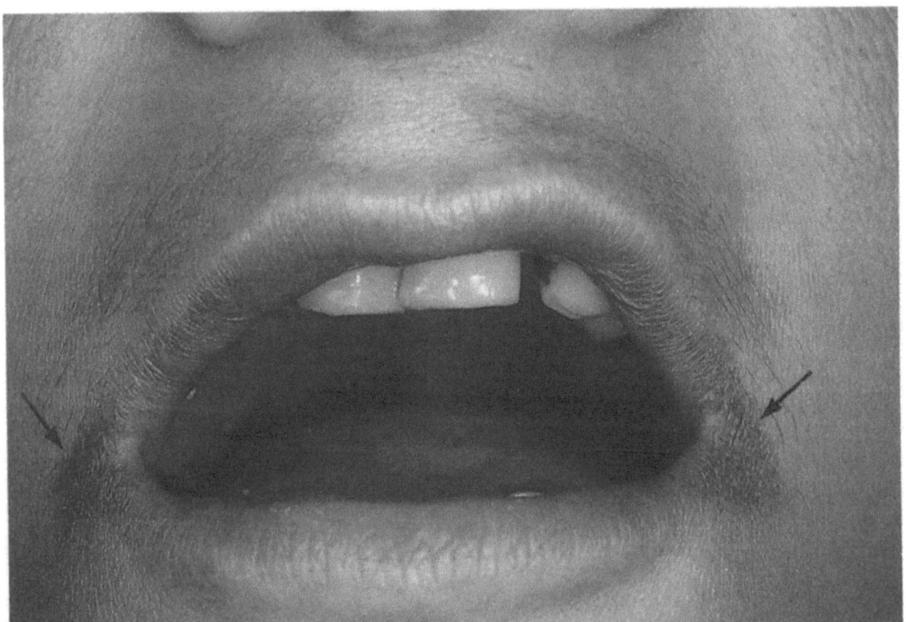

Fig. 1.15. Submucous fibrosis, reduction of the mouth opening and bilateral hyperpigmentation (*arrows*) of the mouth commissures, 33 year old Pakistani female

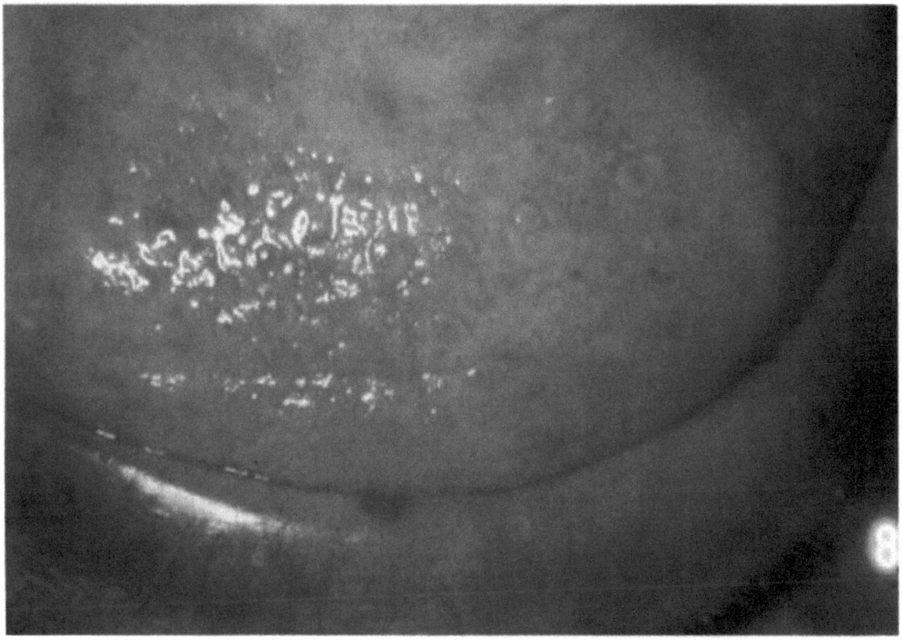

Fig. 1.16. Submucous fibrosis, tongue; atrophy of filiform papillae and reduction in mobility. (Courtesy of Dr. Fali S. Mehta)

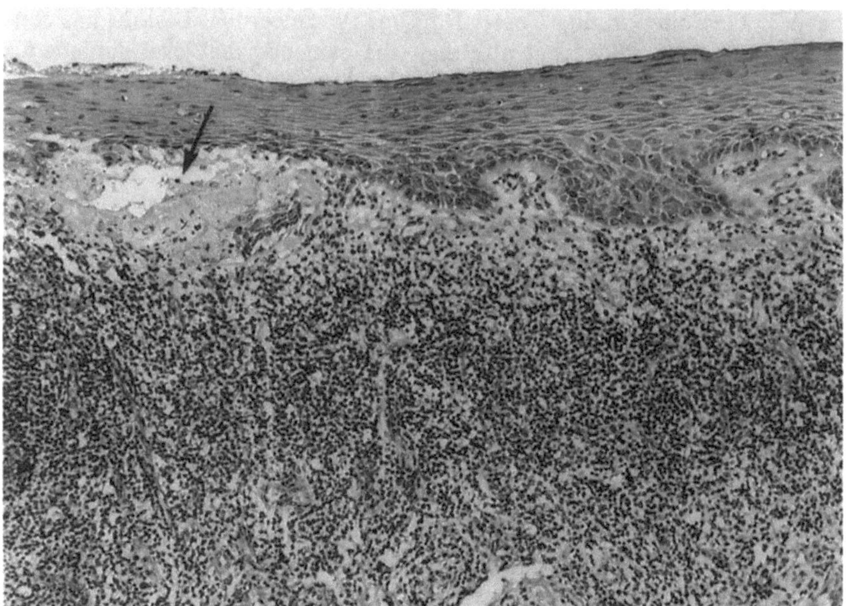

Fig. 1.17. Submucous fibrosis, buccal mucosa; epithelial atrophy, loss of rete peg architecture, chronic inflammation, and beginning subepithelial vesicle (*arrow*), H.&E. stain, ×65

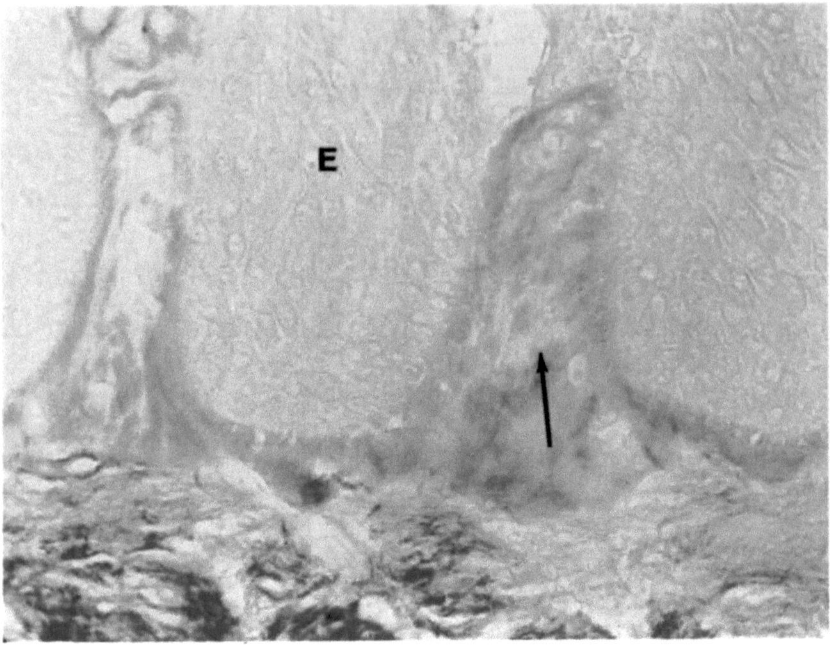

Fig. 1.18. Submucous fibrosis, buccal mucosa, 40 year old Indian female; atypical staining of juxtaepithelial collagen (*arrow*); *E*, epithelium. Rinehart stain, ×350

The W.H.O. Collaborating Center for Oral Precancerous Lesions has concluded after years of study that although the evidence that oral submucous fibrosis predisposes to cancer is not yet absolutely conclusive, it is highly probable that such a relationship does exist [119]. Three facts support this hypothesis:

1. The frequency of oral leukoplakia in submucous fibrosis patients is six to eight times higher than in control groups [124].
2. In South India, almost half of the oral cancer patients also exhibited submucous fibrosis; such a frequency far exceeds the 1.2% of submucous fibrosis in the general population of South India [29, 145, 153].
3. Epithelial dysplasia has been detected at a rate as high as 22.6% among oral submucous fibrosis patients [154].

Such epithelial dysplasia that can proceed to frank carcinoma is shown in Fig. 1.19.

The exact cause of submucous fibrosis remains obscure. As mentioned earlier, some investigators have suggested a hypersensitivity to chili peppers [135, 150]. Wahi believed that tobacco use and vitamin deficiencies produced submucous fibrosis [145]. Shear (1967) and Shian and Kwan (1979) were of the opinion that submucous fibrosis was caused by the betel chewing habit [142, 155].

Ramanathan has offered an alternative hypothesis for the cause of submucous fibrosis. He has expressed the view that submucous fibrosis is the Asian version of sideropenic dysphagia (Plummer-Vinson syndrome), caused by a prolonged period of chronic iron deficiency and/or vitamin B complex deficiency, especially folic acid [156]. Such deficiencies were detected in 10/13 submucous

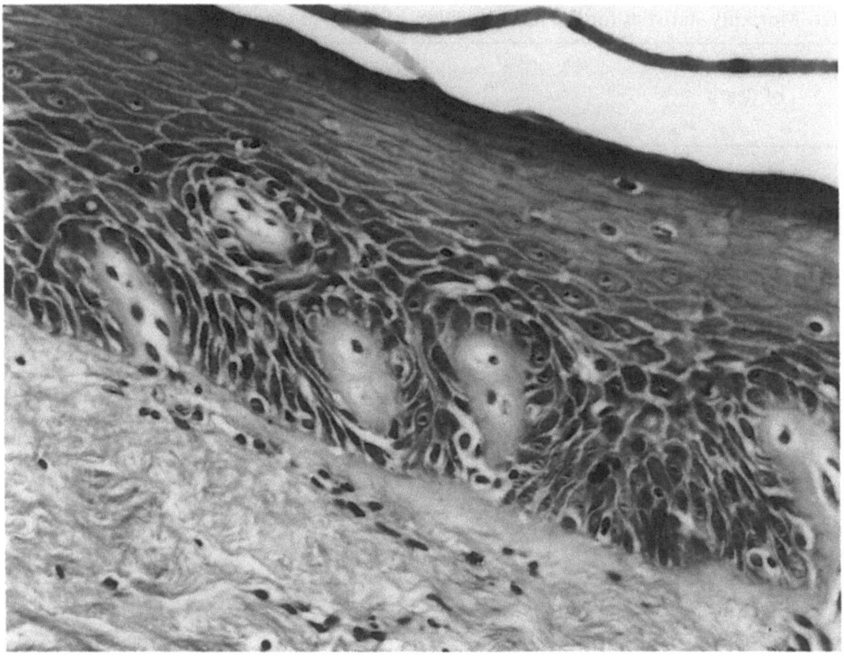

Fig. 1.19. Submucous fibrosis, 33 year old Pakistani female; note the epithelial dysplasia, H.&E. stain, ×350

fibrosis cases that he compiled. Vitamin deficiencies have also been noted in submucous fibrosis cases in the literature: Wahi, 1966 [145], Shear and Lemmer, 1967 [142], Hamner, 1974 [143], and Barnes and Duke, 1975 [157].

While this theory is possible, there must be more factors involved in the etiology of submucous fibrosis, or it would be even more prevalent in parts of the world where iron deficiency and vitamin B complex deficiency are universal. More pathology investigations in depth are needed to gain more accurate insight into the exact cause of submucous fibrosis with enough patients to make these findings statistically significant.

IV. Epidemiology

In 1900 cancer ranked eighth as a cause of death in the United States. Because the successful treatment of infectious diseases has greatly improved during the 82 years interrim from 1900 to 1982, due mainly to antibiotic therapy and national immunization programs, cancer currently ranks second only to heart disease as the most frequent cause of death (Table 1.1). Cancer accounted for 330,730 deaths in 1970 and 396,992 deaths in 1978, reflecting both growth in the elderly American population and more accurate diagnostic modalities [18, 158].

Table 1.1. Mortality statistics for the leading causes of death in the united states – 1978[a]

Rank	Cause of death	Number of deaths	Death rate per 100,000 population	Percent of total deaths
1.	Heart disease	729,510	300.4	37.8
2.	Cancer	396,992	169.9	20.6
3.	Cerebrovascular diseases	175,629	70.8	9.1
4.	Accidents	105,561	45.8	5.5
5.	Pneumonia & influenza	58,319	23.6	3,0
6.	Chronic obstructive lung disease	50,488	12.2	2.6
7.	Diabetes mellitus	33,841	14.2	1.8
8.	Cirrhosis of liver	30,066	13.4	1.6
9.	Arteriosclerosis	28,940	11.1	1.5
10.	Suicide	27,294	11.6	1.4
11.	Diseases of infancy	22,033	12.1	1.1
12.	Homicide	20,432	8.7	1.1
13.	Aortic aneurysm	14,028	5.8	0.8
14.	Congential anomalies	12,968	6.8	0.7
15.	Pulmonary infarction	10,941	4.6	0.6
	Other & Ill-defined	210,606	89.9	10.8
	All causes	1,927,788	809.9	100.0

[a] Source: Vital statistic of the United States (1978)

Three epidemiological measurements are used to arrive at objective measures of cancer illness:

1. Incidence rate: the number of new cases arising during a given time in a specific population, usually measured by counting the number of newly diagnosed cancers in a given year. This is the measure most directly related to cancer risk.

2. Mortality rate: the number of deaths due to the disease occurring during a given time in a specific population.

3. Prevalance rate: the number of cases existing at a given time in a specific population.

The cancer incidence rates by anatomic site in males and females are illustrated by Fig. 1.20. Lung cancer is the most common malignant neoplasm in men (22%), followed by carcinoma of the prostrate (18%) [158]. In women, breast cancer remains the leading site in 1982 (26%), with uterine carcinoma next (13%).

Oral cancer incidence is higher in American men (6%), whereas it is only 2% is women – probably due to the fact that more men still practice tobacco habits than women [158]. Oral cancer accounts for 3% of male deaths and 1% of female deaths (Fig. 1.21). These estimates of the incidence and death percentage of cancer are based upon the National Cancer Institute's Surveillance Epidemiology and End Results (SEER) Program's statistics for 1973–1978.

Excluding carcinoma-in-situ (45,000 new uterine cases annually) and non-melanoma skin cancers (400,000 new cases annually), 835,000 new cancer cases are estimated for 1982. Concurrently, 430,000 cancer deaths are estimated for all sites in 1982 from the on-going cancer-stricken population [158].

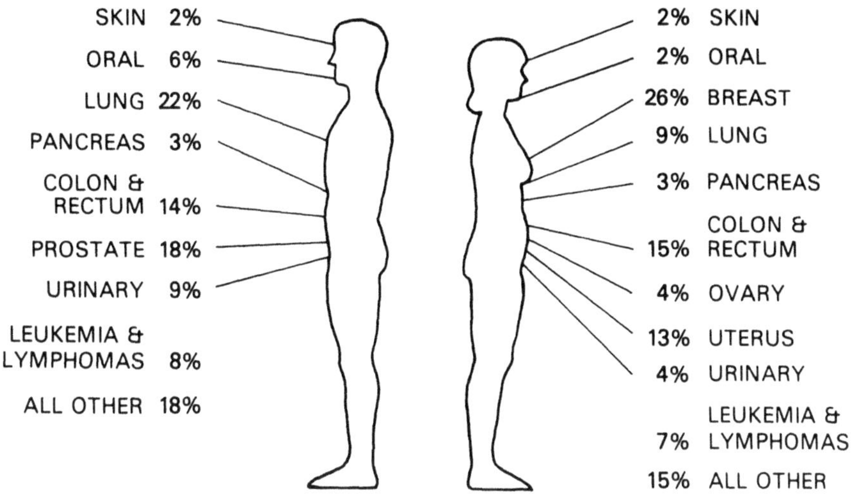

Excluding nonmelanoma skin cancer and carcinoma in situ.

Fig. 1.20. Estimated cancer incidence by anatomic site and sex – 1982. (Source: American cancer society cancer statistics – 1982)

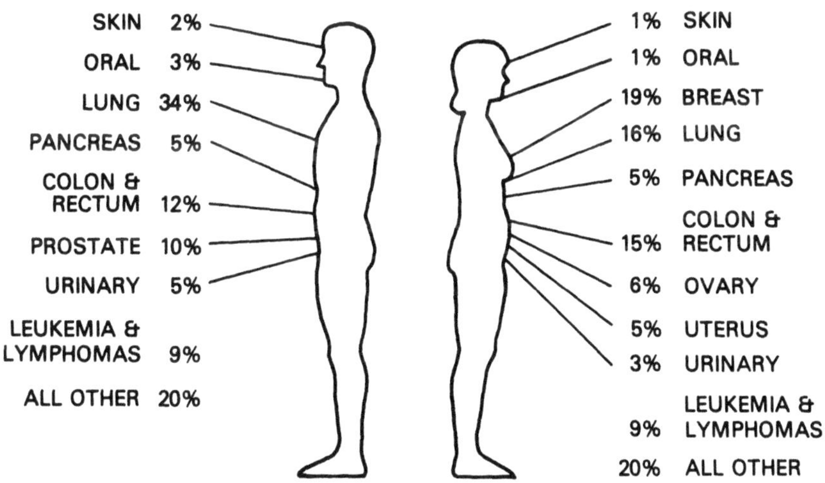

Fig. 1.21. Estimated cancer deaths by site and sex – 1982. (Source: American cancer society cancer statistics – 1982)

Oral cancer will afflict approximately 26,800 Americans annually and will kill about 9,500 each year (Table 1.2). The most common site for oral cancer in both American men and women is the tongue. The incidence and death rates for oral cancer vary among different regions of the world. Table 1.3 depicts the age-adjusted death rates per 100,000 population for oral cancer, based on the 1976–1977 statistical figures from the World Health Statistics Annual [160].

Oral cancer has been one of the two most common cancers reported to the Papua New Guinea Tumor Registry between 1958 and 1970: 668 cases

Table 1.2. Estimated oral cancer incidence and deaths by site and sex – 1982[a]

Site	Estimated oral cancer cases			Estimated oral cancer deaths		
	Total	Male	Female	Total	Male	Female
Lip	4,600	4,100	500	175	150	25
Tongue	4,800	3,200	1,600	2,000	1,400	600
Salivary gland }				700	450	250
Floor of mouth }	9,700	5,800	3,900	525	400	125
Other oral areas }				1,550	1,000	550
Pharynx	7,700	5,500	2,200	4,200	2,900	1,300
Total oral cavity and pharynx	26,800	18,600	8,200	9,150	6,300	2,850

[a] Source: American cancer society cancer statistics (1982)

Table 1.3. International age-adjusted death rates per 100,000 population for oral cancer, 1976–1977[a]

Country	Male	Female
United States	5.8	2.0
Australia	5.3	1.5
Canada	5.3	1.6
Denmark	3.1	1.5
England & Wales	3.7	1.7
Germany	3.5	0.9
Hong Kong	21.2	7.1
Japan	2.2	0.8
Norway	4.3	1.1
Singapore	18.9	6.3
Sweden	3.4	1.4

[a] Source: World health statistics annual (1979–1980)

[161]. Similar to other Southeast Asian countries, this high incidence of oral cancer has been directly related to the introduction of the betel chewing habit to larger regions of that country. Therefore, the most common site for oral cancer among these patients is also the buccal mucosa [161].

Statistical information from Russia indicates that the incidence of oral cancer is higher in their Central Asian republics, as would be expected, than in other regions of the Soviet Union. For example, the age-adjusted incidence rate for oral carcinoma in Uzbek was 2.3, whereas in contrast, the rate was only 0.4 in Byelo-Russia [162]. This difference is attributed to the manner of preparation and degree of use of "nass" in the Central Asian republics. "Nass" is a preparation of tobacco, ash, cotton oil or sesame oil, and lime (plus other desired ingredients according to local choice) that is customarily placed under the tongue. Because clinical cancer often develops where the "nass" quid is held in the mouth, it is firmly believed that a relationship exists between the "nass"

Table 1.4. Oral cancer incidence rates in india

Locality	Year of survey	Author	Oral cancer incidence per 100,000
1. Greater Bombay	(1968–1972)	Jussawalla & Jain [163]	14.7
2. Mainpuri District, Uttar Pradesh	(1968)	Wahi [164]	21.4
3. Ahmedabad, Gujarat	(1974–1976)	Malawalla et al. [165]	25.0
4. Visakhapatnam District, Andhra Pradesh	(1973–1975)	Reddy et al. [166]	9.1
5. Ernakulam District, Kerala	(1969–1977)	Mehta et al. [31]	26.0
6. Srikakulam District, Andhra Pradesh	(1969–1977)	Mehta et al. [31]	14.0

habit and oral cancer [162]. The trend for overall incidence of newly diagnosed oral cancers has statistically risen in Russia from 1.0 in 1962, to 1.7 in 1967, to 2.1 in 1972, to 2.2 in 1973 per 100,000 inhabitants, according to the Registry of Oncological Institutions in Russia [162].

Oral cancer is a much more common tumor in Southeast Asia than elsewhere in the world (e.g. 21.2% in Hong Kong and 18.9% in Singapore versus 2.2% in Japan: see Table 1.3). The world's highest incidence rate for oral cancer is found in India. Example incidence rates per 100,000 population for different studies in various state localities are listed in Table 1.4.

In spite of the fact that it is readily accessible for detection and diagnosis, about 50% of oral cancer cases have already exhibited lymph nodal and/or distant metastases by the time of definitive diagnosis and instigation of treatment. The 5-year survival rate for localized oral cancer is 67%; 30% for regional involvement; and only 14% when distant metastases are present [159].

In 1980 the National Cancer Institute published trends in cancer survival comparing SEER statistics from 1960–1963 to 1970–1973 in white and black patients. Generally speaking, white patients tended to have higher percentages of cancers diagnosed while in the localized stage and were slightly older than black patients. Also, the overall cancer survival experience for white patients was shown to be better than for black patients [167].

For oral cancer, the lack of statistics on black patients did not permit a comparison. However, the trends in oral cancer survival for white male and white female patients are shown in Tables 1.5 and 1.6. It should be pointed out that cancer of the tongue (23% in 1960–1963 to 32% in 1970–1973) and cancer of the pharynx (21% in 1960–1963 to 27% in 1970–1973) showed increases in survival that were statistically significant at the 0.05 level [167].

These survival trends reveal that to cause a significant reduction in cancer mortality, either better cancer treatment methods must be developed and widely utilized, or else cancer must be prevented from developing so that treatment is unnecessary. Major research is needed in both cancer treatment and prevention, with neither one taking precedence over the other.

Table 1.5. Trend in survival for white male oral cancer patients[a]

Site	Number of cases		5-Year relative survival rates (%)	
	1960–1963	1970–1973	1960–1963	1970–1973
Lip	644	331	84	87
Tongue	577	561	23	32[b]
Salivary gland	153	146	55	53
Mouth	727	738	42	40
Pharynx	756	832	21	27[b]

[a] Source: N.C.I. cancer patient survival experience (1980)
[b] Increase in survival statistically significant at the 0.05 level (one-tail test)

Table 1.6. Trend in survival for white female oral cancer patients[a]

Site	Number of cases		5-Year relative survival rates (%)	
	1960–1963	1970–1973	1960–1963	1970–1973
Lip	40	33	88	Too few cases
Tongue	202	272	44	46
Salivary gland	126	118	82	85
Mouth	313	403	50	51
Pharynx	196	331	35	31

[a] Source: N.C.I. cancer patient survival experience (1980)

References

1. Bryan, W.R.: "A Reconsideration of the Nature of the Neoplastic Reaction in the Light of Recent Advances in Cancer Research", J.N.C.I. 24:221–251, 1960
2. Petrov, N.N.: "A New Definition of the Conception of Tumor Growth". In: Pathogenesis and Immuniology of Tumors (Vygodchikov, C.V., ed.), (Pergamon Press: New York, NY), 1959
3. Ackerman, L.V. and del Regato, J.A.: Cancer Diagnosis, Treatment, and Prognosis, Ed. 4, (C.V. Mosby Co.: St. Louis, MO), 1970
4. Miller, E.C. and Miller, J.A.: "Symposium on Immunogenetics and Carcinogenesis; In Vivo Combinations Between Carcinogens and Tissue Constituents and Their Possible Role in Carcinogenesis", Cancer. Res. 12:547–556, 1952
5. Greenstein, J.P.: Biochemistry of Cancer, Ed. 2, (Academic Press: New York, N.Y.), 1954
6. Wiest, W.G. and Heidelberger, C.: "The Interaction of Carcinogenic Hydrocarbons With Tissue Constituents I. Methods", Cancer. Res. 13:246–249, 1953
7. Rusch, H.P.: "Carcinogenesis: A Facet of Living Processes", Cancer. Res. 14:407–417, 1954
8. Hiatt, H.H., Watson, J.D., and Winsten, J.A.: Origins of Human Cancer. Book A. – Incidence of Cancer in Humans, (Cold Spring Harbor Laboratory, Cold Spring Harbor, NY), 1977.
9. Bailar, J.C., III and Hamner, J.E., III: "Summary: NCI Conference on Cancer Prevention – Quantitative Aspects", N.C.I. Cancer Conference: Sept. 25–28, 1978, Reston, VA
10. Southam, C.M.: "The Complex Etiology of Cancer", Cancer. Res., 23:1105–1115, 1963
11. Robbins, S.L.: Pathology, Ed. 3, (W.B. Saunders Co.: Philadelphia, PA.), 1967

12. Hamner, J.E., III: The Effect of X-ray Irradiation on Hydrocarbon Carcinogenesis in the Buccal Mucosa of the Syrian Hamster, (M.S. Thesis – Medical College of Virginia: Richmond, VA), 1964
13. Salley, J.J.: "Effect of Mineral Oil as a Solvent for 9,10-dimethyl-1,2-benzanthracene", J. Dent Res., 34:723, 1955
14. Horton, A.W., Denman, D.T., and Trosset, R.P.: "Carcinogenesis of the Skin. II. The Accelerating Properties of Aliphatic and Related Hydrocarbons", Cancer. Res. 17:758–766, 1957
15. Mottram, J.C.: "Production of Epithelial Tumors by a Combination of Beta Radiation and Painting with Benzpyrene", Amer. J. Cancer 32:76–79, 1938
16. Shubik, P., Goldfarb, A.R., Ritchie, A.C., and Lisco, H.: "Latent Carcinogenic Action of Beta Irradiation on Mouse Epidermis", Nature 171:934–935, 1953
17. Hammond, E.C.: Chapter on "Tobacco" In: Persons at High Risk of Cancer, (Fraumeni J.F. ed.), Ed. 1, (Academic Press: New York, NY), 1975
18. Hamner, J.E., III: Chapter on "Oral Cancer", In: Oral Medicine, (Lynch, M.A., ed.), Ed. 7, (J.B. Lippincott Co.: Philadelphia, PA.) 1977
19. Silverman, S., Jr. and Griffith, M.: "Smoking Characteristics of Patients with Oral Carcinoma and the Risk for Second Oral Primary Cancer", J.A.D.A. 85:637–640, 1972
20. Silverman, S., Jr. and Galante, M.: Oral Cancer, Ed. 4, (Univ. of California: San Francisco, Calif.), 1974
21. Moore, C.: "Cigarette Smoking and Cancer of the Mouth, Pharynx, and Larynx", J.A.M.A. 218:553–558, 1971
22. Wynder, E.L.: Chapter on "Etiological Aspects of Squamous Cancers of the Head and Neck", In: Cancer of the Head and Neck (Rubin P., ed.), Current Concepts in Cancer – Number 30. J.A.M.A. 215:1–124, 1971
23. Wynder, E.L.: "Environmental Factors in Cancer of the Larynx", Cancer 38:1591–1601, 1976
24. Khanolkar, V.R. and Suryabai, B.: "Cancer in Relation to Usages", Arch. Pathol. 40:351–361, 1945
25. Sanghvi, L.D., Rao, K.C.M., and Khanolkar, V.K.: "Smoking and Chewing of Tobacco in Relation to Cancer of the Upper Alimentary Tract", Brit. Med. J. 7:1111–1114, 1955
26. Hirayama, T.: "An Epidemiological Study of Oral and Pharyngeal Cancer in Central and Southeast Asia", Bull. W.H.O. 34:41–69, 1966
27. Malhotra, S.L.: "Geographical Distribution of Gastrointestinal Cancers in India with Special Reference to Causation", Gut. 8:361–372, 1967
28. Jussawalla, D.J. and Deshpande, V.A.: "Evaluation of Cancer Risk in Tobacco Chewers and Smokers: An Epidemiologic Accessment", Cancer 28:244–252, 1971
29. Mehta, F.S., Pindborg, J.J., and Hamner, J.E., III: Oral Cancer and Precancerous Conditions in India, Ed. 1, (Munksgaard: Copenhagen, Denmark), 1971
30. Mehta, F.S., Daftary, D.K., Gupta, P.C., et al.: "Tobacco Habits and Oral Cancer", Science Today 13:27–30, 1978
31. Gupta, P.C., Mehta, F.S., Daftary, D.K., et al.: "Incidence Rates of Oral Cancer and Natural History of Oral Precancerous Lesions in a 10-Year Followup Study of Indian Villagers", Comm. Dent. Oral Epidemiol. 8:287–333, 1980
32. Chin, C.T. and Lee, K.W.: "The Effects of Betel-Nut Chewing on the Buccal Mucosa of 296 Indians and Malays in West Malaysia: A Clinical Study", Brit. J. Cancer 24:427–432, 1970
33. Dunham, L.J. and Herrold, K.M.: "Failure to Produce Tumors in the Hamster Cheek Pouch by Exposure to Ingredients of Betel Quid; Histopathologic Changes in the Pouch and Other Organs by Exposure to Known Carcinogens", J.N.C.I. 6:1047–1067, 1962
34. Dunham, L.J., Muir, C.S., and Hamner, J.E., III: "Epithelial Atypia in Hamster Cheek Pouches Treated Repeatedly with Calcium Hydroxide", Brit. J. Cancer 20:588–593, 1966
35. Sirsat, S.M. and Khandarkar, S.V.: "Histological Changes in the Oral Mucosa of the Wistar Rat Treated with Commercial Lime (Calcium Hydroxide) – An Optical and Submicroscopic Study", Brit. J. Cancer 22:303–315, 1968
36. Cohen, B. and Smith, C.J.: "Aetiological Factors in Oral Cancer: Experimental Investigation of Early Epithelial Changes", Helv. Odont. Acta 2:112–124, 1967

37. Pindborg, J.J. and Renstrup, G.: "Studies in Oral Leukoplakias, II. Effect of Snuff on Oral Epithelium", Acta. Derm. Venereol. 43:271–276, 1963
38. Van Wyk, C.W.: "The Oral Lesion Caused by Snuff", J.D.A.S.A. 21:109–116, 1966
39. Cohen, B., Poswillo, D.E., and Woods, D.A.: "The Effects of Exposure to Chewing Tobacco on the Oral Mucosa of Monkey and Man", Ann. Roy. Coll. Surg. 48:255–273, 1971
40. Hamner, J.E., III: "Betel Quid Inducement of Epithelial Atypia in the Buccal Mucosa of Baboons", Cancer 30:1001–1005, 1972
41. Hamner, J.E., III and Reed, O.M.: "Betel Quid Carcinogenesis in Baboons", J. Med. Prim. 1:75–85, 1972
42. Koop, C.E.: The Surgeon-General's Report on Smoking – 1982, (H.H.S. Publication: Washington, DC), 1982
43. Hutchison, G.B.: Chapter on "Carcinogenic Effects of Medical Irradiation", In: Origins of Human Cancer. Book A. Incidence of Cancer in Humans, (Hiatt H.H., Watson J.D., and Winsten J.A., editors), Ed. 1, (Cold Spring Harbor Laboratories, Cold Spring Harbor, NY) 1977
44. Brues, A.M.: "Radiation as a Carcinogenic Agent", Rad. Res. 3:272–280, 1955
45. Chase, L.P., Toto, P.D., and Magalotti, M.F.: "Radiation-Induced Changes in The Epithelium of the Buccal Mucosa", J. Dent. Res. 40:929–935, 1961
46. Jablon, S.: Chapter on "Radiation", In: Persons at High Risk of Cancer, (Fraumeni J.F., ed.), Ed. 1, (Academic Press: New York, NY), 1975
47. Upton, A.C.: Chapter on "Radiation Effects", In: Origins of Human Cancer Book A. Incidence of Cancer in Humans, (Hiatt H.H., Watson J.D., and Winsten J.A., editors), Ed. 1, (Cold Spring Harbor Laboratories: Cold Spring Harbor, NY), 1977
48. Brill, A.B., Tomonaga, M., Heyssel, R.M.: "Leukemia in Man Following Exposure to Ionizing Radiation: Summary of Findings in Hiroshima and Nagasaki, and Comparison with Other Human Experience". Ann. Intern. Med. 56:590–609, 1962
49. Nishiyama, H., Anderson, R.E., Ishimaru, T., et al.: "The Incidence of Malignant Lymphoma and Multiple Myeloma in Hiroshima and Nagasaki Atomic Bomb Survivors, 1945–1965", Cancer 32:1301–1309, 1973
50. Wood, J.W., Tamagaki, H., Neriishi, S., et al.: "Thyroid Carcinoma in Atomic Bomb Survivors, Hiroshima-Nagasaki", Amer. J. Epidemiol. 89:4–14, 1969
51. Metter, F.A., Hempelmann, L.H., Dutton, A.M., et al.: "Breast Neoplasms in Women Treated with X-rays for Acute Post-Partum Mastitis", J.N.C.I. 43:803–811, 1969
52. Myrden, J.A. and Hiltz, J.E.: "Breast Cancer Following Multiple Fluoroscopies During Artificial Pneumothorax Treatment of Pulmonary Tuberculosis", Can. Med. Assoc. J. 100:1032–1034, 1969
53. Stewart, A. and Kneale, G.W.: "Radiation Dose Effects in Relation to Obstetric X-rays and Childhood Cancers", Lancet 1:1185–1188, 1970
54. Hempelmann, L.H., Pifer, J.W. , and Burke, G.J.: "Neoplasms in Person Treated with X-rays in Infancy for Thymic Enlargement: A Report on the Third Follow-up Survey", J.N.C.I. 38:317–341, 1967
55. Albert, E.R. and Omran, A.R.: "Follow-up Study of Patients Treated by X-ray Epilation for Tinea Capitis", Arch. Environ. Health 17:899–950, 1968
56. Doniach, I.: "Experimental Induction of Tumors of the Thyroid by Radiation", Brit. Med. Bull. 14:181–183, 1958
57. Nicholas, C.W. Jr, Lindsay, W., Sheline, G.E., and Chaikoff, I.L.: "Induction of Neoplasms in the Rat Thyroid by X-radiation of a Single Lobe", Arch. Pathol. 80:177–183, 1965
58. Clark, D.E.: "Association of Irradiation with Cancer of the Thyroid in Children and Adolescents", J.A.M.A. 159:1007–1009, 1955
59. Saenger, E.L., Silverman, F.N., Sterling, T.D., et al.: "Neoplasia Following Therapeutic Irradiation for Benign Conditions in Childhood", Rad. 74:899–904, 1960
60. Socolow, E.L., Hashizume, A., Neriishi, S., et al.: "Thyroid Carcinoma in Man After Exposure to Ionizing Radiation", N.E.J.M. 268:406–410, 1963
61. Farus, J.F., Schneider, A.B., Stachura, M.E., et al.: "Thyroid Malignancy Occuring as a Late Consequence of Head and Neck Irradiation: Evaluation of 1056 Patients", N.E.J.M. 294:1019–1025, 1976

62. McKenzie, A.D.: "The Natural History of Thyroid Cancer. A Report of 102 Cases Analyzed 10 to 15 Years After Diagnosis", Arch. Surg. 102:274–277, 1971
63. Holm, L.E., Lundell, G., and Walinder, G.: "Incidence of Malignant Thyroid Tumors in Humans After Exposure to Diagnostic Doses of Iodine-131. I. Retrospective Cohort Study", J.N.C.I. 64:1055–1059, 1980
64. Sener, S.F. and Scanlon, E.F.: "Irradiation Induced Salivary Gland Neoplasia", Ann. Surg. 191:304–306, 1980
65. Cahan, W.G., Woodard, H.Q., Higinbotham, N.L., et al.: "Sarcoma Arising in Irradiated Bone", Cancer 1:3–29, 1948
66. Sabanas, A.O., Dahlin, D.C., Childs, D.S., and Ivins, J.C.: "Postradiation Sarcoma of Bone", Cancer 9:528–542, 1956
67. Kragh, L.V., Dahlin, D.C., and Erich, J.B.: "Osteogenic Sarcoma of the Jaws and Facial Bones", Amer. J. Surg. 96:496–505, 1958
68. Phillips, T.L. and Sheline, G.E.: "Bone Sarcomas Following Radiation Therapy", Radiology 81:992–996, 1963
69. Garrington, G.E., Scofield, H.H., Cornyn, J., and Hooker, S.P.: "Osteosarcoma of the Jaws", Cancer 20:377–391, 1967
70. Kripke, M.L. and Sass, E.R.: National Cancer Institute Monograph #50: International Conference on Ultravioloet Carcinogenesis. (N.I.H. Publishing: Bethesda, MD), 1977
71. Lane-Brown, M.M. and Melia, D.F.: "A Genetic Diathesis to Skin Cancer", J. Invest. Dermatol. 61:39–41, 1973
72. Gellin, G.A., Kopf, A.W., and Garfinkel, L.: "Malignant Melanoma: A Controlled Study of Possible Associated Factors", Arch. Dermatol. 99:43–48, 1969
73. Gordon, D. and Silverstone, H.: "Deaths from Skin Cancer in Queensland, Australia." In: The Biologic Effects of Ultraviolet Radiation, (Urbach, F., ed.) Ed. 1, (Pergamon Press: New York, NY), 1969
74. Scott, E.L. and Straf, M.L.: Chapter on 'Ultraviolet Radiation as a Cause of Cancer", In: Origins of Human Cancer. Book A – Incidence of Cancer in Humans, (Hiatt, H.H., Watson, J.D., and Winsten, J.A., editors), Ed. 1, (Cold Spring Harbor Laboratories, Cold Spring Harbor, NY), 1977
75. Wogan, G.N.: "Aflatoxin Risks and Control Measures", Fed. Proc. 27:932–938, 1968
76. Oettle, A.G.: "Cancer in Africa, Especially in Regions South of the Sahara", J.N.C.I. 33:383–439, 1964
77. Berg, J.W.: Chapter on "Diet", In: Persons at High Risk of Cancer, (Fraumeni, J.F., ed.), Ed. 1, (Academic Press: New York, NY) 1975
78. Haenszel, W., Kurihara, M., Segi, M., et al.: "Stomach Cancer Among Japanese in Hawaii", J.N.C.I. 49:969–988, 1973
79. Sigurjonsson, J.: "Occupational Variations in Mortality from Gastric Cancer in Relation to Dietary Differences", Brit. J. Cancer 21:651–656, 1967
80. Saffiotti, U., Montesano, R., Sellakumar, A.R., et al.: "Experimental Cancer of the Lung", Cancer 20:857–864, 1967
81. Chu, E.W. and Malmgren, R.A.: "An Inhibitory Effect of Vitamin A on the Induction of Tumors of the Forestomach and Cervix the Syrian Hamster by Carcinogenic Polycyclic Hydrocarbons", Cancer Res. 25:884–895, 1965
82. Rowe, N.H., Grammer, F.C., Watson, F.R., et al.: "A Study of Environmental Influence Upon Salivary Gland Neoplasia in Rats", Cancer 26:436–444, 1970
83. Rogers, A.E., Herndon, B.J. and Newberne, P.M.: "Induction by Dimethylhydrazine of Intestinal Carcinoma in Normal Rats and Rats Fed High or Low Levels of Vitamin A", Cancer Res. 33:1003–1009, 1973
84. Bollag, W. and Ott, F.: "Therapy of Actinic Keratoses and Basal Cell Carcinomas with Local Application of Vitamin A. Acid". Cancer Chemother. Rep. 55:59–60, 1971
85. Shafer, W.G., Hine, M.K. and Levy, B.M.: Oral Pathology Ed. 3, (W.B. Saunders Co.: Philadelphia, PA), 1974
86. Ahlbon, H.E.: "Simple Achlorhydric Anemia, Plummer-Vinson Syndrome, and Carcinoma of the Mouth, Pharynx, and Oesophagus in Women", Brit. Med. J. 2:331–337, 1936
87. Wynder, E.L., Hultberg, S., Jaconsson, F., et al.: "Environmental Factors in Cancer of the Upper Alimentary Tract. A Swedish Study with Special Reference to Plummer-Vinson (Paterson-Kelly) Syndrome", Cancer 10:470–487, 1957

88. Trieger, N., et al.: "The Significance of Liver Dysfunction in Mouth Cancer", Surg. Gynecol. Obstet. 108:230–234, 1959
89. Keller, A.Z.: "The Epidemiology of Lip, Oral, and Pharyngeal Cancers and the Association with Selected Systemic Diseases", Amer. J. Pub. Health 53:1214–1228, 1963
90. Keller, A.Z.: "Cirrhosis of the Liver, Alcoholism, and Heavy Smoking Associated with Cancer of the Mouth and Pharynx", Cancer 20:1015–1022, 1967
91. Wynder, E.L., Bross, I.J., and Feldman, R.: "A Study of the Etiological Factors of Cancer of the Mouth", Cancer 10:1300–1323, 1957
92. Pottern, L.M., Morris, L.E., Blot, W.J., et al.: "Esophageal Cancer Among Black Men in Washington, D.C. (1) Alcohol, Tobacco, and Other Risk Factors", J.N.C.I. 67:777–783, 1981
93. Good, R.A.: Personal Communication
94. Schottenfeld, D., Gantt, R.C., and Wynder, E.L.: "The Role of Alcohol and Tobacco in Multiple Primary Cancers of the Upper Digestive System, Larynx, and Lung: A Prospective Study", Prev. Med. 3:277–293, 1974
95. Rothman, K. and Keller, A.: "The Effect of Joint Exposure to Alcohol and Tobacco on the Risk of Cancer of the Mouth and Pharynx", J. Chronic. Dis. 25:711–716, 1972
96. Kissin, B., et al.: "Head and Neck Cancer in Alcoholics. The Relationship to Drinking, Smoking, and Dietary Patterns", J.A.M.A. 224:1174–1175, 1973
97. Groupe, V. and Salmoiraghi, G.C.: "Alcohol and Cancer Workshop", Cancer Res. 39:2816–2908, 1979
98. Rothman, K.J.: Chapter on "Alcohol", In: Persons at High Risk of Cancer, (Fraumenia J.F., ed), Ed. 1, (Academic Press: New York, NY), 1975
99. Mulvihill, J.J.: Chapter on "Congenital and Genetic Diseases", In: Persons at High Risk of Cancer, (Fraumeni J.F., ed.), Ed. 1, (Academic Press: New York, NY), 1975
100. Hamner, J.E., III and Ketcham, A.S.: "Cherubism: An Analysis of Treatment", Cancer 23:113–1143, 1969
101. Hiatt, H.H., Watson, J.D., and Winsten, J.A.: Origins of Human Cancer. Book B Mechanisms of Carcinogenesis, Ed. 1, (Cold Spring Harbor Laboratory, Cold Spring Harbor, NY)
102. Rowson, K.E.K.: Chapter on "Viruses and Cancer" In: The Biology of Cancer (Ambrose E.J. and Roe F.J.C., editors), Ed. 1, (D. Van Nostrand Co., Ltd.: London, England), 1966
103. Heath, C.W., Caldwell, G.G., and Feorino, P.C.: Chapter on "Viruses and Other Microbes", In: Persons at High Risk of Cancer, (Fraumeni, J.F., ed.), Ed. 1, (Academic Press: New York, NY), 1975
104. Kessler, I.I.: "Prespectives on the Epidemiology of Cervical Cancer with Special Reference to the Herpesvirus Hypothesis", Cancer Res. 34:1091 1110, 1974
105. Aurelian, L., Royston, I., and Davis, H.J.: "Antibody to Genital Herpes Simplex Virus: Association with Cervical Atypia and Carcinoma-in-situ", J.N.C.I. 45:455–464, 1970
106. Catalano, L.W., Jr. and Johnson, L.D.: "Herpesvirus Antibody and Carcinoma-in-situ in the Cervix", J.A.M.A. 217:447–450, 1971
107. Hollinshead, A.C. and Tarro, G.: "Soluable Membrane Antigens of Lip and Cervical Carcinoma: Reactivity with Antibody for Herpesvirus Non-viron Antigens", Science 179:689–700, 1973
108. Hollinshead, A.C., Lee, O., Chretien, P.B., et al.: "Antibodies to Herpes-virus Non-viron Antigens in Squamous Carcinomas", Science 182:713–715, 1973
109. Sabin, A.B.: "Herpes Simplex-Genitalis Virus Non-viron Antigens and Their Implication in Certain Human Cancers: Unconfirmed", Proc. Nat. Acad. Sci. 71:3248–3252, 1974
110. Epstein, M.A., Achong, B.G., and Barr, Y.M.: "Virus Particles in Cultured Lymphoblasts from Burkitt's Lymphoma", Lancet 1:702–703, 1964
111. McAlister, R.M.: "Viruses in Human Carcinogenesis", Prog. Med. Virol. 16:48–85, 1973
112. Henle, G., Henle, W., Cliford, P., et al.: "Antibodies to EB Virus in Burkitt's Lymphoma and Control Groups", J.N.C.I. 43:1147–1157, 1969
113. Pegano, J.S., Huang, C.H., and Levine, P.: "Absence of Epstein-Barr Viral DNA in American Burkitt's Lymphoma", N.E.J.M. 289:1395–1399, 1973
114. Henle, W., Henle, G., Ho, H.C., et al.: "Antibodies to EB Virus in Nasopharyngeal Cancer, Other Head and Neck Neoplasms, and Controls", J.N.C.I. 44:225–231, 1970

115. Levin, M., et al.: "Syphilis and Cancer: Reported Syphilis Prevalence Among 7,761 Cancer Patients", N.Y. State Med. J. 42:1737–1743, 1942
116. Trieger, N., et al.: "Cirrhosis and Other Predisposing Factors in Carcinoma of the Tongue", Cancer 11:357–362, 1958
117. Myer, I. and Abbey, L.M.: "The Relationship of Syphilis to Primary Carcinoma of the Tongue", Oral Surg. 30:678–681, 1970
118. Berenblum, I.: "Irritation and Carcinogenesis", Arch. Pathol. 38:233–244, 1944
119. Kramer, I.R.H., Lucas, R.B., Pindborg, J.J., Sobin, L.H., et al.: "Definition of Leukoplakia and Related Lesions: An Aid to Studies on Oral Precancer". Oral Surg. 46:518–539, 1978
120. Pindborg, J.J., et al.: "Studies in Oral Leukoplakia", Acta Odont. Scand. 21:407, 1963
121. Shedd, D.P.: "Clinical Characteristics of Early Oral Cancer", J.A.M.A. 215:955–956, 1971
122. Mashberg, A.: "Erythroplasia vs. Leukoplakia in the Diagnosis of Early Asyptomatic Oral Squamous Carcinoma", N.E.J.M. 297:109–110, 1977
123. Shafer, W.G. and Waldron, C.A.: "Erythroplakia of the Oral Cavity", Cancer 36:1021–1028, 1975
124. Pindborg, J.J.: Atlas of Diseases of the Oral Mucosa, Ed. 3, (W.B. Saunders Co.: Philadelphia, PA), 1980
125. Schwartz, J.: "Atrophia Idiopathica (Tropica) Mucosae Oris", Presented at the Elventh International Dental Congress, London, England, 1952
126. Joshi, S.G.: "Submucous Fibrosis of the Palate and Pillars", Indian J. Otolaryngol. 4:1–4, 1953
127. Lal, D.: "Diffuse Oral Submucous Fibrosis", J. All-India Dent. Assoc. 26:1–3, 1953
128. Rao, R.V. and Raju, P.R.: "A Preliminary Report on the Treatment of Submucous Fibrosis of the Oral Cavity with Cortisone", Indian J. Otolaryngol. 6:81–83, 1954
129. DeSa, J.V.: "Submucous Fibrosis of the Palate and Cheek", Ann. Otol. Rhinol. Laryngolol. 66:1143–1159, 1957
130. Sharan, J.: "Histopathological Observations on Cases of Submucous Fibrosis of the Oral Cavity", Indian J. Pathol. Bacteriol. 2:150–152, 1959
131. Sirsat, S.M. and Khanolkar, V.R.: "Submucous Fibrosis of the Palate and Pillars of the Fauces", Indian J. Med. Sc. 16:189–197, 1962
132. Rao, A.B.N.: "Idiopathic Palatal Fibrosis", Brit. J. Surg. 50:23–25, 1962
133. Su, I-Pin: "Idiopathic Scleroderma of the Mouth", Arch. Otolaryngol. 59:330–332, 1954
134. Turner, E.P.: Personal Communication (Sited by Pindborg and Sirsat)
135. Pindborg, J.J. and Sirsat, S.M.: "Oral Submucous Fibrosis", Oral Surg. 22:764–779, 1966
136. Millard, P.R.: "Submucous Fibrosis", Brit. J. Dermatol. 78:305–307, 1966
137. Rowell, N.R.: "Submucous Fibrosis of the Mouth", Brit. J. Dermatol. 79:64–66, 1967
138. Kennedy, T.F. and MacDonald, D.G.: "Oral Submucous Fibrosis", Brit. Dent. J. 124:121–122, 1968
139. Moos, K.F. and Madan, D.K.: "Submucous Fibrosis", Brit Dent. J. 124:313–317, 1968
140. Krishnappa, A.: "Submucous Fibrosis", Dent. J. Malaysia Singapore 7:32–36, 1967
141. Pindborg, J.J.: Report on Studies on Oral Leukoplakia in New Guinea and Fiji, submitted to the World Health Organization, 1967
142. Shear, M. and Lemmer, J.: "Histological Features of Oral Submucous Fibrosis", Dent. Pract. 18:49–53, 1967
143. Hamner, J.E., III, Looney, P.D., and Chused, T.M.: "Submucous Fibrosis", Oral Surg. 37:412–421, 1974
144. Pindborg, J.J., Nagpaul, R.K., and Gupta, V.K.: "Frequency of Oral Carcinoma, Leukoplakia, Leukokeratosis, Leukoedema, Submucous Fibrosis, and Lichen Planus in 10,000 Indians in Lucknow, Uttar Pradesh, India", J. Dent. Res. 44:615, 1965
145. Wahi, P.N., Kapor, V.L., Luthra, U.K., and Srivatava, M.C.: "Submucous Fibrosis of the Oral Cavity: Studies on Epidemiology", Bull. W.H.O. 65:793–799, 1966
146. Pindborg, J.J., Mehta, F.S., Gupta, P.C., and Daftary, D.K.: "Prevalence of Oral Submucous Fibrosis Among 50,915 Indian Villagers", Brit. J. Cancer 22:646–654, 1968
147. Zachariah, J., Mathew, B., Varma, N.A.R., et al.: "Frequency of Oral Mucosal Lesions

Among 5,000 Individuals in Trivandrum, South India", J. All-India Dent. Accoc. 38:290–296, 1966
148. Pindborg, J.J.: "Frequency of Oral Submucous Fibrosis in North India", Bull. W.H.O. 32:748–749, 1965
149. Pindborg, J.J., Chawla, T.N., Srivastava, A.N., et al.: "Clinical Aspects or Oral Submucous Fibrosis", Acta Odontol. Scand. 22:678–691, 1964
150. Sirsat, S.M. and Khanolkar, V.R.: "Submucous Fibrosis of the Palate in Diet-Preconditioned Wistar Rats", Arch. Pathol. 70:171–179, 1960
151. Hamner, J.E., III, Mehta, F.S., Pindborg, J.J., and Daftary, D.K.: "Altered Staining Reaction of Connective Tissues in 53 Submucous Fibrosis Patients", J. Dent. Res. 50:388–392, 1971
152. Pindborg, J.J.: "Oral Submucous Fibrosis as a Precancerous Condition", J. Dent. Res. 45:546–551, 1966
153. Pindborg, J.J.: "Is Submucous Fibrosis a Precancerous Condition in the Oral Cavity?", Int. Dent. J. 22:474–480, 1972
154. Pindborg, J.J., Mehta, F.S., and Daftary, D.K.: "Occurrence of Epithelial Atypia in 51 Indian Villagers", Brit. J. Cancer 24:253–257, 1970
155. Shiau, Y.Y. and Kwan, H.W.: "Submucous Fibrosis in Taiwan", Oral Surg. 47:453–457, 1979
156. Ramanathan, K.: "Oral Submucous Fibrosis – An Alternative Hypothesis As To Its Cause", Med. J. Malaysia 36:243–245, 1981
157. Barnes, P. and Duke, P.: "Submucous Fibrosis", Papua-New Guinea Med. J. 18:66–70, 1975
158. Silverberg, E.: "Cancer Statistics, 1982" CA. 32:15–29, 1982
159. A.C.S. Cancer Facts and Figures – 1981, (American Cancer Society: New York, NY), 1981
160. World Health Statistics Annual; 1979–1980
161. Atkinson, L., Clezy, J.K., et al.: The Epidemiology of Cancer in Papua New Guinea, (Star Printery Pty., Ltd.: Erstkineville, Australia), 1974
162. Paches, A.I. and Milievskaya, I.L.: Chapter on "Epidemiological Study of Cancer of the Mucous Membrane of the Oral Cavity in the U.S.S.R." In: Cancer Epidemiology in the U.S.A. and U.S.S.R., Levin D.L., ed., (N.I.H. Publication No. 80-2044: Bethesda, MD.), 1980
163. Jussawalla, D.J. and Jain, D.K.: "Cancer in Greater Bombay." In: Cancer Incidence in Five Continents, vol. III, (I.A.R.C. Scientific Publication No. 15: Lyon, France), 1976
164. Wahi, P.N.: "The Epidemiology of Oral and Oropharyngeal Cancer: A Report of the Study in Mainpuri District, U.P., India", Bull. W.H.O. 38:495–521, 1968
165. Malawalla, A.M., Silverman, S., Jr., Mani, N.J., et al.: "Oral Cancer in 57,518 Industrial Workers of Gujarat, India: A Prevalence and Follow-up Study", Cancer 37:1882–1886, 1976
166. Reddy, C.R.R.M., Prahlad, D., and Ramulu, C.: "Incidence of Oral Cancer with Particular Reference to Hard Palate Cancer with One Million Population in the District of Visakhapatnam", Indian J. Cancer 12:72–76, 1975
167. Myers, M.H. and Hankey, B.F.: Cancer Patient Survival Experience, (N.I.H. Publication No. 80-2148: Bethesda, MD), 1980

Chapter 2. Detection

James E. Hamner, III, and Soli K. Choksi

In the United States, large-scale programs of mass screening for oral cancer have not proven cost effective in terms of societal benefit related to detection cost. A recent, poignant example of this fact is the excellent oral cancer screening program conducted by the State University of New York (Buffalo) and the Roswell Park Memorial Institute in 1978. Of 3,662 persons screened by oral clinical examination, 250 exhibited "abnormalities" and 43 revealed suspicious lesions recommended for biopsy; of these, only one case of cancer was proven [1]. Thus, even such a well-conducted study yielded a detection rate of only 0.027% for that particular population. Sisson reported similar findings in 2,500 persons clinically screened for oral cancer in Chicago [2].

In contrast, the initial epidemiological survey conducted by Mehta, Hamner, and Pindborg on 50,000 rural Indian villagers detected an oral cancer prevalence rate of 0.1% in the Indian states of Kerala and Andhra Pradesh – the highest prevalence rate for oral cancer reported in the world [3]. One must bear in mind, of course, that India has an oral cancer incidence rate of 40–50%, whereas, the United States has only 4–5% [3–5].

While it has been pointed out that the rate of early detection is very low in the usual type of oral cancer screening program, (e.g., screening within dental school clinics, or auto-van clinics for screenings done in shopping centers), this fact is not meant to condemn detection efforts. Careful cancer detection examinations performed routinely on all patients by dentists and dental hygienists are most important as preventive medicine detection measures. These health professionals are the initial and primary front line of oral cancer defense because they are the ones first afforded the opportunity to see and examine potential oral cancer patients.

One other factor should be borne in mind, regarding oral cancer detection. Too often, most screening surveys involve the people least likely to be high risk candidates for oral cancer, namely – the young to middle aged, the healthy well-nourished individual, and the person who is concerned about good health. The actual high risk groups, e.g. the elderly, the nursing home isolated populations, the smoker, the alcoholic, the undernourished poor – these are the persons, who unfortunately through a myriad of circumstances, do not routinely see either a dentist or a physician, unless emergency intervenes. Therefore, most screening efforts miss the most cancer prone persons.

Early warning signs and symptoms that may herald oral cancer include the following:

(1) any ulcerative lesion or irritation that does not heal within two weeks
(2) any swelling or proliferative growth within the oral cavity

(3) any white, red, or speckled patch in the mouth
(4) repeated bleeding without an apparent cause
(5) either pain or numbness in any area of the mouth
(6) loosening of the teeth
(7) difficulty in swallowing
(8) hoarseness in voice

If a patient notices any of these signs or symptoms, he should contact his dentist and physician immediately.

I. Oral Examination

A meticulous, systematic examination of the face, neck, and oral cavity is essential for early detection of oral cancer and oral precancerous lesions. The mouth is one of the most accessible parts of the body, is easy to examine, and often yields significant information, both in regard to local and systemic manifestations of disease. A definite routine should be developed to provide a thorough, careful, yet expeditious examination of the facial/oral structures. The equipment required for an adequate oral examination consists of: tongue depressor, dental mirror, 4″ × 4″ gauze pads, toluidine blue (1%) and acetic acid (1%) for in vivo staining, and adequate light.

1. Facial Structure

Observe the patient carefully for facial asymmetry, swellings, skin ulcerations, nodules, and variations in skin color, texture, and pigmentation.

2. Lymph Nodes

Palpate the submental, submandibular, cervical, preauricular, parotid, and sub-posterior cervical lymph nodes (Fig. 2.1). The cervical chain of lymph nodes is more readily palpable when the overlying tissue, superficial fascia, and platysma muscles are stretched by flexing the patient's neck opposite the side being examined (Fig. 2.2). Extraoral submandibular lymph node palpation can be enhanced by placing the index finger of the opposite hand along the floor of the mouth to fix the myelohyoid muscle (Fig. 2.3).

Notice should be made of any enlargement, firmness, or pain in the lymph nodes.

3. Temporomandibular Joint

The temporomandibular joint should be palpated bilaterally with the fingers of both hands resting over the posterior angles of the mandible, the mandibular

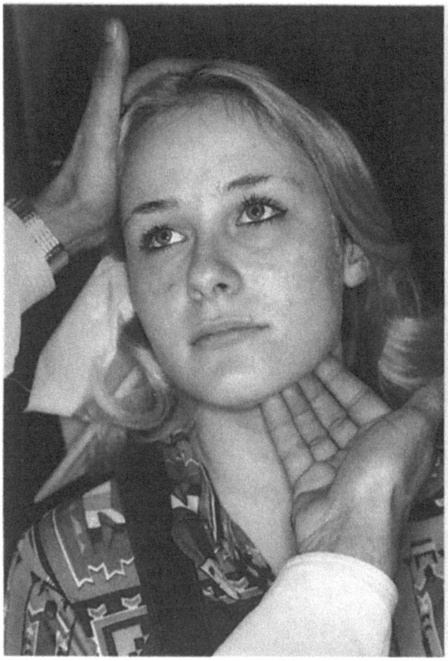

Fig. 2.1

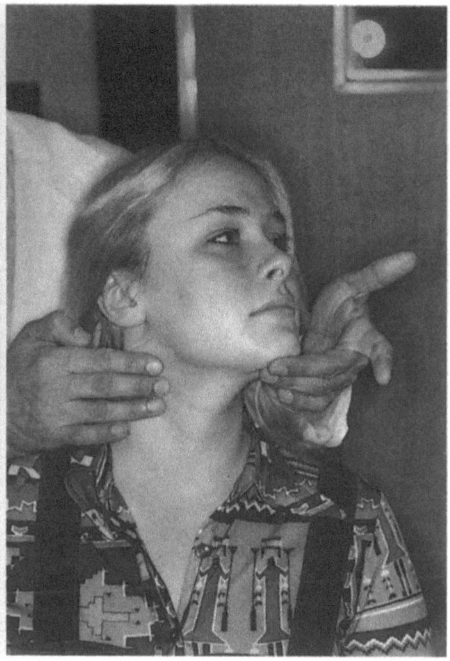

Fig. 2.2

Fig. 2.1. Examination of submental and submandibular lymph nodes

Fig. 2.2. Examination of cervical lymph nodes

condyles, and the T-M joints per se. The T-M joint should be palpated bilaterally with the mouth closed in centric occlusion, then with the mouth opened fully (Fig. 2.4).

Note any asymmetry, swelling, crepitus, pain, or impaired motion.

4. Lips

Both the mucocutaneous and mucosal aspects of the lips are inspected with the mouth opened, then closed. Note the color, texture, and any surface abnormalities. Any thickening, swelling, or induration can be determined by bidigital palpation.

5. Vestibules and Frenums

The maxillary and mandibular vestibules and frenums are examined visually and by digital palpation with the mouth partially open. Color change, swelling, ulceration, or frenum shortening should be noted.

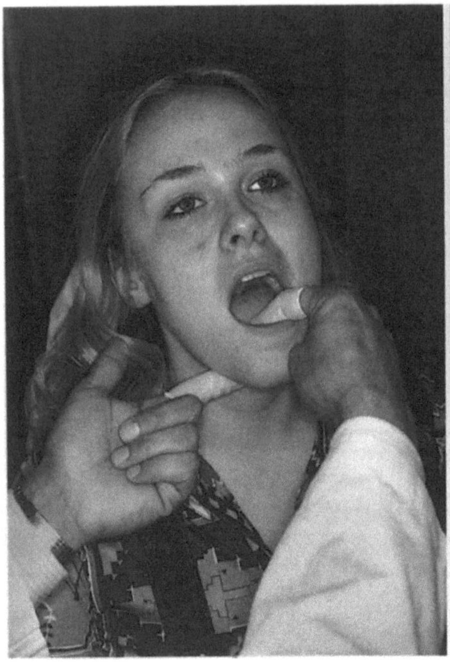

Fig. 2.3

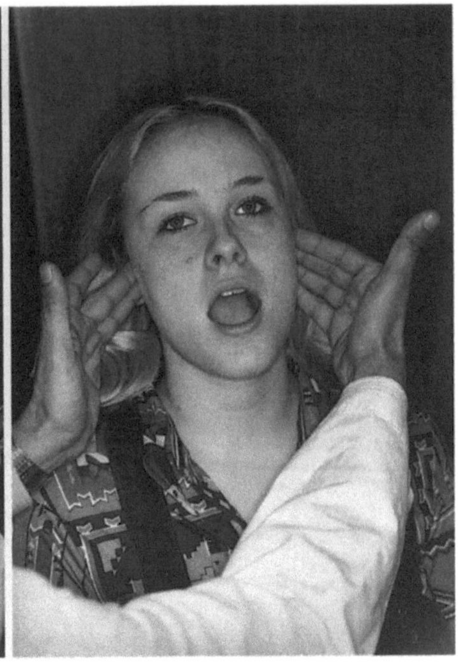

Fig. 2.4

Fig. 2.3. Examination of the sublingual and submandibular glands

Fig. 2.4. Examination of the temporomandibular joint

6. Gingivae

The maxillary and mandibular gingival tissue should be examined for color, swelling, hemorrhage, ulceration, and loss of stippling.

7. Buccal Mucosa and Commissures

With the mouth open, care should be taken to examine the buccal mucosa fully from the commissures back to the anterior pillar. Dental mirrors can be used to retract the cheek, being cautious not to cover any possible lesion with the mirror per se (Fig. 2.5). The orifice of the parotic gland should be noted bilaterally; its patency can be checked by drying the adjacent buccal mucosa, then observing the flow of saliva from the duct opening.

Note any changes in pigmentation, ulceration, swelling, and mobility.

8. Tongue

With the mouth partially open, the dorsal surface of the tongue can be inspected with the tongue at rest to check for any asymmetry, ulcerations, swellings,

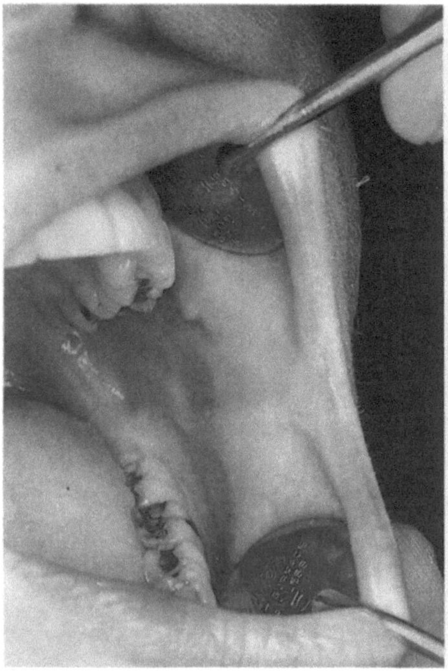

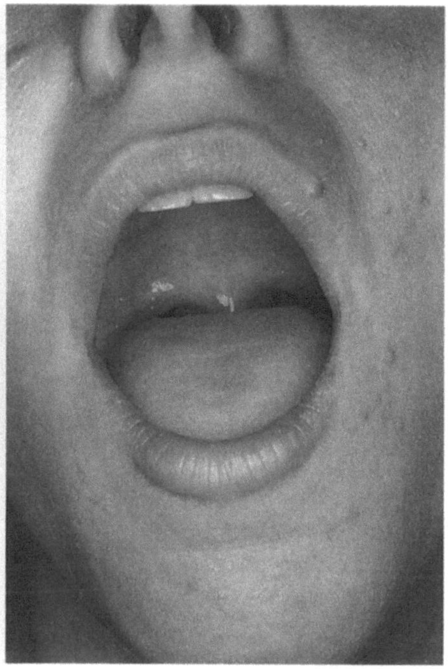

Fig. 2.5 **Fig. 2.6**

Fig. 2.5. Examination of the buccal mucosa and commissure

Fig. 2.6. Examination of the dorsal surface of the tongue

indurated masses, change in the filiform papillae, and change in color or texture (Fig. 2.6).

With a 4×4 inch gauze pad, grasp the tip of the tongue and protrude the tongue forward. Using a slightly warm dental mirror, the base of the tongue and the circumvallate papillae can be observed (Fig. 2.7).

Again using a 4×4 inch gauze pad to grasp the tip of the tongue, the tongue can be moved from side to side to examine the lateral and ventral surfaces (Fig. 2.8). Palpate the tongue bidigitally, as some tumors may occur in deeper tissues and thus not alter the external appearance. Lastly, have the patient touch the tip of his tongue to the palate to check for restriction of mobility.

9. Floor of the Mouth

While the tongue is elevated, the floor of the mouth can be checked for any swellings, ulcerations, or change in color. Next, the entire floor of the mouth should be carefully palpated to identify the submandibular gland and to check for any deeper indurated masses.

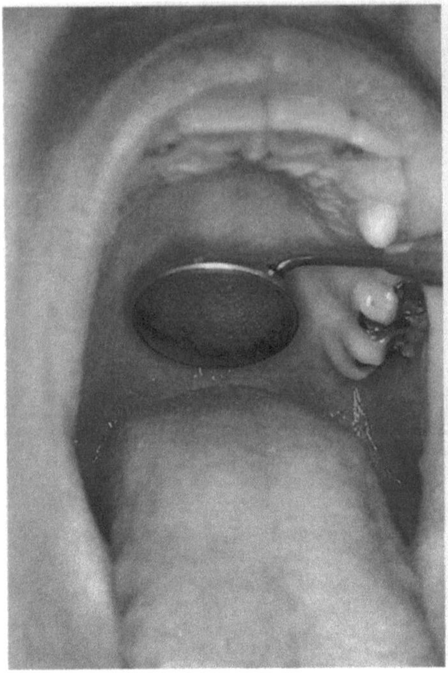

Fig. 2.7

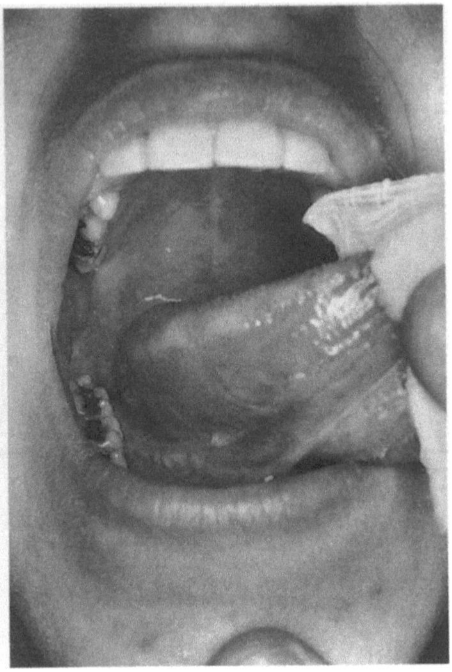

Fig. 2.8

Fig. 2.7. Examination of the base of the tongue and circumvallate papillae

Fig. 2.8. Examination of the lateral border of the tongue

10. Hard and Soft Palates

The hard palate, soft palate, and uvula can best be examined with thc mouth wide open, the head tilted back, and the tongue depressed with a tongue blade. Note any swelling, ulceration, change in color, or asymmetry (Fig. 2.9).

11. Teeth

The teeth are examined clinically and radiographically in an orderly sequence to determine any relationship with soft tissue lesions that might have been previously noted in the oral examination. One or two loosened teeth together is an important finding, because it may signal an undetected cancer involving the underlying bone or maxillary sinuses. Periodontal disease is usually more generalized. Unexplained hemorrhage around the sulcus areas of the teeth, with no provable cause of gingivitis or periodontitis, could be a sign of underlying generalized leukemia. Therefore, the cause of such unknown hemorrhage must be always determined by medical examination, clinical pathological tests, and biopsy.

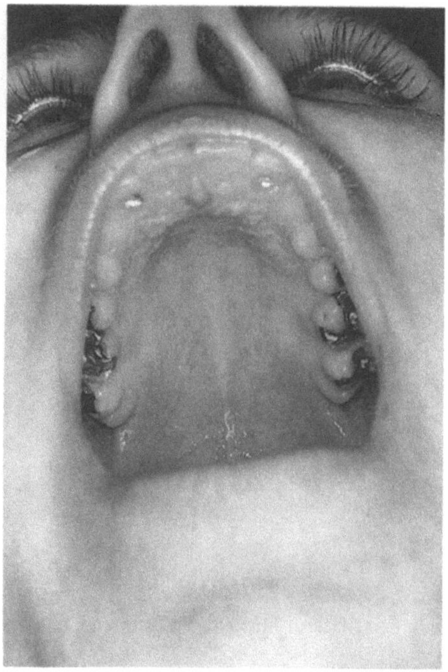

Fig. 2.9. Examination of the palate

II. Toluidine Blue as a Screening Detection Method

Toluidine blue is an acidophilic, metachromatic vital stain that is useful in the detection of small, early squamous cell carcinomas. Figures 2.10 and 2.11 depict the use of this staining technique. A suspected, superficial carcinoma is noted clinically in Fig. 2–10. One percent (1%) toluidine blue is applied to the suspicious area for 60 seconds. Afterwards, the same mucosa is sponged with 1% acetic acid, resulting in a positive concentration of the dye in the malignant site (Fig. 2.11).

In 1964 Niebel and Chomaet described the in-vivo toluidine blue staining test as a means of delineating oral intra-epithelial neoplastic change [6]. Shedd, et al., tested toluidine blue staining in 50 patients with either oral carcinoma or carcinoma-in-situ, successfully demonstrating that both lesions show an affinity for toluidine blue in-vivo. He presumed that this positive staining was due to the high density of nuclear material near the surface of these lesions [7]. In a subsequent study of 62 additional oral cancer patients, Shedd reported similar positive results with no false-negatives, using toluidine blue as an in-vivo staining method for the malignancies [8]. It also facilitated the recognition of inconspicuous second primary tumors.

Strong also found toluidine blue to be a useful tool in detecting oral carcinoma by staining the exposed portion of the tumor, however, it did not delineate the deeper, submucosal extensions of the neoplasm [9].

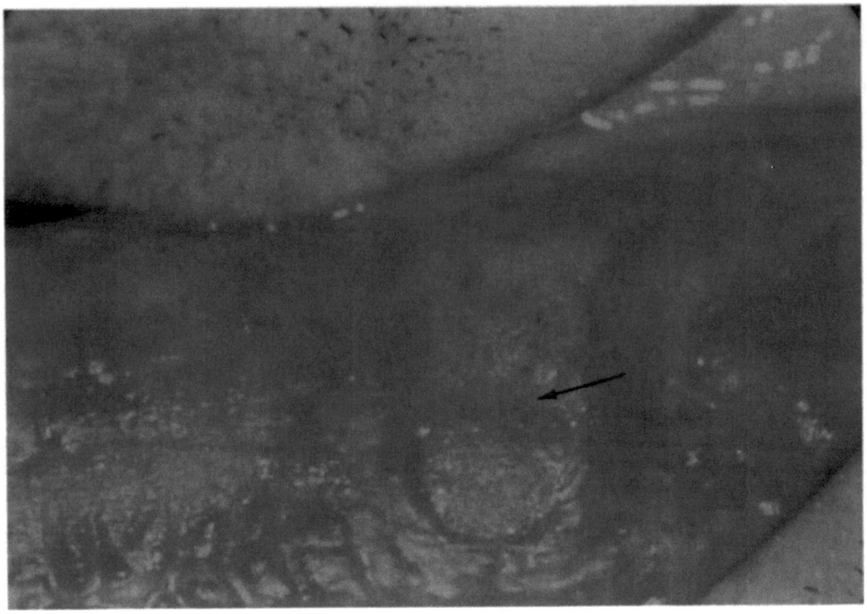

Fig. 2.10. Clinical appearance of carcinoma (*arrow*), right lateral border of the tongue. (Courtesy of Dr. Donald P. Shedd)

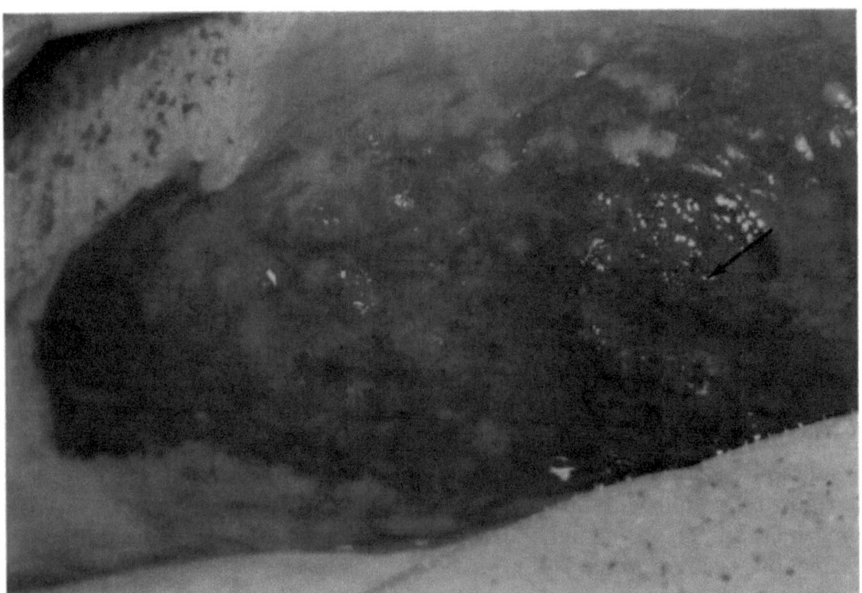

Fig. 2.11. The same cancer stained with toluidine blue (*arrow*). (Courtesy of Dr. Donald P. Shedd)

Contrary opinions have been expressed by other investigators who have felt that due to numerous false-positive and false-negative results, related to inflammatory lesions, the applicability of toluidine blue is limited for cancer detection [10, 11]. Even though Rosen, et al., thought that it was not wholly reliable, he did advocate that it was a quick preliminary screening method that could be used in conjunction with other tests [11].

Mashberg conducted a recent study on Veterans Administration patients to determine the feasibility of using tolonium (toluidine blue) as a mouth rinse to enhance detection of undiscovered oral cancers, after first preforming a thorough clinical examination. One-hundred and five asymptomatic oral lesions (51 cancers and 54 non-malignant lesions) with a persistent history of 10–14 days were evaluated with toluidine blue application staining, tolonium mouth rinse, and biopsy. He reported 2% false-negatives (2/51 cancers) with toluidine blue application in comparison to 5.9% (3/51 cancers) using the toluidine rinse, and 9.3% false-positives (5/54 non-malignant lesions) with toluidine blue application compared to 7.4% (4/54) with the tolonium rinse. He concluded that tolonium rinse does serve as an excellent screening method for detection unapparent oral-pharyngeal cancers, it is a simple expeditious office procedure, and it is inexpensive and harmless for the patient [12].

III. Oral Cytology as a Screening Detection Method

Early investigators enthusiastically described the use of oral exfoliative cytology as a means to screen for oral cancer [13–17]. Other reports stated that the use of oral cytology hastened the biopsy of suspicious lesions, which clinically may not always have the outward appearance of oral cancer, thus leading to an earlier diagnosis of cancers that otherwise would have remained undetected [18, 19].

The equipment needed for taking any oral cytology smear consists of: (1) a wooden spatula or cotton-tipped applicator, (2) glass histologic slides with the patient's name, date, and area of smear on them, and (3) a jar fixative (95% ethyl alcohol and ether, equal parts, or a commercial instant fixative).

Oral smears are collected in the following manner:

1. The lesion or suspected area is cleared of all necrotic material, debris, and/or blood.
2. The area is then scraped vigorously several times with the dull edge of a slightly moistened wooden spatula, using a rolling motion.
3. Next, the scrapings are immediately smeared on the center of two clean, previously marked glass slides, using a circular motion to obtain a thin, uniform smear.
4. The slides are then immediately immersed in the 95% ethyl alcohol/ether, equal parts, fixative to prevent any drying.
5. Lastly, the slides are stained by a modified Papanicolaou-Traut technique, which utilizes Mayer's hematoxylin, orange G, eosin, and light green [20–22].

A cytological interpretation of malignancy would be based on the following criteria, however, not all criteria are necessarily always found in each slide specimen, diagnosed as malignant [23]:

Table 2.1. Cytologic classification (Papanicolaou)

Class I	Normal cytology with an absence of any atypical or abnormal cells
Class II	Atypical cells, but no evidence of malignancy
Class III	Abnormal cells; cytology suggestive of, but not conclusive for, malignancy
Class IV	Cytology strongly suggestive of malignancy
Class V	Cytology conclusive for malignancy

(1) enlarged nuclei
(2) hyperchromatism
(3) variation in nuclear size and shape
(4) multiple, prominent, and irregular nucleoli
(5) abnormal chromatin pattern and distribution
(6) thickening of the nuclear membrane
(7) increased nuclear-cytoplasm ration, due to enlargement of the nucleus
(8) discrepancy in maturation
(9) changes in consistency of staining reaction
(10) lack of distinct cell boundaries

Cytologic diagnosis contains the following possible terms or states: normal, suspicious, inconclusive or inadequate, or malignant. Table 2.1 lists the five classes. The cytological appearance of normal and malignant cells within the oral cavity is compared in Fig. 2.12 and 2.13.

In a comparison of oral biopsy and oral cytology smears, Stahl, et al. also reported that oral cytology did reflect early epithelial atypia seen in oral premalignant and early malignant lesions [24]. Earlier in 1963 he had reported significant correlation between atypical exfoliated cells from chemically-induced tumors in the hamster cheek pouch with atypical histological changes progressing toward malignancy [25].

In 1965, King and Coleman compared the accuracy of oral exfoliative cytology with biopsy and concluded that oral cytology is an accurate methodology in detecting marked epithelial atypia [26]. However, all of these various investigators emphasize that cytologic examination supplements biopsy; it doesn't replace it.

Other analyses of oral cytology as a detection/diagnostic tool often present a contrasting picture to those studies previously described. Shapiro and Gorlin in 1964 examined 404 intraoral lesions by exfoliative cytology, having 92 cases in which histopathologic material was available for direct comparison. In 22 malignancies, 5 were considered cytologically negative for cancer (a false negative rate of 22.7% – very dangerous). In 66 benign lesions, 6 exhibited cytological findings suspicious of cancer (a false positive rate of 9%). In screening modalities, it is the false negative rate that is dangerous because it gives you the erroneous impression of security, when in actuality, cancer is present. Such a false negative rate is the main problem with thermography in accurately detecting breast cancer. Since Shapiro and Gorlin found that their histologically confirmed cases represented less than 25% of all cases, they concluded that negative cytology could not be equated with benignity [27].

In examining 20,360 rural villagers in the Indian states of Kerala and Gujarat, Mehta, et al., discovered 343 clinically detectable leukoplakias and

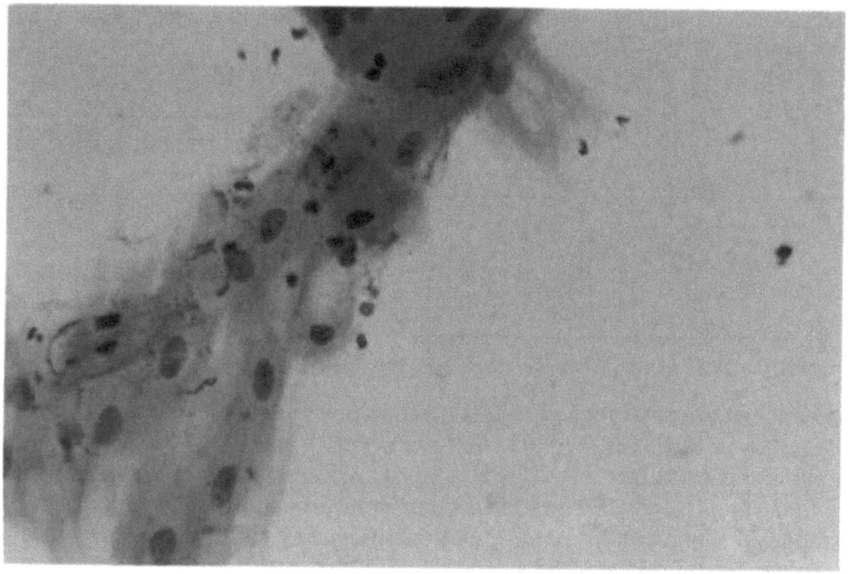

Fig. 2.12. Oral cytology smear, normal superficial squamous cells from the tongue, Papanicolaou stain. (Courtesy of Dr. Fali S. Mehta and Dr. Dinesh K. Daftary)

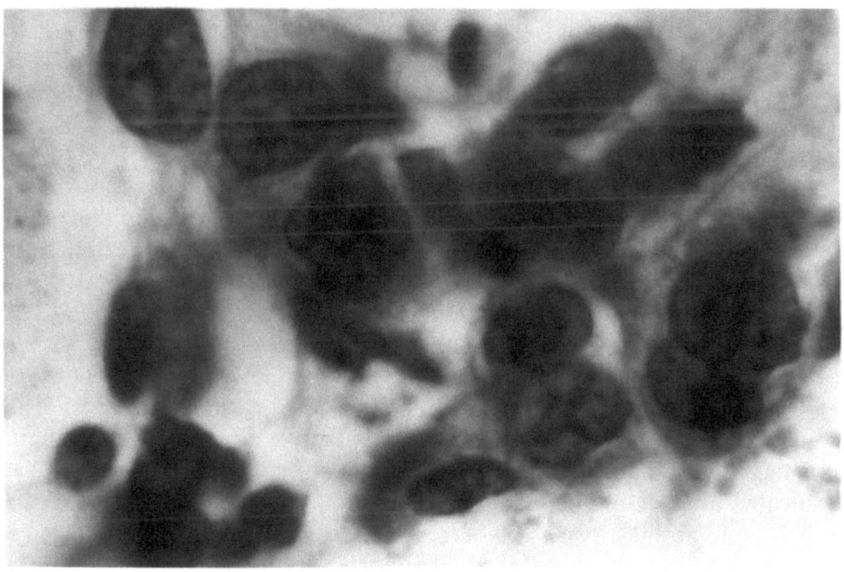

Fig. 2.13. Oral cytology smear, malignant epithelial cells from recurrent epidermoid carcinoma of the tongue, Papanicolaou stain. (Courtesy of Dr. Fali S. Mehta and Dr. Dinesh K. Daftary)

52 cases of submucous fibrosis [28]. Histological and cytological examinations were performed on 269 of these cases (237 leukoplakias, 31 submucous fibrosis cases, and 1 case with both maladies) and comparison of these methodologies is shown in Table 2.2. A correlation of 36 histological epithelial atypias among

Table 2.2. Cytological findings in histological epithelial atypias and non-atypias found in 269 leukoplakias and submucous fibrosis cases[a]

Histological findings	Number of cases	Cytological classification				
		I. (normal)	II. (atypical)	III.	IV.	V.
Atypia	36	23 (63.9%)	13 (36.1%)	–	–	–
Non-atypia	233	229 (98.2%)	4 (1.7%)	–	–	–

[a] Courtesy of Dr. F.S. Mehta. (From Mehta et al. [28])

269 patients with the cytological results on the same patients revealed agreement in only 36.1% of the cases, or a 63.9% false negative rate [28].

In another careful histocytological analysis of carcinoma and epithelial atypia of the palate in cases from the Indian state of Andhra Pradesh, Mehta, et al., reported similar findings. Of the six histologically confirmed palatal carcinomas, only 2 exhibited cytological smear findings consistent with malignancy (a 66.7% false negative rate – in other words, 4 of the 6 carcinomas would have been missed by cytological smear examination). Of the 46 epithelial atypias diagnosed on biopsy, only 6 were diagnosed cytologically (an 87% false negative rate for epithelial atypias) [29].

Even in such an oral cytology advocate as Sandler, if one used the criteria of class IV and V smears as being positive for malignancy, his 1963 study would have missed 73/315 cancers (a false negative rate of 23.2%, which is unacceptable) [16].

Because of the relative scantiness of exfoliation of cells from the surface of oral epithelium, it does not lend itself as accurately to cytological diagnosis as the vaginal or cervical epithelium, which has a much higher rate of exfoliation, thereby leading to more accurate cytological examination and the underlying actual conditions that may exist pathologically.

In conclusion, it is now generally felt that exfoliative oral cytology should be used as an adjunct to biopsy and as an adjunct to clinical follow-up of a previously treated cancer patient. Treatment procedures should *never* be instigated only on the basis of findings from oral exfoliative cytology. When abnormalities suggesting malignancy are found in an oral cytology smear, a biopsy of the smeared area should be taken *immediately* to either to confirm or disapprove the cytologic diagnosis. For these reasons, oral exfoliative cytology is not advocated as beneficial, either in diagnostic accuracy most importantly, or cost-wise, for mass-screening programs in oral cancer.

References

1. Shedd, D.P., Lore, J.M., and Kaufman, S.: "Third Year Implementation Report", (Comprehensive Network Demonstration Project for Head & Neck Cancer, NCI Contract #NO1-CN-55257), 1978
2. Sisson, G.A., et al.: "Annual Report – 1978" (Prototype Comprehensive Network Demonstration Project for Head & Neck Cancer, MCI Contract #NO1-CN65256), 1978

3. Mehta, F.S., Pindborg, J.J., and Hamner, J.E., III: Oral Cancer and Precancerous Conditions in India, Ed. 1 (Munksgaard: Copenhagen, Denmark), 1971
4. American Cancer Society: Cancer Facts & Figures, (A.C.S.: New York, N.Y.), 1981
5. Hamner, J.E., III: "Oral Cancer" Chapter in Lynch, M.A.: Oral Medicine, Ed. 7, (J.B. Lippincott Co.: Philadelphia, PA.), 1977
6. Niebel, H.H. and Chomet, B.: "In-Vivo Staining Test for Delineation of Oral Intra-epithelial Neoplastic Change", J.A.D.A. 68:801–806, 1964
7. Shedd, D., Hukill, P.B., and Bahn, S.: "In-Vivo Staining Properties of Oral Carcinoma", Amer. J. Surg. 110:631–634, 1965
8. Shedd, D.P., Hukill, P.B., Bahn, S., et al.: "Further Appraisal of In-Vivo Staining Properties of Oral Cancer", Arch. Surg. 95:16–22, 1965
9. Strong, M.S., Vaughun, C.W., and Incze, J.S.: "Toluidine Blue in the Management of Carcinoma of the Oral Cavity", Arch Otolaryngol. 87:527–531, 1968
10. Silverman, S. and Galante, M.: Oral Cancer, Ed. 4, (University of California Press: San Francisco, Calif.), 1974
11. Rosen, B., Cornish, M., and Edelson, M.: "Detection of Early Oral Cancer by Toluidine Blue", J. Can. Dent. Assn. 37:347–349, 1971
12. Mashberg, A.: "Tolonium (Toluidine Blue) Rinse – A Screening Method for Recognition of Squamous Carcinoma", J.A.M.A. 254:2408–2410, 1981
13. Sandler, H.C. and Stahl, S.S.: "Exfoliative Cytology as a Diagnostic Aid in the Detection of Oral Neoplasms", J. Oral Surg. 16:414–418, 1958
14. Sandler, H.C.: "The Detection of Early Cancer of the Mouth by Exfoliative Cytology", Acta Cytol. 5:191–194, 1961
15. Sandler, H.C.: "Cytological Screening for Early Mouth Cancer; Interim Report of Veterans Administration Co-operative Study of Oral Exfoliative Cytology", Cancer 15:1119–1124, 1962
16. Sandler, H.C.: "Veterans Administration Co-operative Study of Oral Exfoliative Cytology". Acta Cytol. 7:180–182, 1963
17. Hayes, R.L., Berg, G.W., and Ross, W.L.: "Oral Cytology: Its Value and Its Limitations", J.A.D.A. 79:649–657, 1969
18. Folsom, T.C., White, C.P., Bromer, L., Canby, H.F., and Garrington, G.E.: "Oral Exfoliative Cytology: Review of the Literature and Report of a Three Year Study", Oral Surg. 33:61–74, 1972
19. Allegra, S.R., Broderick, P.A., and Corvese, C.T.: "Seven Year Oral Cytology Screening Program in the State of Rhode Island: Analysis of 6,448 Cases", Acta. Cytol. 17:42–48, 1973
20. Papanicolaou, G.N.: Atlas of Exfoliative Cytology (Harvard University Press: Cambridge, Mass.), 1954
21. Mehta, F.S.: Early Detection of Oral Cancer and Precancerous Lesions (Tata Institute of Fundamental Research Press: Bombay, India), 1973
22. Alling, C.C. and Secord, R.T.: "A Technique for Oral Exfoliative Cytology", Oral Surg. 17:668–676, 1964
23. Medak, H., McGrew, E.A., Burlakow, P., and Tiecke, R.W.: Atlas of Oral Cytology Ed. 1, (P.H.S. Publication No. 1949: Washington, D.C
24. Stahl, S.S., Sandler, H.C., and Cahn, L.H.: "The Significance of Dyskaryotic Cells in Exfoliative Cytology", Acta Cytol. 8:73–79, 1964
25. Stahl, S.S.: "Correlation of Cytodiagnosis and Biopsy in the Evolution of an Experimentally Induced Carcinoma", Oral Surg. 16:985–993, 1963
26. King, O.H. and Coleman, S.A.: "Analysis of Oral Exfoliative Cytologic Accuracy by Control Biopsy Technique", Acta Cytol. 9:351–354, 1965
27. Shapiro, B.L. and Gorlin, R.J.: "An Analysis of Oral Cytodiagnosis", Cancer 17:1477–1479, 1964
28. Mehta, F.S., Daftary, D.K., and Sahiar, B.E.: "A Correlative Histocytological Study of Epithelial Atypia in Leukoplakic and Submucous Fibrosis Lesions Amongst Indian Villagers in a Mass Screening Programme", Indian J. Cancer 7:18–23, 1970
29. Mehta, F.S., Sahiar, B.E., Daftary, D.K., Gupta, P.C., and Pindborg, J.J.: "A Correlative Histocytological Study of Carcinoma and Epithelial Atypia of the Palate Among Indian Reverse Smokers: Brit. J. Cancer 26:230–233, 1972

Chapter 3. Diagnosis

James E. Hamner, III

The vast majority of malignant tumors of the head and neck area are epidermoid carcinoma, which accounts for over 90% of all such malignant cases [1–4]. Therefore, it will receive most of our diagnostic emphasis in this chapter. It is not the primary intention of this portion to discuss all of the various potential neoplasms that can involve the head and neck region. However, in addition to the significance attached to epidermoid (squamous cell) carcinoma, discussions regarding the diagnosis of basal cell carcinoma, malignant melanoma, odontogenic tumors, salivary gland tumors, and fibro-osseous lesions will be included.

Once oral cancer has advanced far clinically and lymph nodal metastasis has occurred, it possesses one of the poorest 5-year survival rates of all forms of cancer. Conversely, oral cancer should readily lend itself to early detection and diagnosis by the alert clinician, since it is easily accessible for examination and produces definite signs and symptoms [5].

Early diagnosis is the greatest single factor in successfully combating oral cancer, provided proper treatment is instigated as soon as the patient has been properly evaluated. It has been estimated that cancer mortality could be reduced by one-third, if its initial signs and symptoms were correctly recognized by early diagnosis and prompt, effective therapeutic measures were carried out [6].

I. Epidermoid Carcinoma

Epidermoid (squamous cell) carcinoma is the most common malignant tumor of the oral cavity, pharynx and larynx. Excluding the lips, epidermoid cancer is detected as a primary lesion most commonly on the tongue, floor of the mouth, alveolar mucosa, palate and buccal mucosa-in that order of frequency [1, 5, 7].

The usual chief complaint of the oral cancer patient is that of a "sore" or "irritation" in the mouth. Pain occurs later, often when the lesion has become either ulcerated and secondary infection has taken place, or when sensory nerve tissue has become involved. Occasionally, a patient will seek dental or medical advice because a swelling ("lump") has been noticeable in his neck. Such swelling usually represents a reactive lymph node affected by either infection or metastases.

Silverman found the most frequent asymptomatic patients to be those involved with carcinoma of the floor of the mouth (29%). The most common

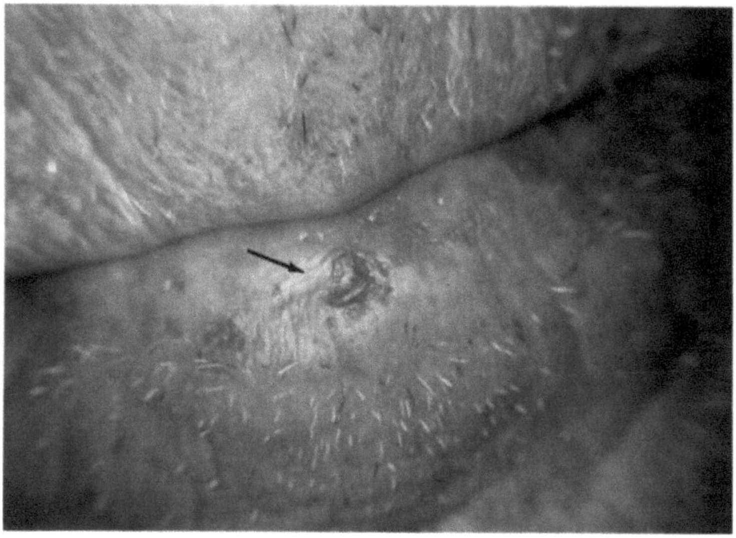

Fig. 3.1. Epidermoid carcinoma (*arrow*), lower lip, 58-year-old Caucasian male

symptom was pain (60%), and the most common signs were swelling and ulceration [8, 9].

A patient presented with the following signs should be suspected as a prime candidate for oral cancer: a chronic ulcer that does not heal, a hard lesion with rolled indurated borders, a lesion that is fixed to deeper tissues, a red velvety lesion, a speckled white lesion, an exophytic lesion, or painless lymphadenopathy.

1. Carcinoma of the Lip

Lip carcinoma is a frequent tumor, comprising 25 to 30% of all oral cancers. The vast majority (95%) develop on the vermilion border of the lower lip, often between the midline and the commissure. In the United States there is a marked predilection for males, the ratio being 14:1; whereas, in Sweden the ratio of males to females with lip cancer is 1:1, probably due to the high incidence of Plummer-Vinson syndrome in that nation. Lip cancer usually strikes older persons (50–70 years of age), people having ruddy complexions and outdoor occupations, and Caucasians. It is a very rare tumor among Negroes. The lesion can occur in exophytic, ulcerative, or verrucal forms, but the ulcerated form is more frequent and carries a greater malignant potential. It commonly presents as a localized, indurated white area which may be ulcerated and crusted with form rolled borders (Fig. 3.1). The prognosis for lip cancer is excellent since it is easily detectable, readily operable, and has a delayed incidence of metastatic spread [1, 5, 10].

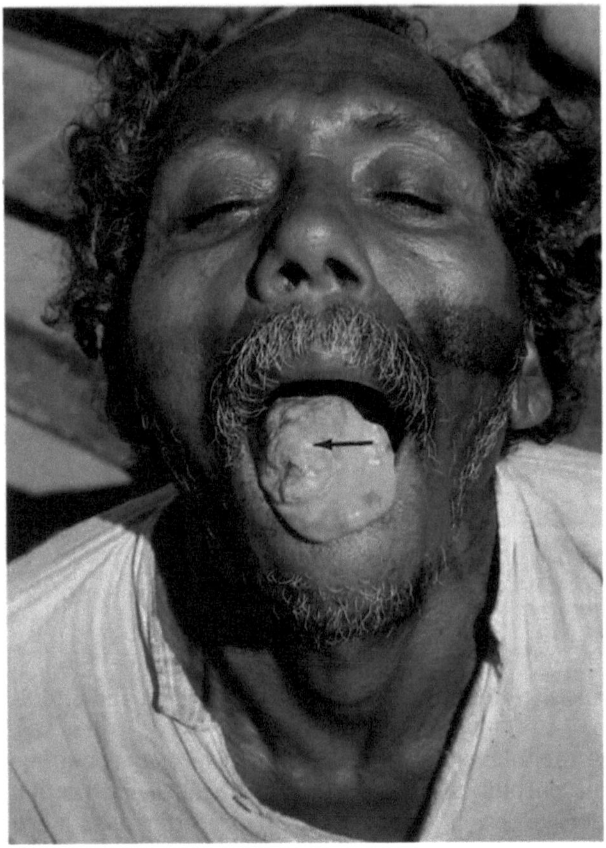

Fig. 3.2. Exophytic epidermoid carcinoma (*arrow*), dorsum and right lateral surfaces of the tongue, 55-year-old Indian male. (Courtesy of Dr. Fali S. Mehta)

2. Carcinoma of the Tongue

This neoplasm is the most important intraoral tumor in terms of incidence and equals the total of other intraoral tumors of all sites. This tumor also predominates among American men at a 4:1 male to female ratio. The usual age range is 50 to 70 years, although cases have been reported in younger individuals. The most frequent site of occurance is the lateral border of the middle-third of the tongue. In the anterior two-thirds of the tongue it commonly presents as a painless mass, whereas pain is the most common symptom connected with a carcinoma of the posterior one-third of the tongue. Dysphagia and lymphadenopathy may also be noted. The lesion itself appears as either a focal thickening or painless ulceration, which develops a firm, rolled border. Later, either an exophytic or an infiltrative pattern emerges leading to a fungating ulcerative mass (Fig. 3.2) or deep infiltration through muscle, respectively. For unexplainable reasons, except for the denial syndrome, patients often delay in seeking consultation and proper treatment, undoubtedly contributing to the high incidence of regional lymph node metastases. Carcinoma of the tongue is a highly lethal tumor with a poor prognosis for advanced cases. Reported

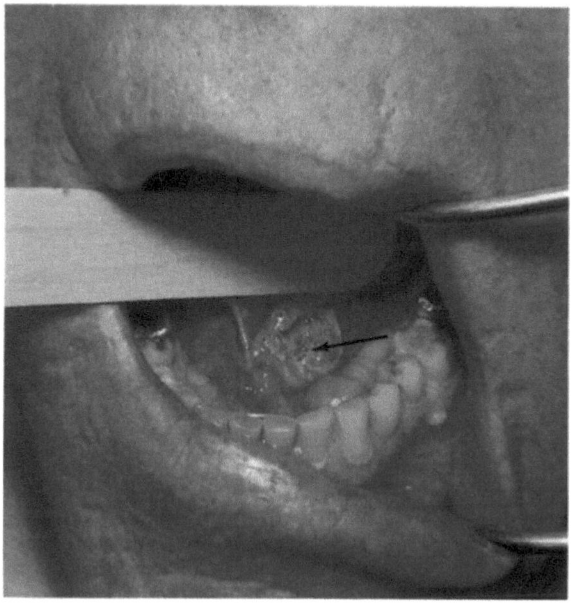

Fig. 3.3. Ulcerative carcinoma (*arrow*), anterior floor of the mouth, 51-year-old Caucasian male

5-year survival rates have varied from 14 to 70%, determined by tumor location, degree of malignancy, population sampled, extent of metastasis, and modalities of therapy [1, 4, 7, 11].

3. Carcinoma of the Floor of the Mouth

Correa's investigation reported that this cancer is the second most common intraoral tumor [12]. Likewise, it occurs more often in men (5:1 male to female ratio) who are in the 50 to 60-year age bracket. The anterior floor of the mouth appears to be involved more frequently than the posterior floor. Leffal and White report it to be the most common intraoral site for epidermoid carcinoma in Negroes [13]. The early lesions can be quite innocuous, appearing as a red or white raised patch or even an ulceration. Fixation and induration develop (Fig. 3.3), and the lesion usually follows an infiltrative pattern. Firmness is the first symptom; pain develops later. Carcinoma in this site is usually a moderately well-differentiate neoplasm. Metastases are common, and bilateral regional lymphatic spread can occur. The metastases do not transpire as early as in cases of carcinoma of the tongue, and therefore the prognosis is somewhat better (18–50% 5-year survival rate) than for carcinoma of the tongue [5–7].

4. Carcinoma of the Alveolar Mucosa and Gingiva

This cancer is seen most typically in men over 60 years of age. It is more frequently discovered on the mandibular gingiva (2:1) than on the maxillary

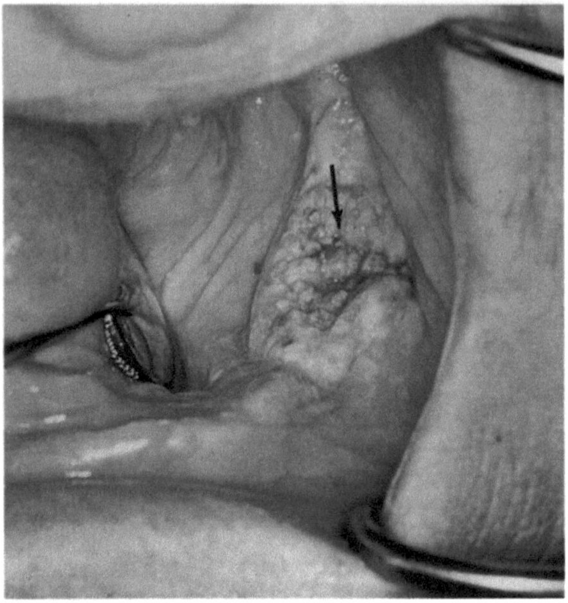

Fig. 3.4. Eroding carcinoma (*arrow*), alveolar mucosa, 80-year-old Caucasian male. (Courtesy of Dr. Jens J. Pindborg)

alveolar mucosa and classically is seen in the mandibular molar area. Often this tumor occurs on edentulous ridges in which it may mimic epulis fissuratum. It appears usually as a small nodular outgrowth with a roughened surface, which advances into an exophytic mass with an erosive ulcerated center (Fig. 3.4). This tumor may also initially appear as a leukoplakic patch or a small ulcer. Metastases spread first to the submandibular lymph nodes in most cases. Brown reported a 52%, 5-year survival rate for carcinoma of the mandibular ridge in contrast to only 45% for carcinoma of the maxillary alveolar mucosa. It is usually well-differentiated and has a 5-year survival rate similar to that of carcinoma of the floor of the mouth [5, 6, 14].

5. Carcinoma of the Palate

This cancer is rarely seen in the United States, but it is a common neoplasm in India, especially in the state of Andhra Pradesh and other areas where the reverse smoking habit is practiced (see Fig. 1.7). American investigations of palatal carcinoma indicate that the soft palate appears to be affected three times more often than the hard palate, with the malignancy frequently occurring at the junction of the soft and hard palates. Again, men are affected more often (3:1) than women, and it is a tumor most often discovered in persons over 55 years of age. The granular exophytic growth can cause a problem with denture retention, which is a frequent presenting complaint. When the tumor occurs on the soft palate, pain is an early symptom; dysphagia and trismus follow later. Customarily, this tumor is a moderately well-differentiated

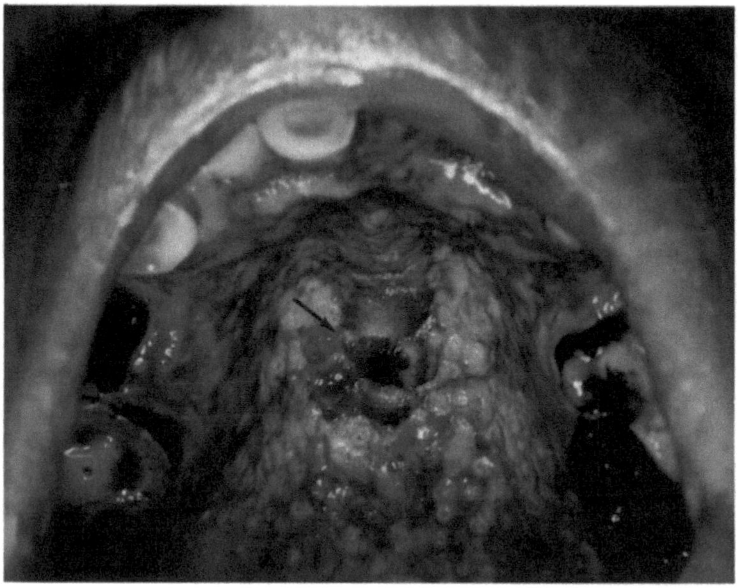

Fig. 3.5. Carcinoma (*arrow*) of the palate arising in an area of leukokeratosis nicotina palati, 52-year-old-Indian female. (Courtesy of Dr. Soli K. Choksi)

epidermoid carcinoma that usually metastasizes to the deep cervical lymph nodes. In prognosis for 5-year survival, carcinoma of the hard palate is more favorable than carcinoma of the soft palate [5, 6, 15–17].

Figure 3.5 illustrates the clinical appearance of epidermal carcinoma of the palate arising in a concurrent area of leukokeratosis nicotina palata in a 52 year old Indian female, who practiced reverse "chutta" smoking.

6. Carcinoma of the Buccal Mucosa

Buccal mucosal epidermoid carcinoma comprises only 8% of the intraoral carcinomas in the United States [1, 5, 6]. However, it is much more common in areas of the world where the betel-chewing or snuff-dipping habits are practiced [15]. In the United States buccal carcinoma is seen more frequently in men than in women (4:1), who usually are over 50 years of age. In India the occurrence of buccal carcinoma is more nearly equal in males and females and may be seen at an earlier age [6, 15, 18, 19]. This tumor can appear in one of three forms: exophytic, ulcerative-infiltrating, or verrucal. The exophytic type is often associated with leukoplakia and develops into a fungating, erythematous mass with indurated borders in the full-blown lesion (Fig. 3.6). This particular case was a 56 year old Indian male, who had two tobacco habits: betel quid with tobacco and "bidi" smoking. The ulcerative form is less common and infiltrates the submucosa and deeper musculature. The verrucal form will be discussed as a separate entity. Buccal carcinoma is usually a moderate to well-

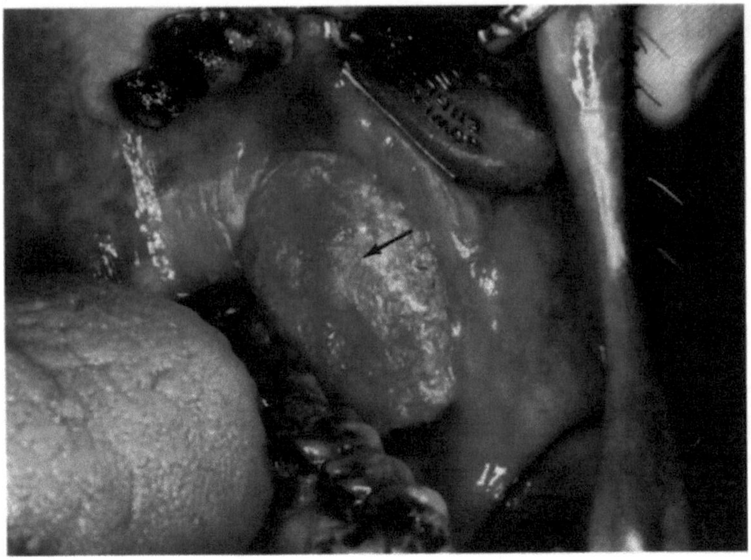

Fig. 3.6. Exophytic epidermoid carcinoma (*arrow*) of the buccal mucosa, 56-year-old Indian male. (Courtesy of Dr. Denish K. Daftary)

differentiated tumor which metastasizes to the submandibular lymph nodes or deep cervical chains. O'Brien and Catlin noted that 64% of their 248-patient study had either extension of tumor beyond the buccal mucosa or metastases at the time of admission for treatment [20]. Indian investigations have reported a late development of metastatic spread in most betel-quid induced carcinomas, which characteristically appear clinically as slow-growing tumors. The prognosis is good, provided treatment is adequate, producing a 60 to 75% 5-year survival ratc [15, 18].

7. Verrucous Carcinoma

Verrucous carcinoma is a separate clinicopathological type of low-grade epidermoid carcinoma, which grows in a slow relentless fashion and may eventually kill the patient by distinctive extension to vital areas. Lesions, which have a similar morphology and natural history, are also seen on the dorsum of the hand, penis, vulva, scrotum, larynx, and nasal fossa. It is difficult to assess the frequency of verrucous carcinoma, since it is often lumped with epidermoid carcinoma. This tumor is closely associated with a history of using chewing tobacco or snuff. It resembles in many ways the exophytic type of buccal mucosal carcinomas seen in betel quid chewers in Southeast Asia [5, 15].

Verrucous carcinoma is most frequently detected in the mandibular buccal sulcus, the buccal mucosa, and the adjacent alveolar mucosa. In Jacobson and Shear's study of 168 such cases, it was found that 58% were located on the buccal mucosa [21]. It usually occurs in elderly individuals, but differs from

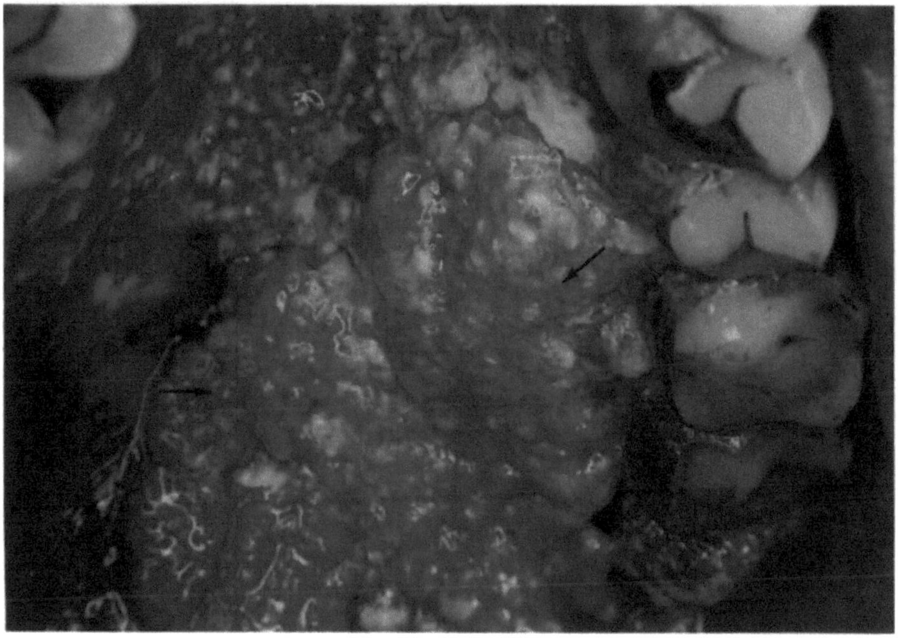

Fig. 3.7. Verucous carcinoma (*arrows*) of the palate, 62-year-old Negro female

the typical epidermoid carcinoma in sex distribution, being seen more frequently in women (male/female ratio is 2:3). It usually presents as a bulky, soft mass composed of multiple papillary excrescences with deep fissures (Fig. 3.7). Color varies from white to red, depending upon the degree of keratinization. Ulceration is not common, but can occur on the tips of the papillary projections. The tumor grows more often by lateral spread than by deep invasion, but underlying bone destruction can occur with time. Also, the tumor eventually can penetrate the cheek and extend over the external skin as a fungating mass [10, 22]. Histologically, the tumor appears as a papillary mass of well-differentiated squamous epithelial folds. Cellular atypia is not usually seen. Prognosis is good with a 75% 5-year survival rate in most cases following proper therapy [19, 21].

8. Histopathology

Epidermoid carcinoma usually appears histopathologically as masses, sheets, islands, or cords of malignant squamous cells, which proliferate downward into the connective tissue and muscular layers (Fig. 3.8). The microscopic pattern shows wide variation depending upon the degree of cellular differentiation. A well-differentiation carcinoma tends to resemble normal squamous epithelium in many ways. The malignant cells consist of peripheral cuboidal cells, spinous cells, and granular cells which are still capable of producing keratin, forming

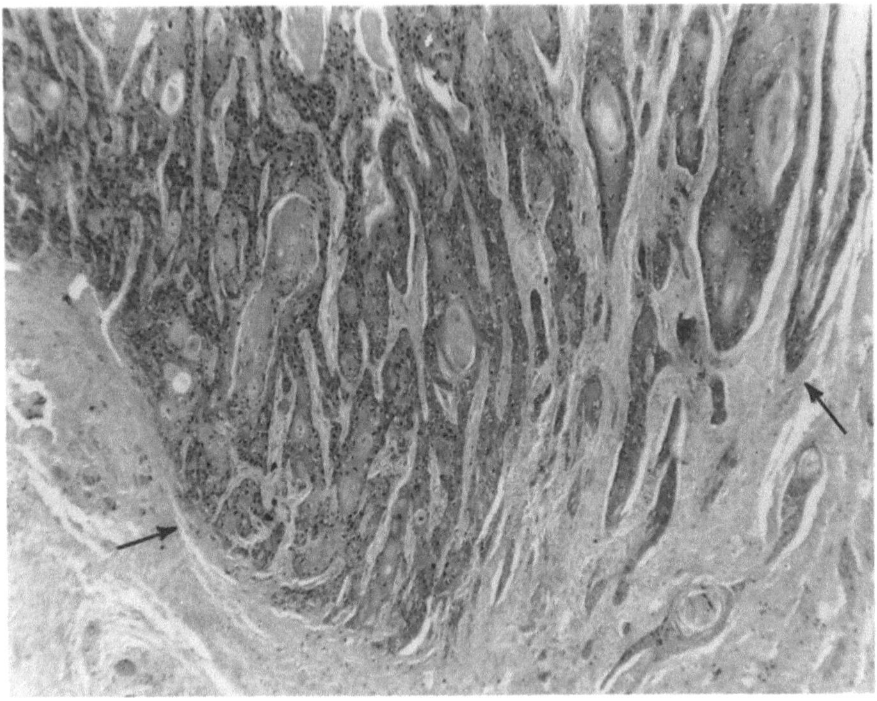

Fig. 3.8. Epidermoid carcinoma; note the sheets and cords of invading malignant cells (*arrows*). H. & E. stain, ×65

the characteristic keratin pearls (Fig. 3.9). Mitotic activity is usually minimal, and the mitotic divisions are normal. These tumors appear to push into the underlying lamina propria, which typically reacts with a chronic inflammatory response.

Moderately-differentiated carcinomas (Fig. 3.10) demonstrate a greater variety in histological composition with variations in malignant cell size, shape, and nuclear morphology. The staining reaction of the cells may vary considerably, also. Mitotic activity is more pronounced, and both normal and abnormal mitotic divisions occur. Keratin pearls may be present, but are not as conspicuous as in well-differentiated carcinoma.

The poorly-differentiated carcinoma exhibits little if any keratin production ability in its malignant cells, which show marked morphological variance, hyperchromatic bizarre nuclei, and frequent abnormal mitotic divisions. Invasion of the underlying tissue is rapid and extensive, projecting downward as extending nests or islands of malignant cells which often retain little cellular cohesion (Fig. 3.11).

The American Joint Committee recommends utilization of Broder's classification for grading epidermoid tumors, as follows:

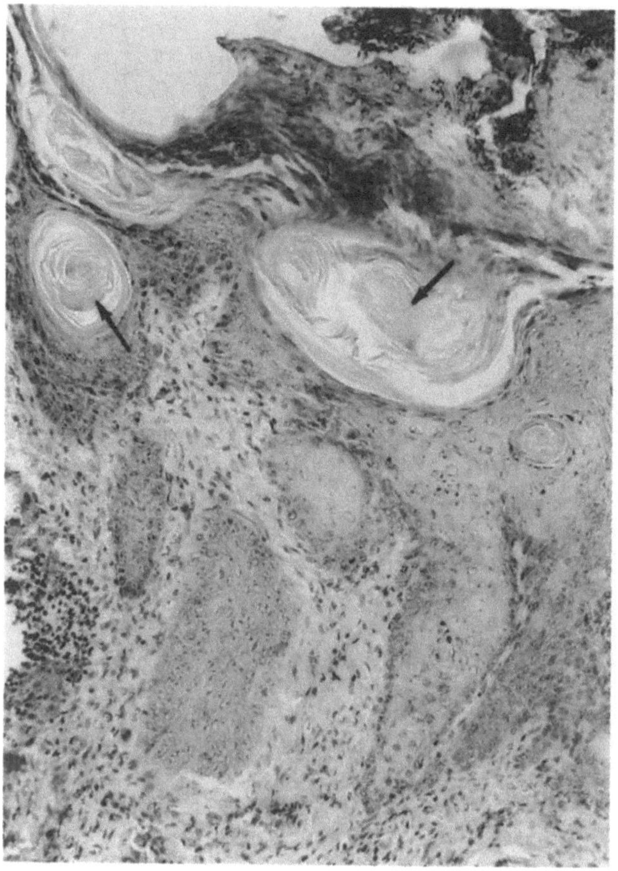

Fig. 3.9. Well-differentiated epidermoid carcinoma exhibiting keratin pearl formation (*arrows*). H. & E. stain, ×160

Tumor Grade (G)

G1	Well-differentiated
G2	Moderately well-differentiated
G3–G4	Poorly to very poorly-differentiated
	Use whichever indicator is most appropriate (term or G + number)

A Grade 1 tumor would have 75 to 100% well-differentiated cells, and Grade 4 could have only 10 to 25% of its cells as well-differentiated [2, 5].

However, most pathologists would rather convey an idea of the relative histological malignant degree to the oncologist by the use of well, moderate, or poor tumor differentiation. Some individuals believe that a numerical grading may give the therapist an erroneous impression, since a Grade 1 carcinoma of the tongue with multiple fixed lymph node metastases would have a worse prognosis than a Grade III localized tumor with no lymph node metastases and negative radioisotope scans.

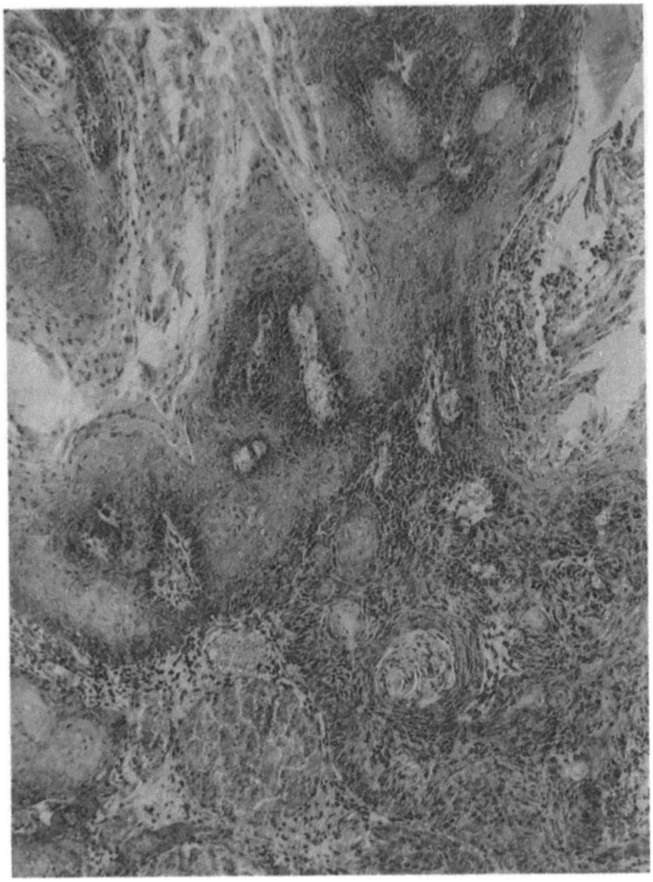

Fig. 3.10. Moderately-differentiated epidermoid carcinoma, buccal mucosa. H. & E. stain, ×120

9. Metastasis

Metastasis from oral cancer occurs chiefly through the lymphatic channels to involve the regional lymph nodes. Distant metastases have been most frequently reported in the lungs, liver, vertebrae, and brain in 10–55% of patients suffering from epidermoid carcinoma. Death is usually due to direct local complications from the primary lesion or distant metastases, bronchopneumonia, or respiratory or cardiac failure.

II. Carcinoma-in-situ

Carcinoma-in-situ is a histopathological entity in which the epithelial layers exhibit malignant morphology, but the lesion has not broken the basement membrane and invaded the subjacent lamina propria. The clinical appearance

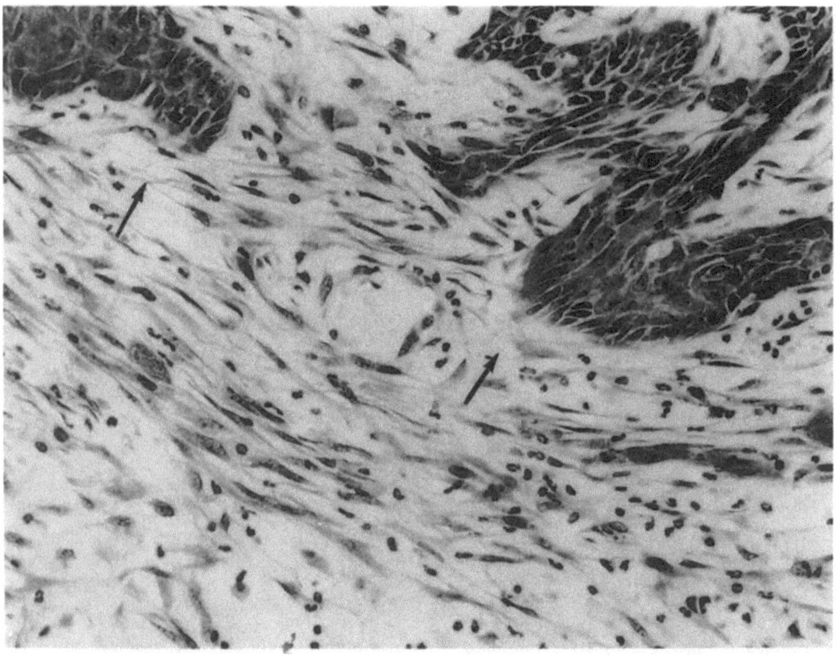

Fig. 3.11. Poorly-differentiated epidermoid carcinoma with invading nests of malignant cells (*arrows*). H. & E. stain, ×250

can vary from shiny atrophic patches to leukoplakia to erythroplakia. Carcinoma-in-situ has received considerable emphasis in its relationship to the development of frank carcinoma in the uterine, cervix, skin, larynx, esophagus, and gastrointestinal tract [5, 10].

Microscopically, the lesion demonstrates complete disorientation of cells throughout all epithelial layers, yet the basement membrane remains intact. The change from normal to atypical epithelium is quite abrupt with variations in cellular size and shape, loss of rete pegs, hyperchromatic bizarre muclei, and loss of cellular cohesion (Fig. 3.12).

Koss suggested that a definition limiting epithelial change to involve all layers was too restrictive. As an alternative, he defined carcinoma-in-situ as the presence of significant cellular abnormalities distributed vertically through the epithelial profile [23]. Thus, the presence of surface flattening of squamous cells in a hyperkeratotic or hyperparakeratotic fashion would not impede this diagnosis (Fig. 3.13).

III. Basal Cell Carcinoma

It is an established fact that an etiological relationship exists between sunlight exposure and skin cancer, as epidermiological studies of individuals in the South-

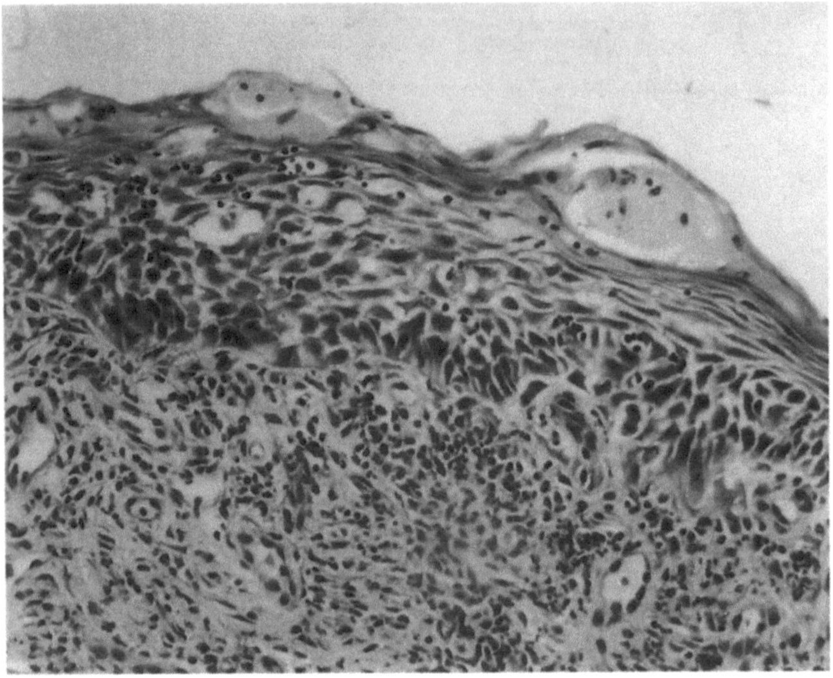

Fig. 3.12. Carcinoma-in-situ. H. & E. stain, ×190

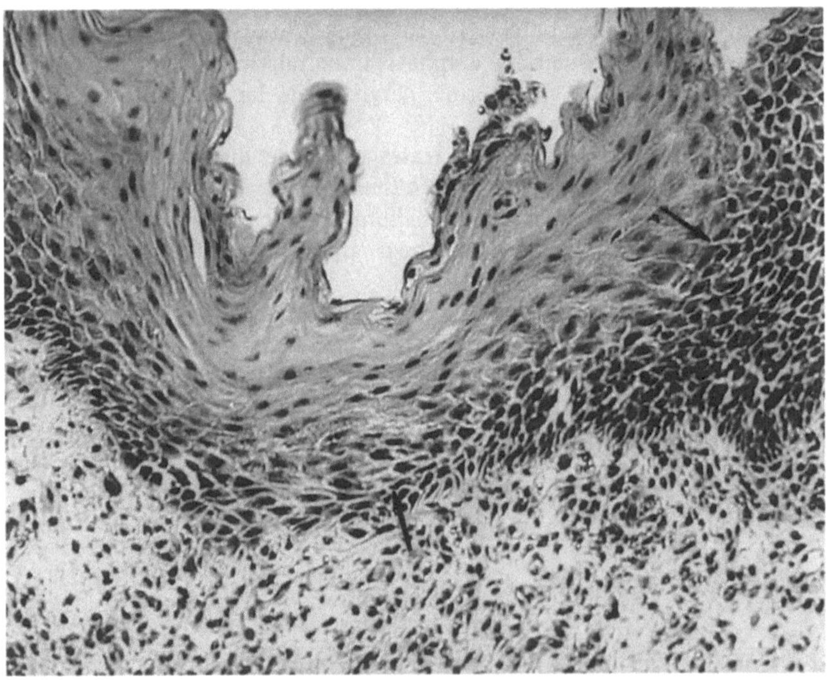

Fig. 3.13. Carcinoma-in-situ; note the abrupt change in epithelium (*arrows*). H. & E. stain, ×200

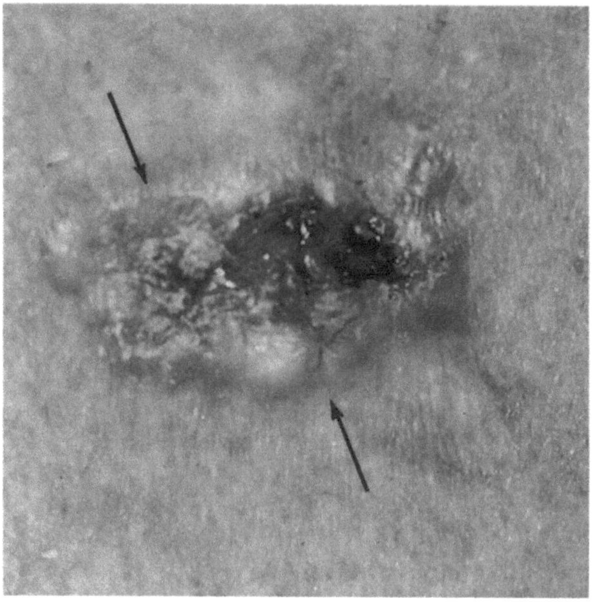

Fig. 3.14. Basal cell carcinoma exhibiting a smooth, indurated rolled border (*arrows*)

western United States or persons in outdoor occupations have confirmed [24–27].

The basal cell carcinoma usually occurs on hair-bearing skin surfaces, and the middle third of the face (the periorbital region) is the most common site. Although this tumor can occur in children and young persons, it is more frequently detected in the 30 to 40-year-old age bracket. Probably because of working vocation, basal cell carcinoma is found more often in men than in women. Since this neoplasm does not arise from oral mucosa, it is not seen within the oral cavity [10, 28, 29].

Clinically, the lesion begins as a small elevated papule which ulcerates, heals, breaks down again, and repeats the cycle as it slowly enlarges. Later, the crusting ulcer develops a rolled, smooth border, indicating that the tumor cells are spreading laterally underneath the skin (Fig. 3.14). The adjacent and deeper tissue are slowly infiltrated by tumor cells, which eventually can erode through bone or cartilage [29].

Histopathologically, the tumor appears as nests, islands, or sheets of similar malignant cells with large, oval deeply basophilic nuclei, scanty cytoplasm, and indistinct cell membranes (Fig. 3.15). The periphery of the cell nests is composed of well-polarized tumor cells, which closely resemble basal cells in the skin. The basal cell is pluripotential, and thus it can form hair, sebaceous glands, sweat glands, or keratin under normal circumstances. Often malignant tumor cells make an abortive attempt to form similar structures (note arrow in Fig. 3.15).

The prognosis for basal cell carcinoma is good when treated early and adequately by either surgical removal or radiation therapy. Some lesions are persistent, resist therapy, and tend to recur. This tumor rarely metastasizes, yet it can be lethal by tissue destruction and erosion into vital structures.

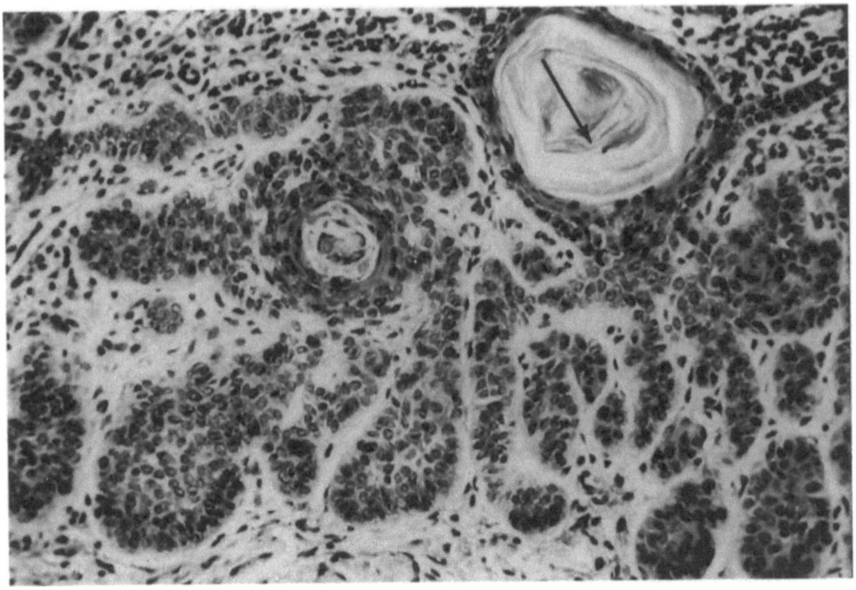

Fig. 3.15. Basal cell carcinoma; note the keratin formation (*arrow*) typical of such multipotential cells. H. & E. stain, ×200

IV. Malignant Melanoma

Excluding non-melanoma skin cancer, malignant melanoma represents only 2% of all cancers by incidence. In the United States this statistic means that approximately 16,700 new melanoma cases can be expected for 1982 (out of 835,000 new cancer cases), and nearly 5,000 deaths from melanoma will result [1, 30]. Over 50% of melanomas occur in persons 15 to 50 years of age, and with more leisure time to spend exposed to the sun the trend is toward a younger age incidence each year [31, 32]. In comparing the 5-year relative survival rates from 1960–1963 to 1970–1973 for malignant melanoma, Myers and Hankey found an upward trend in white males from 51% to 62% and in white females from 68% to 75%. These figures were statistically significant at the 0.05 level [11].

Malignant melanoma constitutes approximately 20% of all primary cancers of the skin. It principally affects Caucasians, expecially those persons with light

Fig. 3.16. Lentigo-maligna melanoma of the nose (*arrows*). (Courtesy of Drs. A.J. Sober, T.B. Fitzpatrick, M.C. Mihm, and W.H. Clark)

Fig. 3.17. Superficial spreading melanoma of the back; note the irregular knotched border (*arrow*). (Courtesy of Drs. A.J. Sober, T.B. Fitzpatrick, M.C. Mihm, and W.H. Clark)

Fig. 3.18. Deeply invasive nodular melanoma of the leg (*arrows*). (Courtesy of Drs. A.J. Sober, T.B. Sober, T.B. Fitzpatrick, M.C. Mihm, and W.H. Clark)

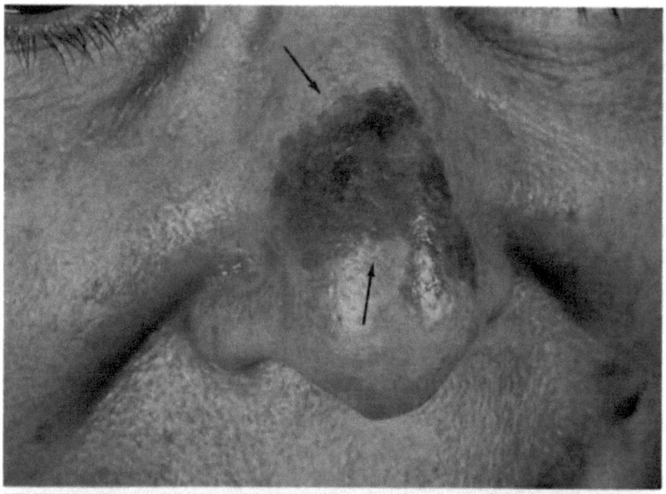

Fig. 3.16

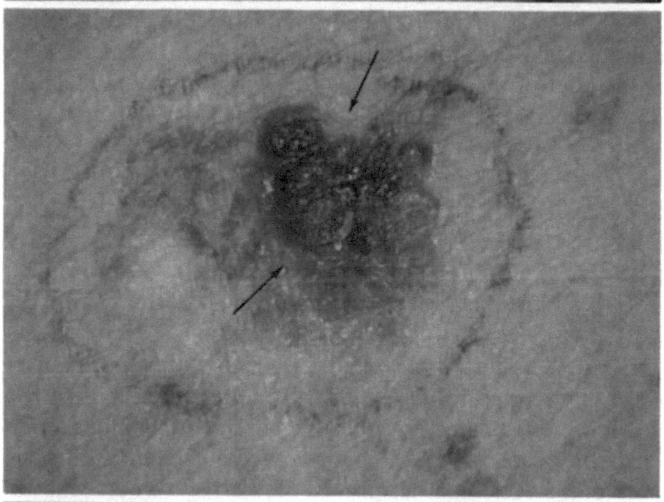

Fig. 3.17

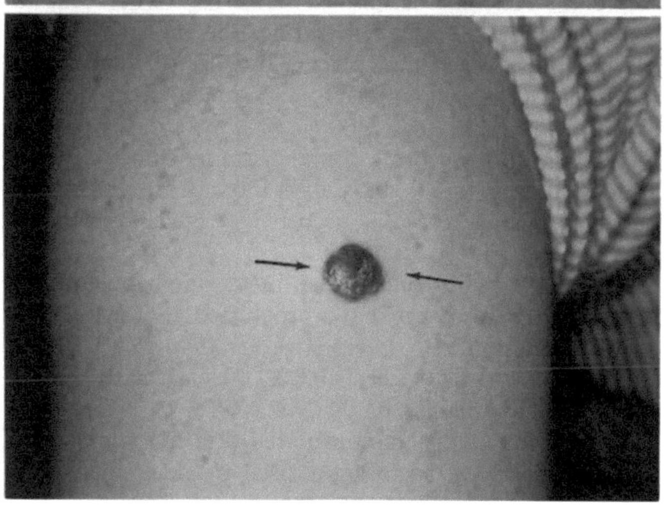

Fig. 3.18

hair, blue eyes, and fair skin. The incidence increases at lower latitudes because of high ultraviolet light flux. Seventy percent of the most common, lethal melanomas occur during 20 to 60 years of age [32, 33].

The traditional clinical description of malignant melanoma, (i.e., an enlarging dark pigmented lesion which ulcerates, crusts, and bleeds easily) actually apples to melanomas which have already invaded the skin deeply, metastasized widely, and naturally have a very poor prognosis.

Melanoma is a rare tumor within the oral cavity. Chaudhry reviewed 105 cases in the literature, and Trodahl added 42 cases from the Armed Forces Institute of Pathology files. Even in this nondermal anatomical site, melanoma occurs with twice the frequency in men as in women with an average case incidence of 50 years of age. It exhibits a definite predilection for the maxillary alveolar ridge and palate (80% of the reported cases). Because it is often diagnosed late, it appears as a deeply pigmented lesion which ulcerates and bleeds easily.

The only hope for better survival rates is early clinical detection. Clark et al. have described three types of malignant melanoma which are distinguished by clinical and histopathological appearance which correlate with their biological behavior. These are in order of increasing lethality: lentigo-maligna melanoma (LMM; Fig. 3.16); superficial spreading melanoma (SSM; Fig. 3.17); and nodular melanoma (NM; Fig. 3.18). SSM and LMM may exist for a long time in a superficial growth phase with little tendency to metastasize before deep invasion into the skin occurs. Thus, cure by surgical excision is possible during the prolonged superifical growth phase. As the level of local skin invasion increases, the prognosis becomes poorer. Nodular melanoma behaves in a much more lethal fashion, acting as an invasive neoplasm from the onset and does not exhibit superifical, preinvasive growth [32, 36, 37].

From 208 cases of melanoma Clark and Fitzpatrick have established a correlation between death and survival rate and the level of histological invasion (Table 3.1). In level I all tumor cells are above the basement membrane. In Level II tumor cells penetrate the basement membrane and extend into the papillary body, but not to the reticular dermis. In Level III, tumor cells fill the papillary dermis extending to, but not penetrating, the reticular dermis. In Level IV, tumor cells extend between the collagen bundles of the reticular dermis. In Level V, melanoma cells penetrate into the subcutaneous fat [32, 36, 37].

The percent distribution for all three forms of malignant melanoma by level is shown in Table 3.2. This finding was a study of 1,130 cases of melanoma in Caucasians. The higher percentage of cases occurred at Levels III and IV [38].

A marked improvement in mortality rate is seen in melanomas which are diagnosed at Level II invasion before they have progressed to Level III. If surgery is performed when the lesion is at Level II rather than Level III, the mortality rate is reduced from 35.2 to 8.3% (see Table 3.1). Hence, early diagnosis is absolutely critical in malignant melanoma.

The clinical features of malignant melanoma of the skin are summarized in Table 3.3. Three positive signs have been emphasized to aid immensely in

Table 3.1. Correlation of level of melanoma invasion with mortality

Tumor invasion level	Mortality rate (%)	Median survival time (years)	Percent of total 208 melanomas
Level II	8.3	1.50	17
Level III	35.2	2.08	33
Level IV	46.1	2.25	35
Level V	52.0	1.83	12

Courtesy of Dr. W.H. Clark and Dr. T.B. Fitzpatrick, Massachusetts General Hospital Data

Table 3.2. Malignant melanoma. Percent distribution by level

Level	Number of cases	(%)
II	309	27
III	349	31
IV	357	32
V	79	7
Unknown	36	3
	1,130	100

Courtesy of Dr. T.B. Fitzpatrick, Massachusetts General Hospital Data

Table 3.3. Clinical features of cutaneous melanoma [39]

Type	Location	Median age (year)	Duration of premetastatic lesion	Border	Color
1. Lentigo maligna	Usually on sun-exposed surfaces: head and neck (less commonly, on hands and legs)	70	Usually 5–15 years	Flat	Various shades of brown and black; frequent hypopigmentation (regression)
2. Superficial spreading	All body surfaces	47	1–7 years	Palpable	Various shades of brown and black; gray and pink common.
3. Nodular	All body surfaces	50	Months-2 years	Palpable	Uniform blush black

the early clinical diagnosis of cutaneous malignant melanoma [32, 39, 40]. In order of importance these signs are:

1. Variegated Color. This phenomenon is a common clinical characteristic of malignant melanoma, especially the superficial spreading type. Shades of red, white, and blue portend malignancy in a brown or black pigmented lesion. Shades of blue connote the most ominous sign.

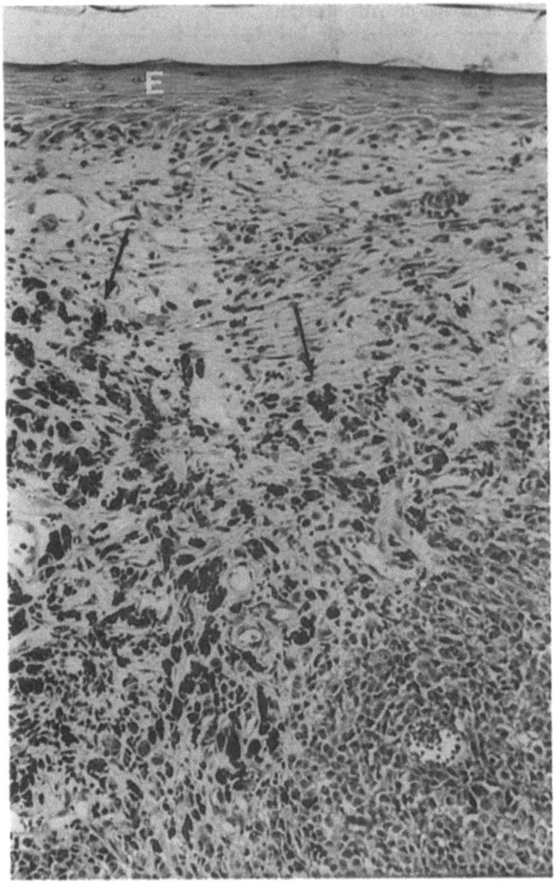

Fig. 3.19. Malignant melanoma. *E,* epithelium; *arrows,* melanoma cells. H. & E. stain, ×65

2. Irregular Border. This sign is seen most often as a notch in the border of the lesion (see Fig. 3.17).

3. Irregular Surface. Irregular elevations are present in many melanomas and may be either seen or palpated; however, some nodular melanomas may present with a smooth surface.

Histopathologically, the typical malignant melanoma extends from the dermal-epidermal junction into deeper connective tissue for varying distances. Tumor cells may vary, appearing either epitheloid, fusiform, or nevus-like in shape. The atypical melanocytes have large open nuclei, prominent nucleoli, and pinkish-tan cytoplasm with numerous granules [32, 40, 41]. Figure 3.19 shows the disrupted epithelium and melanoma cells deeper in the lamina propria. A higher magnification (Fig. 3.20) reveals malignant cells arranged in a closely packed alveolar pattern. In most cases the melanoma cells are packed with melanin granules. However, in some patients, melanin may either not be prominent, or it may be absent altogether. On fresh, unfixed tumor tissue, stains for activated tyosinase or dihydroxphenylalanine (dopa) oxidase will usually be positive for most melanomas.

Prior to the recent emphasis and educational efforts to stress early clinical diagnosis prior to Level III invasion, the historical prognosis for malignant

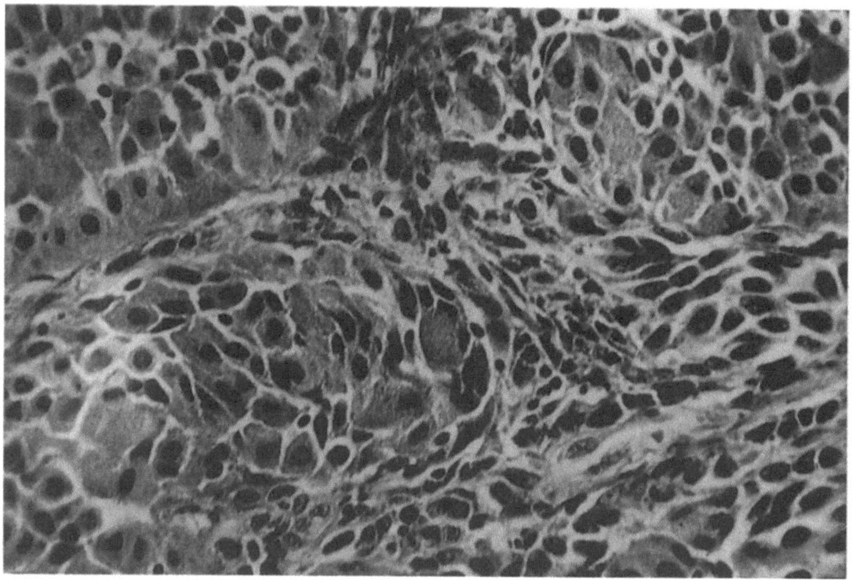

Fig. 3.20. Malignant melanoma cells arranged in a clustered, alveolar pattern. H. & E. stain, ×350

melanoma was nortoriously poor. For example, in his study of oral cavity melanoma cases, Chaudhry reported only a 5% 5-year survival rate [34]. The survival rates now have been greatly improved, as shown in Table 3.1, for all melanomas, because they are now being picked up much earlier, prior to metastasis.

Treatment of the early lesion consists of adequate surgical excision with wide margins. The invasive lesion that has penetrated deeper required more radical surgical resection with lymph nodal dissection. Intradermal BCG immuniotherapy has been used as adjuvant therapy with varying success [42, 43]. All melanoma patients should receive very careful follow-up.

V. Odontogenic Tumors

Odontogenic tumors as a group are quite uncommon and are of interest mainly as an academic entity, yet must be recognized correctly for diagnostic reasons. When viewed in the broad context of significant numbers of various types of cancer, the ameloblastoma and the calcifying epithelial odontogenic tumor (which are the two most aggressive odontogenic tumors) are extremely rare neoplasms. They are even rare when considered in the narrower category of oral neoplasms. It has been estimated that odentogic tumors probably constitute less than 1% of all jaw cysts and tumors, and thus, they are an insignificant cause of oral cancer [5, 10, 44, 45].

Many classifications for odontogenic tumors have been attempted, each with its own deficiencies. One pathological classification is shown in Table 3.4. In

Table 3.4. Pathologic classification of odontogenic tumors

I. *Ectodermal origin*
   (1) ameloblastoma
   (2) adenomatoid odontogenic tumor (adenoameloblastoma)
   (3) calcifying epithelial odontogenic tumor (Pindborg Tumor)

II. *Mesodermal origin*
   (1) odontogenic fibroma
   (2) odontogenic myxoma
   (3) ossifying fibroma
   (4) cementifying fibroma
   (5) cemento-ossifying fibroma
   (6) central fibroma

III. *Mixed origin*
   (1) ameloblastic fibroma
   (2) ameloblastic odontoma
   (3) odontoma
      (A) compound type
      (B) complex type
   (4) ameloblastic fibrosarcoma

this chapter, we shall dwell more on the ameloblastoma and the calcifying epithelial odentogenic tumor because these two entities are of greater importance due to their undoubted neoplastic activity. Diagnostic features of the other odontogenic tumors will also be discussed except for the ossifying fibroma, cementifying fibroma, cemento-ossifying fibroma, and the central fibroma, which will be covered under the section on benign fibro-osseous lesions.

1. Ectodermal Origin

(A) Ameloblastoma

Ameloblastoma is the best known odontogenic tumor. In 1965 Stanley and Diehl added 195 cases from the Armed Forces Institute of Pathology and National Institutes of Health files to the 1,036 cases of ameloblastoma reported earlier by Small and Waldron from the English scientific literature and their own files to make a total of 1,231 reported cases at that time [45, 46]. Currently, most investigators consider that the ameloblastoma has a varied origin, conceivably being derived from either: (A) cell rest remnants of either the dental lamina or Hertwig's sheath (epithelial rests of Malassez); (B) epithelium from dentigenous cysts; (C) disturbances of the developing enamel organs; (D) basal cells of the surface epithelium of the jaws; or (E) heterotropic epithelium in other parts of the body, especially the pituitary gland [10, 44, 46–50].

The statistical clinical picture for ameloblastoma is presented in Table 3.5. Ameloblastoma occurs approximately evenly between the sexes. Racial specificity is difficult to evaluate; however, in Small and Waldron's review there was

Table 3.5. Ameloblastomas of the jaws. Statistical analysis of the literature [10]

		Number	%
Total cases		1,036	
Sex (987 cases)			
Male		514	52
Female		473	48
Race (594 cases)			
Caucasian		371	
Negro		121	
Chinese		71	
Egyptian		15	
Indian		15	
Filipino		1	
Average age at time of report	38.9 years		
Average duration of tumor	5.8 years		
Average age at time of discovery	32.7 years		
Site of growth (925 cases)			
Mandible		752	81
Maxilla		173	19
Structural characteristies (465 cases)			
Cystic (includes those called cystic and solid)		365	78
Solid		100	22
Location			
Mandible			
Molar-ramus area		170	70
Premolar area		49	20
Symphysis area		27	10
Maxilla			
Molar area		21	47
Antrum and floor of nose		15	33
Premolar area		4	9
Canine area		4	9
Palate		1	2

a 3:1 predominance of occurence in Caucasians over Negroes. While ameloblastoma may occur at any age, over half of them are discovered between the ages of 20 and 40 years, with an average age at onset of 33 years. The tumor has arisen in the mandible in 81% of the reported cases compared to 19% in the maxilla. Most of these tumors (70%) are found in the manulibular molar-ramus area [44, 45, 51, 52].

The classical radiographic description of an ameloblastoma depicts it as a multilocular, cyst-like central jaw lesion (see Fig. 3.21). Such an appearance is suggestive, rather than pathognomonic, since many oral lesions (e.g. odontogenic cysts, aneurysmal bone cyst, cherubism, etc.) can present radiographically in an identical manner. Ameloblastoma may also appear as a unilocular radiolucency [5, 10, 44, 47, 53].

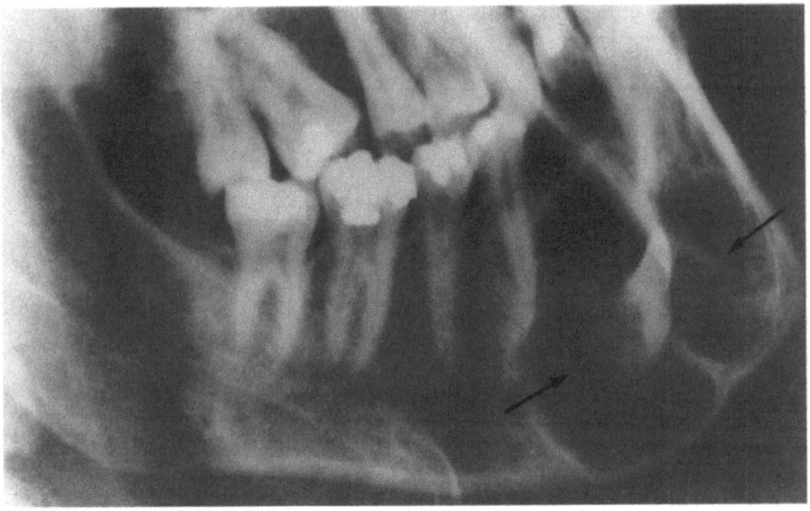

Fig. 3.21. Radiographic appearance of ameloblastoma; note the multilocular, cystic areas (*arrows*). (Courtesy of Division of Stomatology, School of Dental and Oral Surgery, Columbia University, New York, NY)

Histopathologically, this tumor is characterized by ameloblastic cells comprising the periphery of strands or islands in a fibrous connective tissue stroma. It usually follows one of two predominant patterns, namely, the follicular pattern or the plexiform pattern, although on occasion both patterns may be seen in the same tumor.

The follicular ameloblastoma tends to resemble the enamel organ with the outer cells similar in appearance to the inner dental epithelium. The center portion of the epithelial island contains a loose, delicate network of cells, similar to the stellate reticulum (Fig. 3.22). Squamous metaplasia of epithelial cells within the stellate reticulum-like central area has given rise to the term acanthomatous ameloblastoma (Fig. 3.23). Cystic degeneration can occur within the follicle areas and the stroma per se. Figure 3.24 demonstrates such cystic change, leaving clear spaces in some of the follicles, lined by flattened epithelial cells [5, 10, 44, 47, 49].

The plexiform pattern ameloblastoma exhibits irregular masses and strands of epithelial cells, which resemble ameloblasts or basal cells (Fig. 3.25). Cystic degeneration of the central portion is common [10, 44, 49].

On occasion, marked transformation of the cytoplasm of the ameloblastic cells takes place, producing large, coarse granular-appearing cells (Fig. 3.26) [54–56]. Hodson noted that the periodic acid – Schiff reaction of these granular cells was variable with scanty or no glycogen and fat being present [57]. Other investigators found this tumor relatively inert [55, 58].

In the spindle-cell variety of the ameloblastoma (Fig. 3.27], the ameloblastic cells have undergone metaplastic change and closely resemble epithelial spindle cells.

Various studies have reported the apparent development of ameloblastoma from the wall of a dentigerous cyst: Sonesson (26%), Bernier and Tiecke (33%)

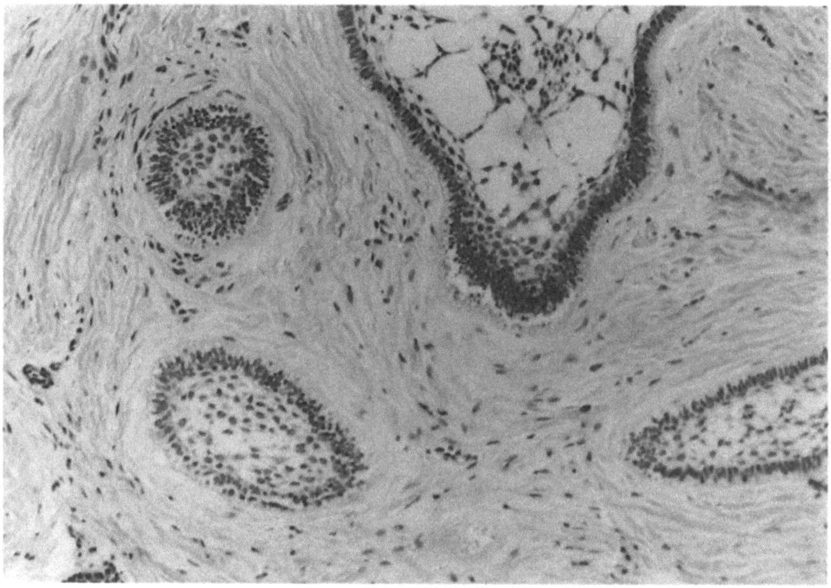

Fig. 3.22. Follicular pattern ameloblastoma. H. & E. stain, ×65

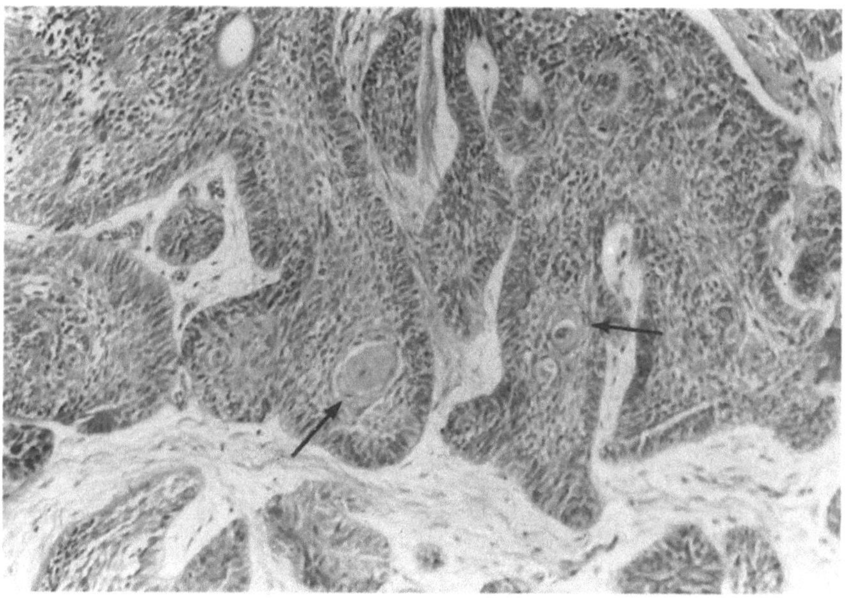

Fig. 3.23. Acanthomatous ameloblastoma; note the squamous metaplasia and formation of keratin (*arrows*). H. & E. stain, ×65

and Stanley and Diehl (15%) [46, 50, 59, 60]. Figure 3.28 illustrates the histopathologic appearance of an ameloblastoma arising in the lining wall of a follicular cyst.

The occurance of occasional "malignant" ameloblastoma cases with metastases has raised much skepticism and debate. In their analysis of 33 such amelo-

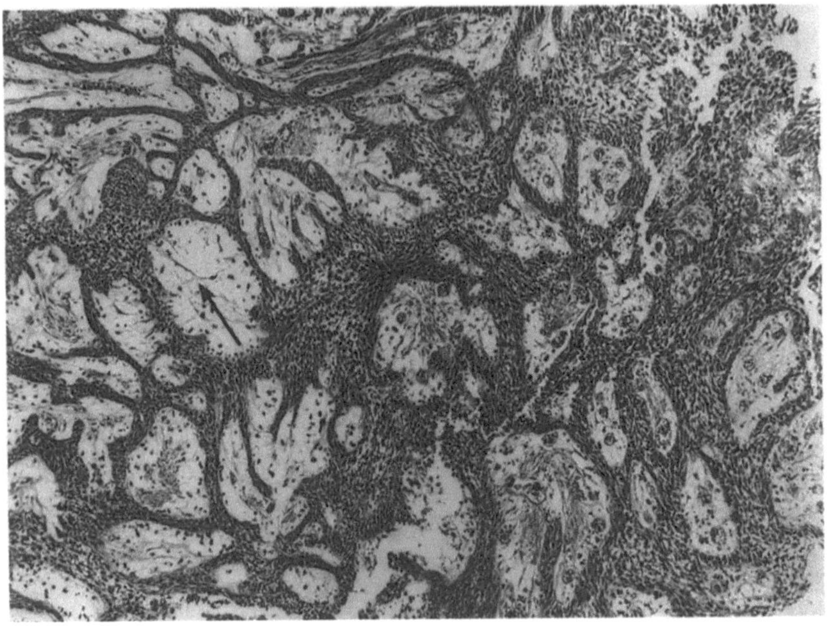

Fig. 3.24. Cystic degeneration (*arrow*) in an ameloblastoma. H. & E. ×65

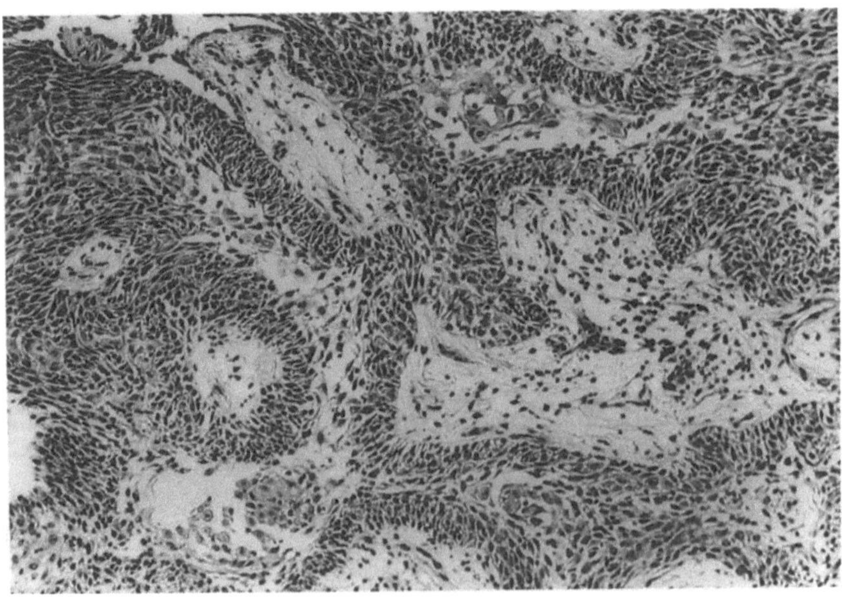

Fig. 3.25. Plexiform pattern ameloblastoma. H. & E. stain, ×100

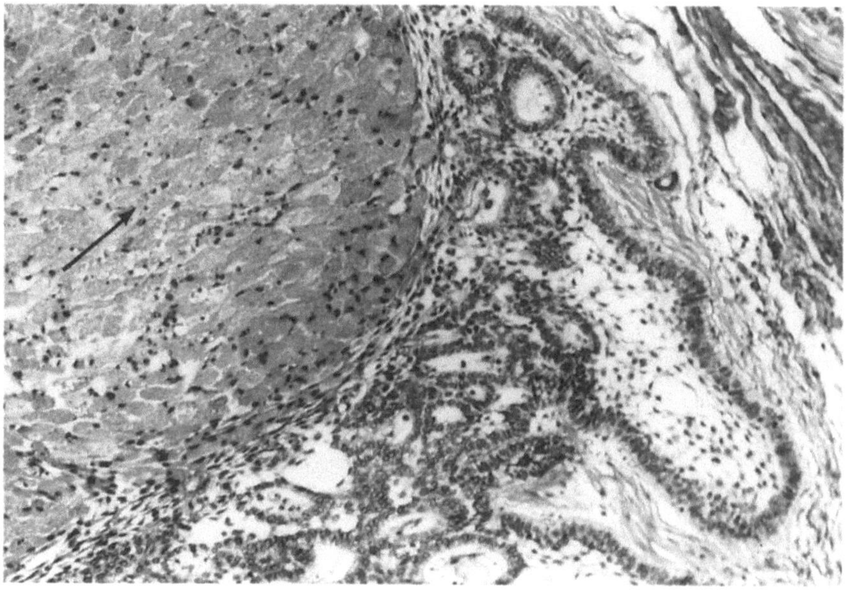

Fig. 3.26. Granular cell type (*arrow*) ameloblastoma. H. & E. stain, ×65

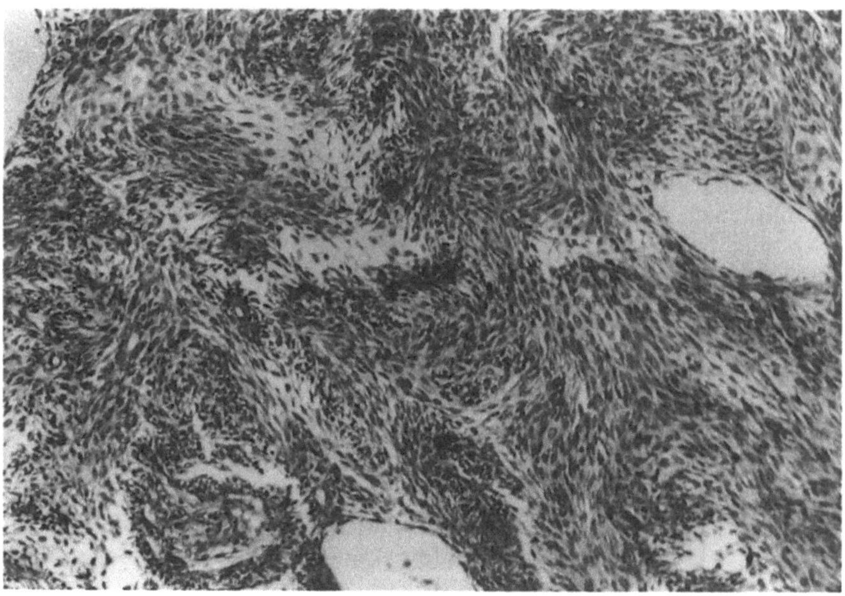

Fig. 3.27. Spindle cell type ameloblastoma. H. & E. stain, ×150

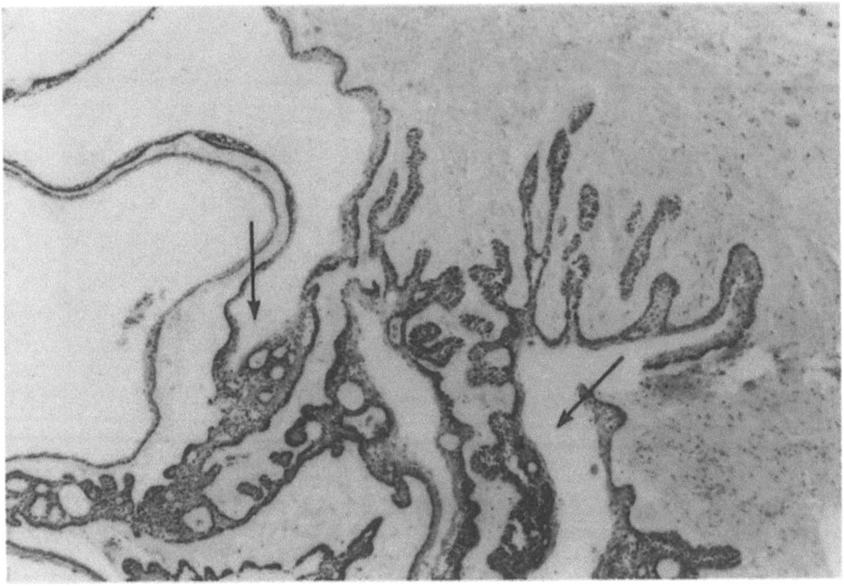

Fig. 3.28. Ameloblastoma (*arrows*) arising from the wall of a dentigerous cyst. H. & E. stain, ×35

blastoma cases, Small and Waldron concluded that 12/33 were unacceptable, and a number of the remaining 21 were doubtful due to lack of photographic evidence [45]. Following the period covered by Small and Waldron's review, 13 years later in 1968 Carr and Halperin reported in their review of the literature on "malignant ameloblastoma" that only 4 additional cases were proven malignant, and 12 reported cases were possibly malignant, and 5 of the reported cases were doubtfully malignant [61]. Lee and others have pointed out that often even demonstrable lung "metastatic lesions" are a result of aspiration implantation, since many of these reported lesions are located in the lungs where aspirated foreign bodies often lodge [62]. However, the well-documented cases of Tsukada et al. [56], Hoke and Harrelson [63], Sugimura et al. [64] and Vorzimer and Perla [65], do demonstrate that the ameloblastoma may spread by lymphatics, blood stream, or airway.

Many types of treatment have been employed for ameloblastoma including conservative and radical surgery, radiotherapy, chemicals, or electrocautery [10, 44, 62]. Surgical resection remains the treatment of choice. Table 3.6 illustrates the results of a comprehensive study by Becker and Pertl on therapeutic practices for ameloblastomas in 1967 [66]. Radical surgical resection yielded the best results – only a 4.5% recurrence rate compared to radiotherapy 41.6%, and conservative surgery (59.1%). They also found that the solid form of aneloblastoma had a higher recurrence rate than the cystic form [66]. Because the ameloblastoma is considered highly radio-resistant, this form of therapy is not advocated [10, 67].

The prognosis of ameloblastoma in terms of survival is good because it is essentially a local problem. Death seldom ensues unless vital structures are

Table 3.6. Comparison of therapeutic results in treating ameloblastoma [66]

Treatment	Number of patients	Tumor recurrence
1. radiotherapy	36	41.6% [a]
2. conservative surgery	120	59.1%
3. radical surgery	98	4.5%

[a] Postradiation sarcoma killed an additional 25% of these treated patients

involved. However, it does often present both comestic and rehabilitation problems and challenges because of its local aggressive destruction of hard and soft tissues, producing disfigurement and difficulties in speech, chewing, and swallowing.

(B) Adenomatoid Odentogenic Tumor (Adenoameloblastoma)

This tumor is an uncommon odontogenic tumor. In 1970 Giansanti, Someren, and Waldron reported slightly over 100 cases in their review of the literature [68]. In the last decade this number has increased by almost half with the addition of Courtney and Kerr's 20 new cases, plus numerous individual case reports [69–71]. It has been known by a wide variety of names, e.g. ameloblastic adenomatoid tumor, adenoamelo-blastoma, cystic complex composite odentoma, glandular ameloblastoma, etc. However, most authorities now agree with Philipen and Birn's argument that the best descriptive title should be adenomtoid odentogenic tumor [72].

The clinical features of this tumor are derived from Giansanti's review. The age range for occurrence is 4–43 years, however, more than 90% of the patients have been between the ages of 12 and 30 years at the time of tumor detection. It is more common in females than males (64% versus 36%). The adenomatoid odentogenic tumor customarily presents as a slow-growing, painless mass. In 75% of the patients it is associated with an unerupted tooth, most often a maxillary cuspid or anterior tooth. The site of occurrence is far greater in the maxilla (65%) compared to the mandible (35%), and 76% of all cases occur from the cuspid area anteriorly [10, 44, 68].

Radiographically, the adenomatoid odentogenic tumor is seen as a radiolucent, unilocular lesion, often resembling a dentigerous cyst or lateral periodontal cyst, with scattered areas of radio-opague calcifications (see Fig. 3.29). This tumor expands the cortical plate of bone, but is not invasive [44, 53].

The tumor cells per se appear histologically as a highly regular polyhedral epithelial type cell with prominent dark vesicular nuclei and a minimum of cytoplasm. The growth pattern of these tumor cells varies from nests, whorls, and rosettes to cells of columnar or cubiodal type arranged in a duct-like adenomatoid configuration. Three distinct features are: the round duct-like structures, lined by a single layer of columnar cells whose nuclei are polarized away from the lumen (see Fig. 3.30). As the tumor matures, an eosinophilic hyaline material is broken down, and hollow cell masses that resemble ducts are formed. Distinct

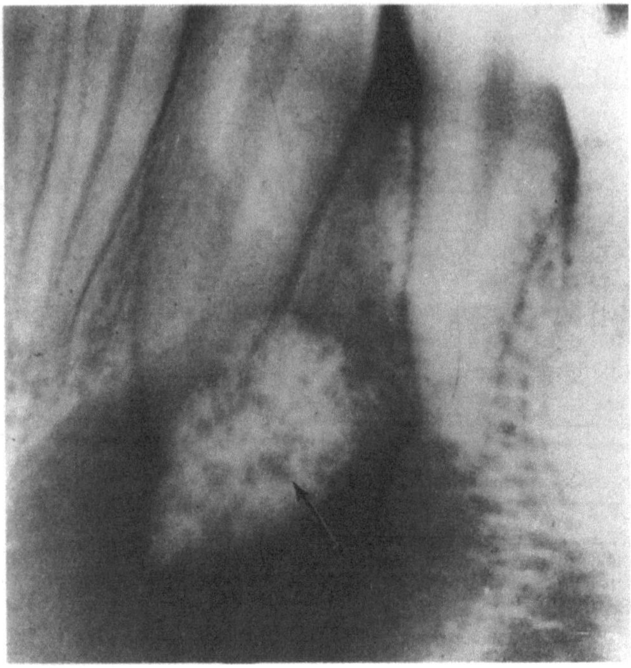

Fig. 3.29. Radiographic appearance of the adenomatoid odontogenic tumor, mandibular cuspid and first premolar region; note the area of calcification (*arrow*). (Courtesy of Armed Forces Institute of Pathology)

duct-like spaces may not be detected in each case and are not required for the diagnosis of this tumor. A second feature is the presence of PAS (periodic acid – Schiff) positive-staining eosinophilic, amorphorus filling material within the duct spaces. Third, focal areas of calcifications, may be randomly scattered throughout the tumor. These calcifications stain positive for calcium with the von Kossa stain [5, 10, 73]. The periphery of the tumor is almost invariably encapsulated by fibrous tissue, making its surgical removal by curettement easy.

Several possibilities have been suggested as the origin of the adenomatoid odentogenic tumor, however, universal agreement does not exist. Lucas, Stafne, Miles, and Gorlin and Chaudhry postulated origin from the preameloblast, based on morphologic and histochemical studies [74–77]. Shear thought that this tumor arose from ondontogenic epithelium before histodifferentiation [78]. Spouge advocated origin from the inner enamel epithelium as a "preameloblastoma" [73]. Ultrastructural studies with electron microscopy indicate an enamel organ origin [71, 79–81]. This tumor was found to contain cells resembling preameloblasts, the stratum intermedium, and the stellate reticulum. Hatakeyama and Suzuki have also described a fourth type of cells of the enamel organ, namely cells resembling the outer enamel epithelium [81]. Histochemical and ultrastructural evidence indicates that the eosinophilic granulo-fibrillar material in the duct-like spaces is amyloid [71, 80, 82]. The duct-like structures are now thought to be formed as a result effect of the secretory activity of the tumor cells, rather than a degenerative process [71, 82].

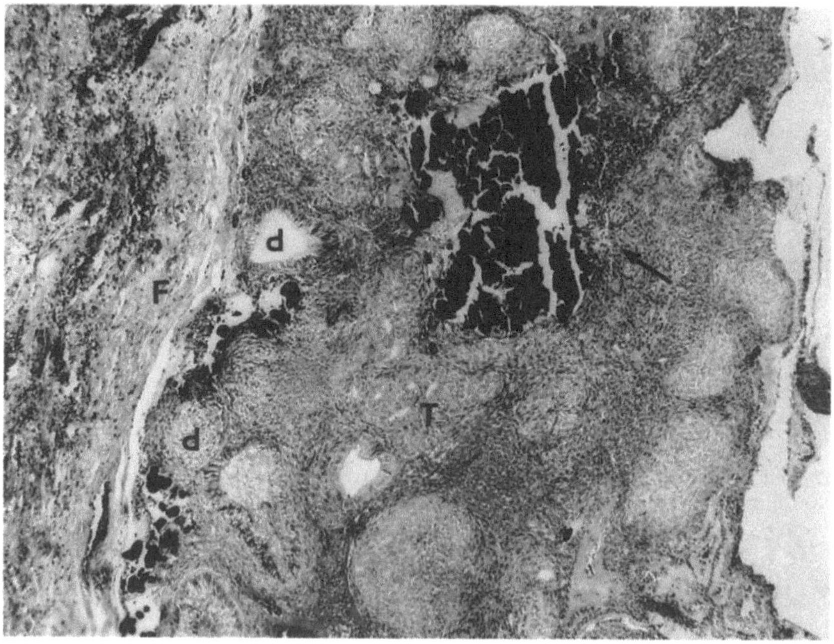

Fig. 3.30. Adenomatoid odontogenic tumor with ductlike structures (*d*); tumor cells (*T*); fibrous capsule (*F*), and calcifications (*arrow*). H. & E. stain, ×65

Because of its fibrous encapsulation, the adenomatoid odontogenic tumor responds well to surgical curettage; no cases of recurrence have been reported [5, 10]. It does not act in a local invasive or aggressive fashion.

(C) Calcifying Epithelial Odontogenic Tumor

The calcifying epithelial odontogenic tumor was first described as an entity by Pindborg in 1955 [83]. Approximately 50 cases now exist in the reported literature.

From this data, the following clinical profile appears. The age range at this time of diagnosis for this tumor is 12–78 years, with an average age of 42 years. There is no sex predilection (26 females: 24 males). Approximately 75% arose arose in the mandible versus the maxilla, and the majority of them were in the premolar-molar area of the jaws, associated with an embedded or unerupted tooth, similar to the ameloblastoma. The calcifying epithelial odontogenic tumor presents as a painless swelling and grows by expansion of the surrounding bone. It can be invasive, destructive, and locally recurrent. The degree of reported aggressivenes varies – some were markedly aggressive, whereas the case reported by Langer had a 40 year duration, the one described by Stimson had a 17 year history, and the case noted by Gardner recurred 31 years after the original surgical treatment. This tumor usually occurs as a central lesion in bone; however, several extra-osseous cases have been described [10, 44, 83–85].

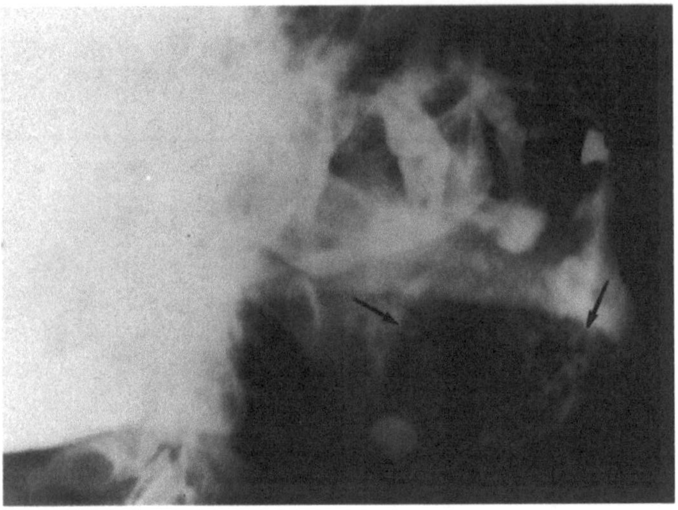

Fig. 3.31. Radiographic appearance of a large calcifying epithelial odontogenic tumor (*arrows*), lateral head film. (Courtesy of the Armed Forces Institute of Pathology)

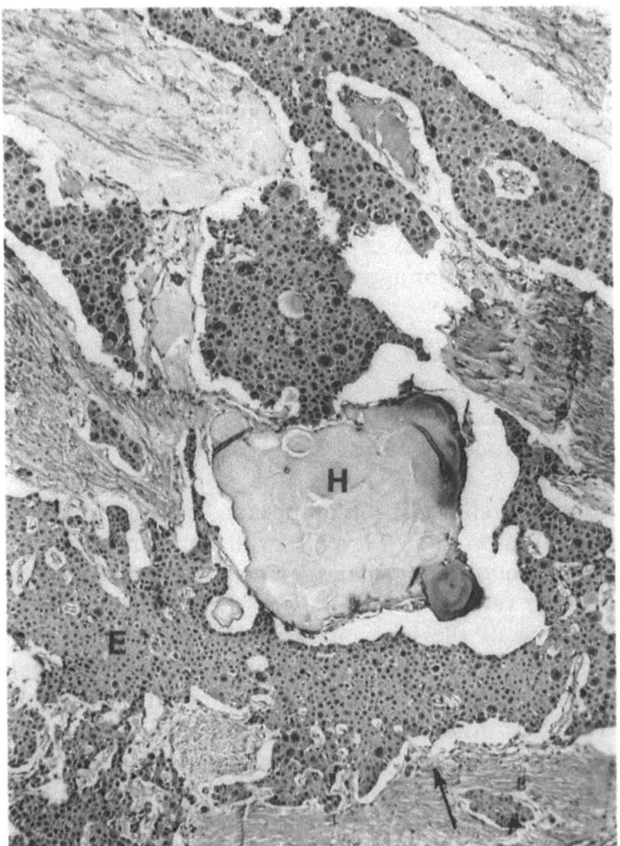

Fig. 3.32. Calcifying epithelial odontogenic tumor cells (*E*); spherical eosinophilic homogenous substance (*H*); and Liesegang ring calcifications (*arrow*). H. & E. stain, ×65

Table 3.7. Comparison of epithelial odontogenic tumors

	Ameloblastoma	Adenomatoid odontogenic tumor	Calcifying epithelial odontogenic tumor
1. Incidence	comprises approximately 1% of all oral tumors and cysts	approximately 150 reported cases	approximately 50 reported cases
2. Age of occurrence	20–40 years (50% of cases)	12–30 years (90% of cases)	12–78 years ($\bar{X}=42$)
3. Sex incidence	male: female ratio is equal	females > males ratio (64%: 36%)	male: female ratio is equal
4. Location	mandible > maxilla (molar ramus area)	maxilla > mandible (anterior-cuspid area)	mandible > maxilla
5. Radiographic	multilocular radiolucency	1–2 cm diameter radiolucency with small masses of calcification	radiolucency with radio-opaque islands
6. Signs/symptoms	swelling; destructively invasive; "locally malignant" with few true proven metastases	expands cortical bone, but is not invasive	swelling with local invasive destruction
7. Treatment	surgical resection with adequate margins	curettement	surgical resection with adequate margins

The radiographic appearance of the calcifying epithelial odontogenic tumor consists of a diffuse or circumscribed radiolucency, most often with a scattering of radio-opague calcifications throughout the tumor (see Fig. 3.31) [10, 44, 84].

Four distinctive microscopic features are evident in diagnosing this odontogenic tumor. First is the presence of sheets of large polyhedral epithelial cells within a scanty connective tissue stroma. The nucleus is vesicular usually with distinct nucleoli, while the cytoplasm is eosinophilic and homogenous. Distinct intercellular bridges are often present. Second is development of an intracytoplasmic homogenous substance. Third is occassional calcification of the spherical homogenous substance in the Liesegang ring fashion. Fourth is the rupture of cell walls, leaving calcified areas of the homogenous substance within the stroma [5, 10, 83–85]. These histopathologic characteristies are exhibited in Fig. 3.32.

Pindborg noted that the homogenous substance produced a strong PAS-positive reaction [85]. Vickers, et al., suggested that this material was amyloid after demonstrating amyloid's presence with the methyl violet stain [86]. This work was later confirmed by Ranlox and Pindborg and Gardner [87, 88]. Using histochemical stains and polarized light, Gon theorized that the epithelial cells comprising this tumor are identical to the cells of the stratum intermedium of the enamel organ [89].

Since the calcifying epithelial odontogenic tumor behaves in a fashion similar to the ameloblastoma, is locally invasive, and tends to recur locally, it should be treated by careful surgical resection with adequate margins [10].

A comparison of selected pertinent features of the three epithelial odontogenic tumors is given in Table 3.7.

2. Mesodermal Origin

(A) Odontogenic Fibroma

The odontogenic fibroma is a rare, benign central mesodermal tumor of odontogenic origin which may be found in either the maxilla or mandible [10]. Some investigators have lumped the odontogenic fibroma and odontogenic myxoma into a single entity, the "myxofibroma"; for example, Zimmerman and Dahlin's study of 26 such cases in the Mayo Clinic files [90]. For our diagnostic purposes, the two will be discussed separately.

Clinically, the salient features of this tumor are a gradual progressive enlargement of the affected jaw and facial deformity, usually unaccompanied by pain. Often there is a resultant displacement of the adjacent teeth in the affected area. The tumor's presence may be manifested for periods varying from several weeks to several years before the patient seeks treatment [90–93]. Zimmerman and Dahlin found that is 67% of their reported cases of odontogenic "myxofibroma" patients were between 10 and 29 years of age [90]. Bhaskar stated that this particular tumor commonly occurs in patients under 20 years of age [94]. The ages on the five cases in Hamner's analysis were 8, 8, 19, 23, and 73 years respectively [91]. The sexes appear to be affected equally [10, 44].

The mesodermal portion of the tooth germ (the dental papilla, the dental follicle, or later, the periodontal membrane) has been suggested as the origin of the odontogenic fibroma [10, 44, 91, 93, 95]. It is frequently associated with missing, unerupted, or partially erupted teeth.

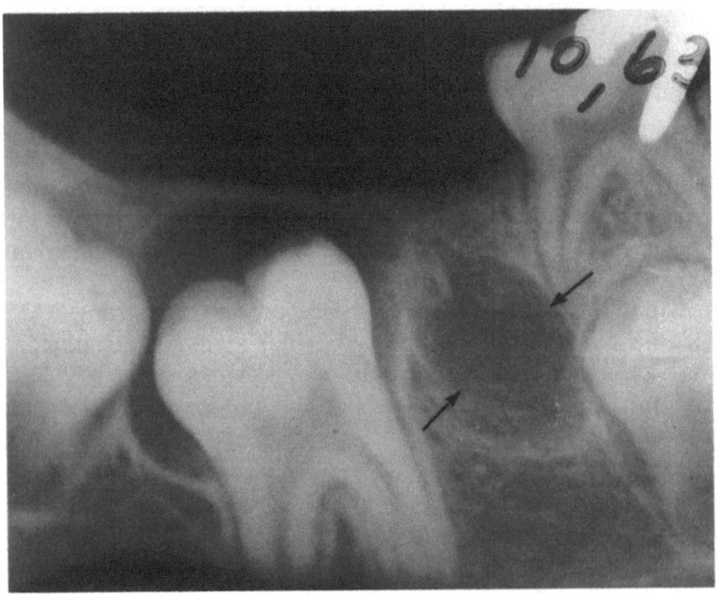

Fig. 3.33. Odontogenic fibroma (*arrows*) in the mandible of an 8-year-old Caucasian female

The radiographic appearance of the odontogenic fibroma is nonspecific. On roentgenograms the lesion appears as a well-defined radiolucency simulating a unilocular ameloblastoma or an odontogenic cyst. The margins may become scalloped, and gracile straight trabeculae have been described in the central portion [91–93, 76, 97]. Figure 3.33 shows an odontogenic fibroma as a rounded, well-defined radiolucency located subjacent and distal to the deciduous left mandibular second molar. It appears to be associated with the dental follicles of either the unerupted permanent first molar or second premolar in an 8 year old white girl.

Histopathologically, this tumor is composed predominantly of mature collagenous fibers with numerous interspersed fibroblasts. The connective tissue cells may have a stellate, triangular, or cunciform shape, resembling the young cells found in the dental papilla. Small nests, remnants, or tiny strands of inactive odontogenic epithelium support the odontogenic theory of its genesis (see Fig. 3.34) [91–93, 97].

Since this is a benign fibrous type tumor, simple enucleation with thorough curettage is the treatment of choice. However, surgical inaccessibility and/or massive size may necessitate resection of the involved area. It does not tend to recur, however, Heimdal et al., reported an example that recurred 9 years after initial surgical treatment at age 20 in a female patient [93]. The recurrent tumor did not act in an aggressive fashion.

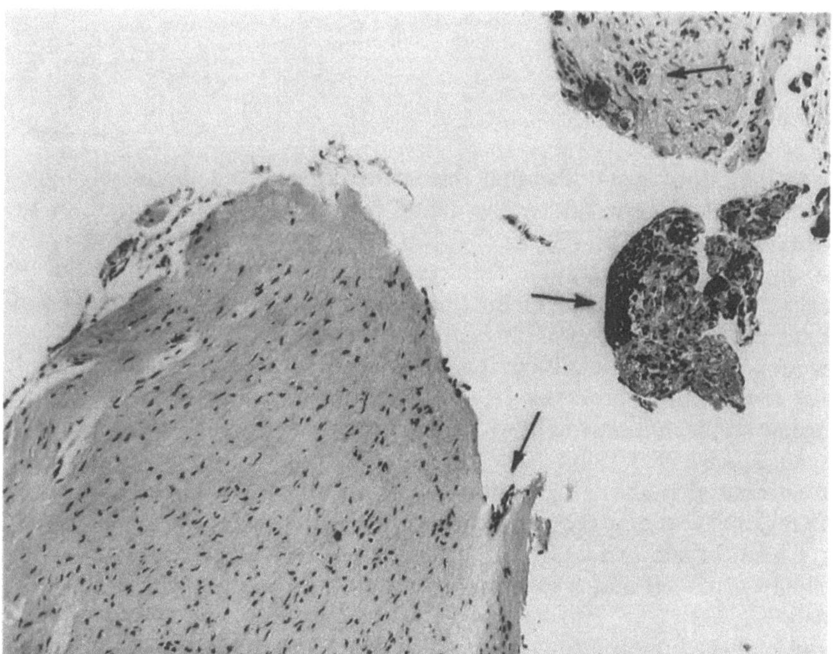

Fig. 3.34. Odontogenic fibroma; note the inactive remnants of odontogenic epithelium (*arrows*). H. & E. stain, ×92

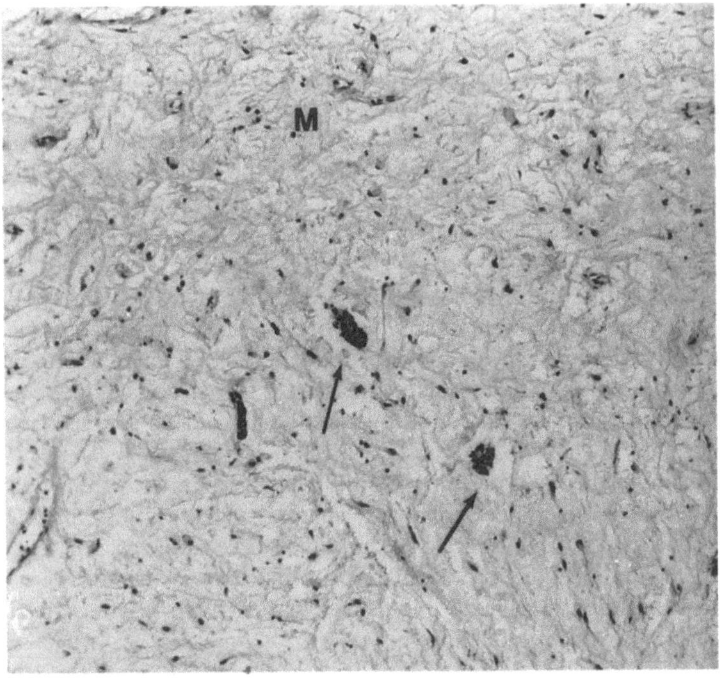

Fig. 3.35. Odontogenic myxoma, 19-year-old Caucasian male. *M*, myxomatous stroma; *arrows*, inactive odontogenic epithelium. H. & E. stain, ×92

(B) Odontogenic Myxoma

Similar to the odontogenic fibroma, this tumor arises from the mesenchymal portion of the tooth germ (either the dental papilla, the dental follicle, or the periodontal membrane) [10, 93].

The clinical and radiographic features mimic those just described for the odontogenic fibroma. The chief distinction between these two mesodermal odontogenic tumors is their histopathological appearance.

The odontogenic myxoma is composed of loosely arranged spindling, stellate cells with long fibrillar processes [10, 98–100]. Occassionally, nests of inactive odontogenic epithelium are found within the tumor matrix, but are not necessary for diagnosis (see Fig. 3.35).

Ultrastructural studies of the odontogenic myxoma have provided evidence that the myxoblast tumor cell is a secretory cell that secretes the loose, mucoid matrix. Chemical and histochemical investigations have demonstrated that the intercellular matrix contains excessive amounts of acid mucopolysaccharides [101–107].

Because of the odontogenic myxoma's ability to infiltrate and destroy bone, it requires more extensive surgical treatment than the odontogenic fibroma. Surgeons have advocated both en bloc resection of the involved bone and/or careful and thorough curettage to eradicate this tumor. Because of its high recurrence rate (approximately 25%), some clinicians have favored a bloc resection, although both surgical approaches have been successful. The procedure of choice should depend on the extent of the lesion, its anatomical site, and the aggressiveness of each individual lesion [107–111].

3. Mixed Origin

(A) Ameloblastic Fibroma

The ameloblastic fibroma is a true "mixed tumor" of odontogenic origin, characterized by the simultaneous proliferation of both the ectodermal and mesodermal components of the tooth germ. Proliferation occurs before these tissues develop the potential to form enamel, dentin, and cementum. Hence, no calcifed dental tissues are found in the tumor [112].

It is an uncommon odontogenic neoplasm, which often affects children and young adults and occurs with equal frequency in both sexes [10, 44]. In Gorlin's analysis of 43 cases, he found that the vast majority of patients with this tumor were between 5–20 years of age [44]. It arises most often in the premolar-molar region of the mandible and presents clinically as an asymptomatic enlargement of the buccal and/or lingual cortical plates of bone [112]. As the tumor enlarges it expands and thins, but rarely perforates the cortical plates [44, 112, 113].

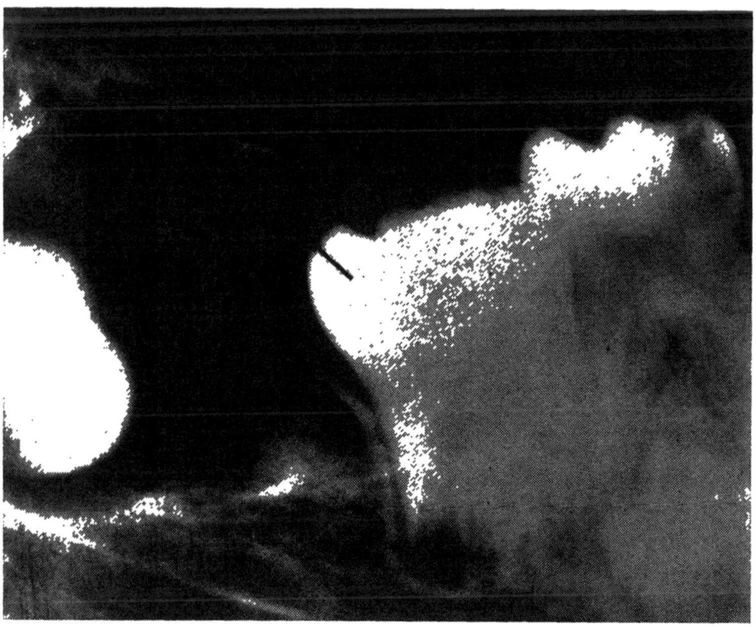

Fig. 3.36. Ameloblastic fibroma presenting as a multilocular radiolucency (*arrows*) displacing the partially formed mandibular first and second molars in a 6-year-old female. (Courtesy of the Armed Forces Institute of Pathology)

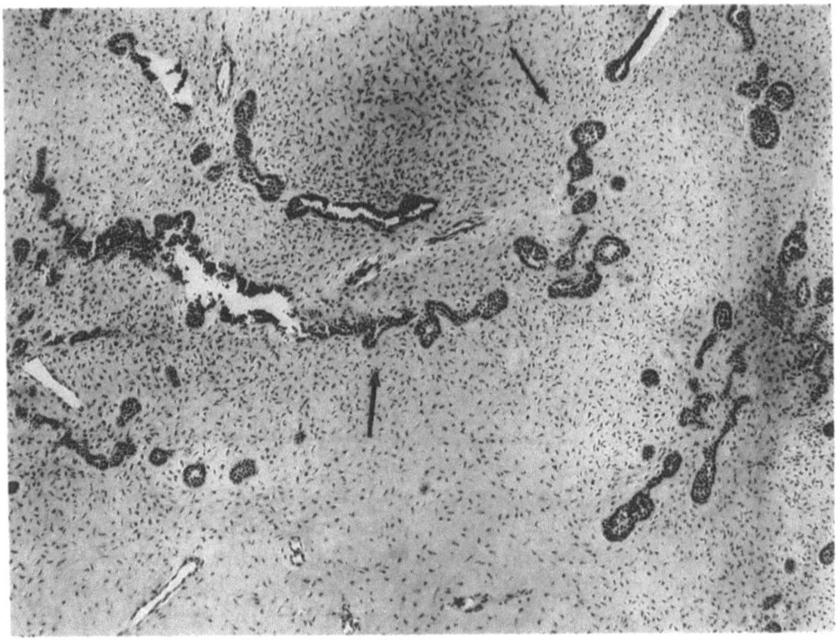

Fig. 3.37. Ameloblastic fibroma; note the epithelial nests and strands of tissue (*arrows*). H. & E. stain, ×35

Radiographically, the ameloblastic fibroma appears as a central, unilocular, or multilocular radiolucent osseous defect, indistinguishable from an odontogenic cyst or an ameloblastoma (Fig. 3.36) [10, 112]. As the tumor enlarges, it tends to push aside adjacent structures, so that not infrequently it is associated with malposed or displaced teeth.

Microscopically, the epithelial component of the ameloblastic fibroma consists of nests, cords, and strands of cuboidal or columnar cells in an arrangement which often bears a striking similarity to dental laminae or primitive enamel organs. The mesenchymal portion of the tumor is composed of delicate, young, fibrous connective tissue resembling the dental papilla (see Fig. 3.37).

A rare variant of the ameloblastic fibroma in which the connective tissue component of the tumor contains large granular cells with eosinophilic staining cytoplasm (Fig. 3.38) has been described in case reports by Couch, Waldron, and Gorlin [44, 114, 115]. In 1978, White and his associates added four additional cases to the literature [116]. The ages of these patients were 53, 55, 59, 50, 50, 50, 55, and 65 in the four respective reports. Seven of the eight cases occurred in the mandible, one in the maxilla. Treatment was conservative, and none recurred. The initial reports suggested that the granular cell component of the tumor represented an aging or degenerative alteration in the typical ameloblastic fibroma [44, 114, 115]. However, in their histopathologic and electron microscopic analysis of their four cases, White et al., concluded that there was no evidence to support the theory that this is a degenerative phenomenom, since the granular cells exhibited regular nuclei and no signs of degeneration

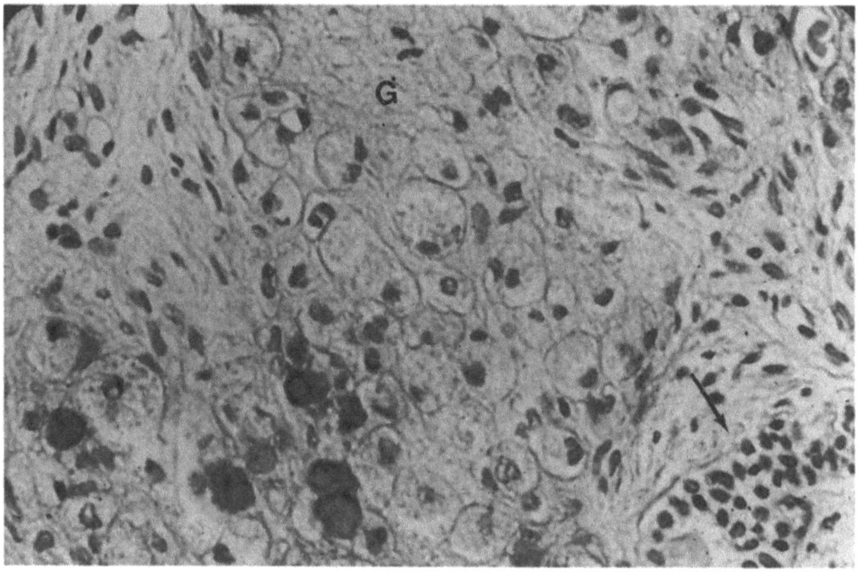

Fig. 3.38. Granular-cell variant of the ameloblastice fibroma. *G*, granular cells; *arrow*, epithelium. H. & E. stain, ×115

[116]. Also, their ultrastructural studies revealed that the granular cells were of connective-tissue origin, contained many lysosome-like particles, and resembled the cells found in the granular cell myoblastoma [116]. Thus, it may well be a separate entity.

For many years conservative surgical treatment for the ameloblastic fibroma has been advocated, since it apparently exhibited scant evidence of recurrence [10, 44]. Carr reported a case of recurrent ameloblastic fibroma in 1970, and Trodahl's review of the Armed Forces Institute of Pathology's cases suggested that this tumor could show aggressive behavior [117, 118]. Addition recurrences were also reported by Huebsch and Stephenson and Tanaka, et al. [119, 120]. The largest (2,072 grams) tumor and longest history of persistent recurrence of an ameloblastic fibroma (23 years) was reported by Sawyer et al., as one of his two recurrent cases [121]. Therefore, it is advocated that thorough surgical removal of this tumor be carried out in a conservative fashion, with careful periodic follow-up to check for recurrence. A definitive diagnosis to separate the ameloblastic fibroma from the ameloblastoma is an absolute necessity to prevent unwarranted surgical mutilation, especially since most cases of this tumor involve children. Table 3.8 compares the characteristics of these two entirely different tumors.

(B) Ameloblastic Odontoma

Ameloblastic odontoma is an uncommon odontogenic tumor of mixed origin, having both epithelial and mesenchymal components. It has been reported in the literature under a variety of names including odontoblastoma [44], ada-

Table 3.8. Comparison of ameloblastic fibroma and ameloblastoma

	Ameloblastic fibroma	Ameloblastoma
1. Mean ($\bar{x}$) presenting age at time of treatment	14 years[a]	33 years
2. Site	maxilla or mandible premolar or molar area	most often mandibular 3rd molar area
3. Growth in bone	by expansion – slow	by infiltration – more aggressive
4. Response to conservative curettage	excellent	30–50% recurrence
5. Histology	composed chiefly of young, fibrous tissue, resembling dental papilla, with nests and strands of ameloblastic epithelium	composed chiefly of ameloblastic epithelium with a mature fibrous stroma; squamous metaplasia and cystic features may be present

[a] Mean age for granular cell ameloblastic fibroma = 55 years

Table 3.9. Comparison of surveys on ameloblastic odontoma

		Gorlin's survey	Hooker's survey
Number of cases		28	26
Age	Range	1–40 years	0.5–39 years
	Mean	11.95 years	11.5 years
Male	Female ratio	13:15	20: 6
Maxilla	Mandible ratio	17:11	13:13

manto-odontoma [10], calcified mixed odontogenic tumor [122], and soft and calcified mixed odontoma [123]. Ameloblastic odontoma is the preferred name because the tumor is formed from odontogenic epithelium which as differentiated to the stage of forming mature ameloblasts that deposit enamel matrix; the matrix in turn induces the mesenchymal component to lay down dentin, cementum, and bone in a random fashion. This tumor is of particular interest to both the dentist and the pediatrician, since it is one of the more frequently occurring odontogènic tumors in children [67, 124].

Table 3.9 compares Gorlin's survey (composed of his own case plus those cases reported in the earlier literature which he thought belonged in this diagnostic category) with Hooker's survey (26 cases obtained from the files of the Armed Forces Institute of Pathology [AFIP]). Most of their findings are similar. Hooker was able to apply uniform diagnostic criteria to all of his cases by having the opportunity to examine each of the patient histories, microscopic sections, radiographs, and follow-up data [125, 126].

The ameloblastic odontoma has been shown to occur in patients from age 6 months to 40 years. The majority of these lesions have been found in younger persons (mean age, 11.5 years); 19 of Hooker's 26 reported patients were children under 16 years of age. Incidence is approximately equal in maxilla and

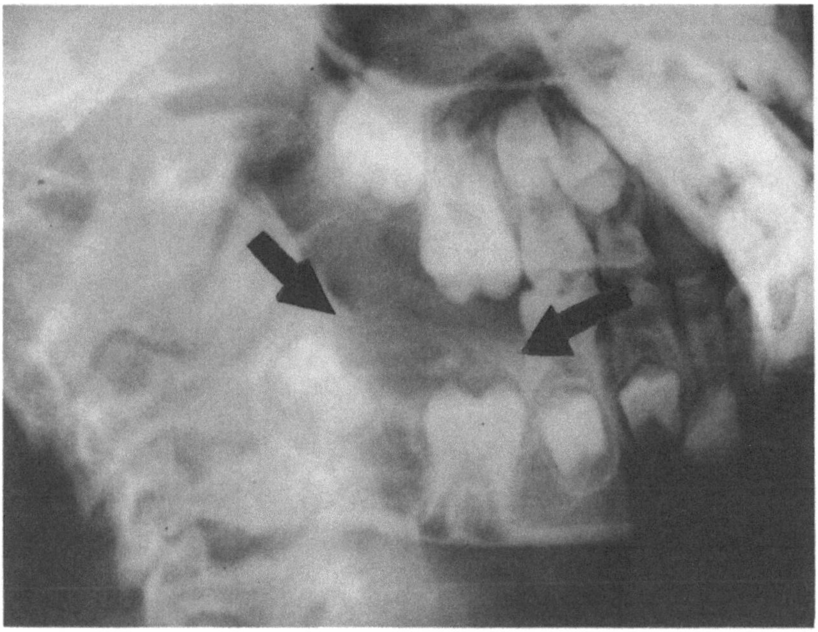

Fig. 3.39. Radiographic appearance of an ameloblastic odontoma (outlined by *arrows*) in the mandible of a 7-year-old male

mandible. Men and women appear equally affected when the natural male bias of the AFIP military population is considered [125, 126].

Ameloblastic odontomas tend to grow at a slow rate as expansile, destructive, central lesions within either jaw and are capable of attaining huge size. Swelling, mild pain, altered occlusion, and delayed eruption of teeth are common presenting local symptoms. Occurrence is most likely in the molar-premolar area of the jaws [124].

Stafne describes the radiographic appearance of ameloblastic odontoma as a well-defined radiolucent cavity in bone within which are varied amounts of radiopaque material representing malformed dental structures. Hooker states that all of the ameloblastic odontomas in his series were associated with impacted or embedded teeth [53, 126]. Figure 3.39 illustrates an ameloblastic odontoma occurring in the mandibular molar region of a 7 year-old boy. It, too, is closely associated with an embedded first molar tooth.

The microscopic appearance of an ameloblastic odontoma may run the gamut of odontogenic tissues in varied arrangements: ameloblastic epithelium, enamel matrix, enamel, dentin, osteodentin, cementum, bone, stellate reticulum, pulpal tissue, and stromal connective tissue. Attempts at small tooth formation similar to a compound odontoma may be present, or the mineralized tissues may be randomly arranged as in a complex odontoma. In conjunction with either of these mineralized forms is the characteristic diagnostic component: rosettes, islets, or strands of proliferating odontogenic epithelium, or both which give it its descriptive name: ameloblastic odontoma [124–126]. Histologic exam-

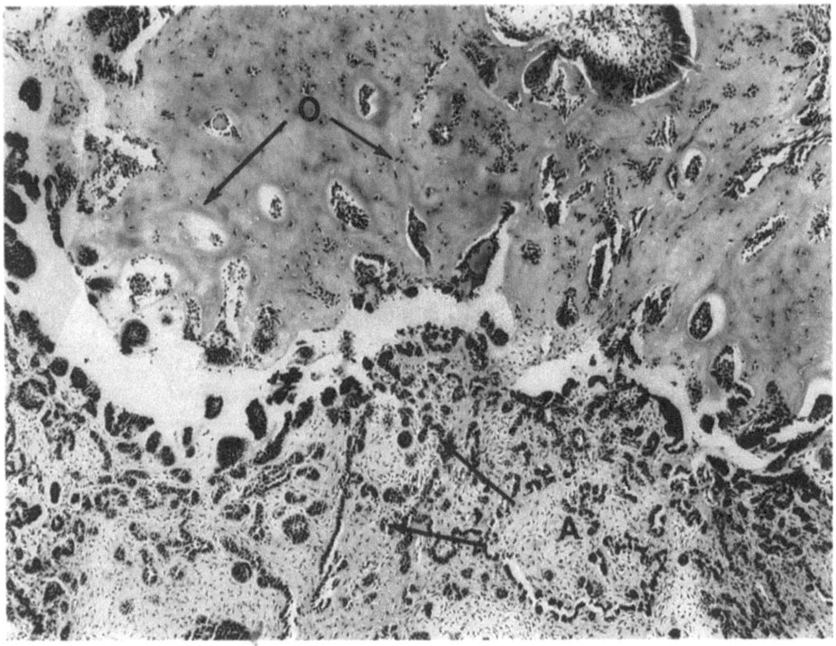

Fig. 3.40. Ameloblastic odontoma. *A*, ameloblastic epithelial rosettes; *O*, osteodentin. H. & E. stain, ×65

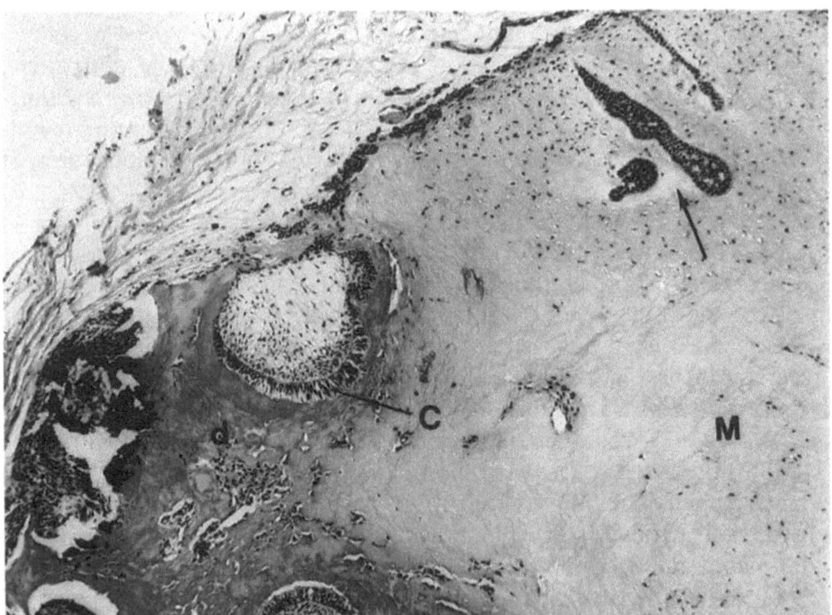

Fig. 3.41. Ameloblastic odontoma. *C*, columnar ameloblastic epithelium inducing dentin formation (*d*); *M*, myxomatous area; *arrow*, epithelial nest and strand. H. & E. stain, ×63

ples of this tumor are depicted in Fig. 3.40 and 3.41, demonstrating the epithelial component and the hard mesodermal tissues.

Slootweg's extensive analysis of the interrelationship of mixed odontogenic tumors concluded that: (A) the ameloblastic fibroma does represent a separate entity that does not develop into a more differentiated odontogenic tumor; and (B) the ameloblastic odontoma is an immature complex odontoma [127]. He also postulated that age-related factors determine whether an aberrant development of the odontogenic tissues exhibits a hamartomatous or a neoplastic nature [127].

With a larger number of authentic ameloblastic odontomas studies by adequate follow-up, it is now evident that this tumor is best managed by adequate conservative surgery after accurate pathologic diagnosis. Careful surgical curettage of all of the tumor and capsule fragments is required because peripheral tissue is often the site of the more active proliferating ameloblastic component. Archard reported no recurrence within five years in a patient with a large ameloblastic odontoma (2.5 cm in diameter) following thorough curettage [128]. None of the tumors in the 26 cases in Hooker's series of ameloblastic odontoma recurred after adequate curettage [126]. Likewise, 3 year follow-up on each of our two cases of this tumor revealed normal healing and tooth development with no tumor recurrence [124].

(C) Odontoma

In an odontoma the epithelial and mesenchymal components have reached the stage of complete differentiation, resulting in the formation of both enamel and dentin. These hard tissues are deposited in an abnormal pattern because the odontogenic cells per se have not reached a normal state of morphodifferentiation [10]. Since the tumor is composed of several types of tissue, it has been termed as "composite". In addition, the term compound composite odontoma is used when the tumor forms in such a manner as to bear superficial anatomic similarity to normal teeth. If the calcified tissues are arranged in an irregular mass with no morphological similarity even to rudimentary teeth, it is called a complex composite odontoma.

Clinically, it is usually found in young children, but it may persist into adult life. Most often, it remains a small symptomatic lesion, but occassional cases can attain large size, producing a painless expansion of bone and displacement of teeth [122, 129].

On x-ray, odontomas can appear either as irregular radio-opaque masses often situated between the roots of teeth with a radiolucent periphery, or else as a number of tiny, tooth-like, radio-opaque structures. Usually these tumors, also, are associated with unerupted or impacted teeth, as illustrated in Fig. 3.42.

Histologically, the odontoma may contain enamel or enamel matrix, dentin, pulp tissue, and cementum which may appear either in an admixture fashion, such as Fig. 3.43, or as morphologic, i.e., structures resembling single-rooted teeth. A connective tissue capsule surrounds the tumor [10, 122].

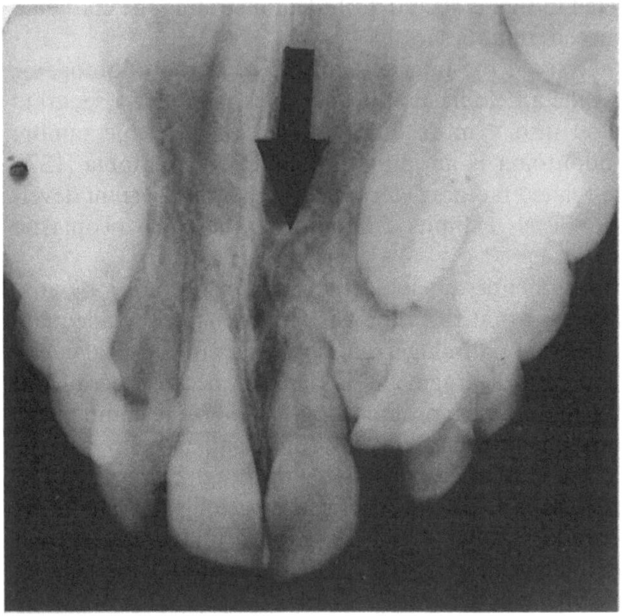

Fig. 3.42. Complex odontoma (*arrow*) in the anterior right maxillary region of a 10-year-old female, causing impaction of the right lateral incisor

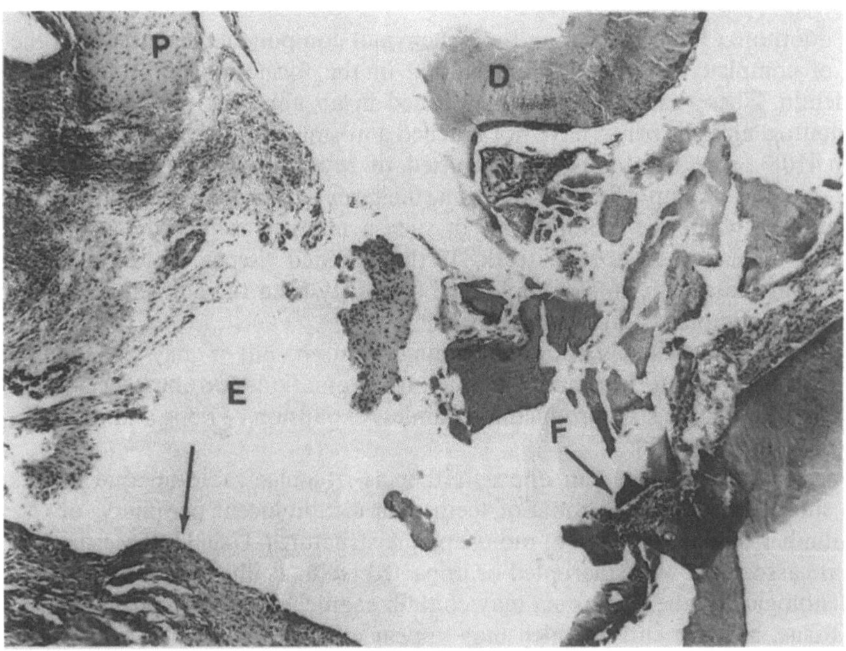

Fig. 3.43. Complex odontoma with an admixture of enamel (*E*); dentin (*D*); pulpal tissue (*P*); and fibrous tissue (*F*). H. & E. stain, ×63

Treatment consists of careful surgical removal, and recurrence is unlikely. Gould reported an interesting three-year follow-up in his large complex odontoma case in a 14 year-old boy in whom remodeling of normal anatomy and extensive tooth movement occurred over this time-span, in spite of gross displacements and tissue destruction [129].

(D) Ameloblastic Fibrosarcoma

The ameloblastic fibrosarcoma is an extremely rare, locally malignant odontogenic tumor [10, 44]. In their 1977 update of Lieder et al.'s earlier 1972 substantial review of the literature on ameloblastic fibrosarcoma, Howell and Burkes recorded 22 authenicated cases of this tumor in the literature at that time and added two cases of their own [130–140]. Adekeye and his associates added another case from Nigeria in 1978, making a total of 25 cases to date [141]. Debate still exists in regard to the true malignant nature of this neoplasm, and Gorlin has commented that the evidence reported for certain of these cases is not always convincing [44].

From the paucity of case materials that is available, the following typical clinical picture emerges. Apparently, the ameloblastic fibrosarcoma occurs most frequently from the second to the fourth decades, occurs without predilection for either sex or race, and is seen slightly more often in the mandible than the maxilla [130, 140]. Gorlin states that in most patients suffering from this tumor, pain proceeded the noticeable clinical swelling and helped significantly to differentiate this neoplasm from most other odontogenic tumors [44].

Radiographically, its appearance is not diagnostically specific, but resembles that of an extensive, rapidly-growing, poorly defined, destructive bony neoplasm [10, 133].

Histopathologically, it is composed of highly cellular connective tissue with scattered strands of inactive odontogenic epithelium. The fibroblasts can appear quite anaplastic, especially after local recurrences of the tumor. "Ghost" cells, similar to the ones seen in a keratinizing and calcifying odontogenic cyst, as well as irregular deposits of dentin and enamel have also been recorded [10, 44, 130, 134, 140].

Howell and Burkes' analysis of reported cases concluded that 19/24 patients exhibited recurrence of the tumor, and of these 19 persons with recurrence, 6 (32%) died as a result of their disease [130]. As far as can be determined, none of the current 25 total cases in the literature have exhibited metastatic lesions, resulting from the original tumor. Yet, from the local aggressiveness and 32% mortality rate in recurrent cases, it is evident that this tumor can be fatal.

The primary mode of therapy is radical surgical resection, since recurrence after initial treatment connotes a very grave prognosis. The questionable malignant transformation of benign odontogenic tumors to locally malignant ones does not justify the use of such extensive, radical surgical procedures for all odontogenic tumors. Careful attention must be paid to each one's clinical history and behavior and also to any change in the histologic appearance of a lesion that recurs from the fairly normal original histopathological characteristics toward a more cellular, less mature pattern. Radiation therapy is contraindicated, since it does not elicit an effectual response in this neoplasm [10, 130, 137]. A chemotherapy regimen of cytoxan, actinomycin, and vincristine appeared to cause a positive response in controling one reported case with N.E.D. (no evidence of disease) for three years, but a similar attempt for another patient failed because of the patient's intolerance to the chemical medication [130].

VI. Fibro-Osseous Lesions

The fibrous connective tissues of the periodontal membrane are composed chiefly of collagen fibers, mucopolysaccharides, and oxytalan fibers. Within this versatile ligament surrounding every tooth are mesenchymal blastic cells possessing the capacity to form cementum, alveolar bone, and fibrous tissue (Fig. 3.44) [142].

1. Fibro-Osseous Jaw Lesions of Periodontal Membrane Origin

Under pathologic conditions such blastic cells are capable of producing tumors composed of either cementum, lamellar bone, fibrous tissue, or any combination of these three tissues. Such lesions may be referred to as tumors of periodontal membrane origin [143].

The difficulty of differential diagnosis in determining tumors of periodontal membrane origin from tumors of medullary bone origin – namely, fibro-osteoma, osteoblastoma "cherubism", giant cell tumor, aneurysmal bone cyst, "brown tumor" of hyperparathyrodism, and Paget's disease – has long been recognized. Differentiation between tumors of medullary bone origin is important because the latter tumors usually behave in a more aggressive fashion, even though they are benign. The absolute proof of medullary bone origin in the group of tumors (listed above) is yet to come forth. One classification, separating the fibro-osseous lesions according to origin, is illustrated in Table 3.10.

In 1968, Fullmer and Lillie reported a previously undescribed connective tissue fiber in the human periodontal membrane and gingiva, naming it the oxytalan fiber because of its resistance to acid hydrolysis [144]. Since their discovery, oxytalan fibers have been reported in dental granulomas, radicular cysts, and ameloblastomas [145, 146]. Because the reported fibers were found in odontogenic tissues, Hamner and Fullmer postulated that perhaps oxytalan fibers could serve as a positive marker for lesions of periodontal membrane origin. If this proved correct, obtaining a positive stain for oxytalan fibers, using the monopersulfatealdehyde fuchsin-Halmi method in a problem lesion would indicate periodontal membrane origin. After analyzing 42 cases of fibro-osseous jaw lesions of odontogenic and nonodontogenic origin by the use of histochemical stains for oxytalan fibers, collagen fibers, mucopolysaccharide content, and elastic fibers, they found fibers in most fibro-osseous jaw lesions

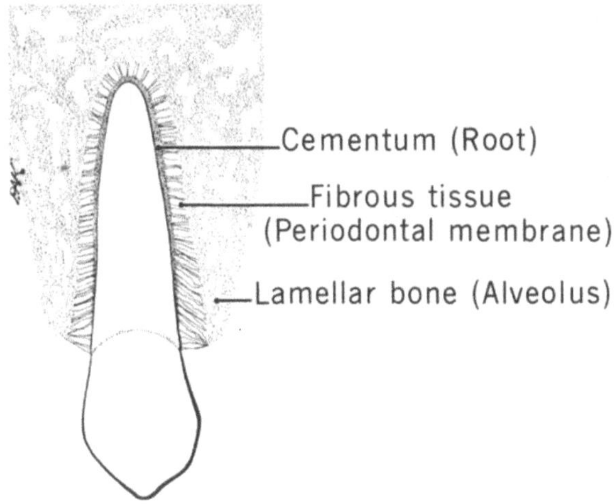

Fig. 3.44. Multipotentiality of the periodontal membrane

Table 3.10. Fibro-osseous lesions of the jaws

I. *Benign tumors*	
(A) *Periodontal membrane origin*	(4) fibrous dysplasia
(1) cementifying fibroma → cementoma	(5) giant cell tumor, active or benign
(2) ossifying fibroma	(6) aneurysmal bone cyst
(3) cemento-ossifying fibroma	(7) hyperparathyroidism jaw lesion
(4) fibroma	(8) Paget's Disease
(B) *Medullary bone origin*	II. *Malignant tumors*
(1) fibro-osteoma	(1) osteosarcoma
(2) active juvenile ossifying fibroma	(2) chondrosarcoma
(3) cherubism	(3) fibrosarcoma

that stained by the oxytalan method, regardless of origin, provided mature collagen fibers were present. They concluded that the demonstration of oxytalan fibers in a lesion does not constitute conclusive evidence of periodontal memgrane origin of the tumor [147].

(A) Cementoid Lesions

Cementoid lesions have been studied extensively in the past (Table 3.11). It should be emphasized that all these surveys, with the exceptions of Bernier's and Chaudlhry's series, were performed using only radiographs without a correlation of histologic material and radiographs from the same patients. Therefore, it is not certain that all the lesions included in the other surveys were definitely cementoid lesions [148–153].

Statistical analysis of the combined data from the 377 cases reported in Table 3.11 yields the following information for a "typical cementoid lesion": patient age range = 17–82 years (mean age = 39.01 years); sex ratio = 38 male to 339 female patients; racial ratio = 77 Caucasians, 207 Negroes, and 4 Mon-

Table 3.11. Previous cementoma studies

Survey	No. of cases	Age (years) Range	Mean	Sex male: female	Race caucasian: negro	Site occurrence mandible: maxilla	Multiple lesions
Stafne [148]	35	20–62	43	10:25	–	33:2	Yes
Zegarelli and Ziskin [149]	50	20–68	40	0:50	17:33	43:7	Yes–64%
Bernier and Thompson [150]	15	23–57	37	7:8	–	14:1	Yes
Scannel [151]	19	–	39	3:16	–	16:3	Yes–25%
Fontaine [152]	228	20–68	38.2	14:214	53:171 [a]	207:21 [a]	Yes–67.5%
Chaudhry et al. [153]	30	17–82	36.9	4:26	27:3	28:2	Yes–83%

[a] Includes four Mongols

gols; occurrence site – 341 patients with mandibular lesions and 36 patients with maxillary lesions, and 59.5% of all patients had multiple lesions.

Hamner's extensive Armed Forces Institute of Pathology analysis of 249 cases of periodontal membrane lesions revealed 148/249 to be cementoid tumors. These clinical findings are shown in Table 3.12 [143].

The age for cementoid lesions was 8 to 69 years with a mean age ($\bar{x}$) of 36.35 years. The age figures represent the patient's age at the time of tumor discovery or treatment, not onset of tumor.

Cementoid lesions were more prevalent in females than males (61%) in spite of bias due to a predominantly male military sampling group. One hundred and nine Caucasian patients (76%) exhibited one or more cementoid lesions in comparison with 29 Negro patients (20%) and 5 Mongol patients (4%). The 35 non-Caucasians represented 24% of the patients which is greater than the proportion of non-Caucasians in the general population (11.4% according to the 1960 U.S. Census).

The majority of cementoid lesions were located in the mandible. One hundred and seventeen patients (79%) had mandibular tumors, while only 31 patients (21%) had maxillary tumors. Lesions were found in both the anterior and posterior regions of each jaw; however, the premolar-molar area was the more common site (80% and 82% for the mandible and maxilla, respectively).

Multiple cementoid lesions appear to be more common than the 27/148 cases would indicate. In many instances full-mouth radiographs were not taken on the patient, and the clinical history was limited to only the one lesion in question with no comment concerning the other areas of each jaw. Multiple lesion incidence among Caucasians and Negroes was about equal, but considering the percentage of Negroes in the entire cementoid lesion group (20%) in relation to the sample population, the percentage of multiple cementomas in Negroes is definitely higher.

Three maxillary giant cementoid lesions occurred in males (1 Caucasian and 2 Negroes). Giant lesions were defined as those tumors, excluding true

Table 3.12. Clinical findings – cementoid lesions [143]

1. Age range	8–69 years (137/148 cases recorded age)	
2. ($\bar{x}$) age	36.35 years (137/148 cases recorded age)	
3. Racial incidence	109 Caucasian (76%), 29 Negro (20%), 5 Mongol (4), (5 not listed)	
4. Sexual incidence	52 males (39%), 81 females (61%), (15 not listed)	
5. Location	mandible–117 cases (79%)	21 anterior area (20%) 84 posterior area (88%) (12 not listed)
	maxilla – 31 cases (21%)	5 anterior area (18%) 22 posterior area (82%) (4 not listed)
6. Multiple lesions	27/148 cases (18%) – (1 maxillary case, 23 mandibular cases, 3 both jaws cases)	
	Caucasian – 13/27	3 males 10 females
	Negro – 12/27	0 males 12 females
	Mongol – 1/27	0 males 1 females
7. Giant lesions	3/148 cases (2%) – (1 Caucasian male, 2 Negro males, all lesions in the maxilla)	
8. True cementomas	15/148 cases (10%) 3 maxillary cases, 12 mandibular cases)	
	Caucasian – 12/15	6 males 6 females
	Negro – 2/15	1 male 1 female
	Mongol – 1/15	0 males 1 female
9. Cementomas	81/148 cases (55%) – (14/81 maxilla (19%), 66/81 mandible (81%)	
10. Cementifying fibroma	67/148 cases (45%) – (16/67 maxilla (24%), 51/67 mandible (76%)	

cementomas, involving the space occupied by two teeth, or being larger than 2×2 cm. Fifteen "true cementomas" (10%) were discovered in the series of 148 cementoid lesions. Twelve of these occurred in Caucasian patients, two in Negro patients, and one in an American Indian. Male and female incidence was equal.

The solid cementoma was seen more often (55%) than the cementifying fibroma (45%). Both stages of the cementoid lesion occurred more frequently in the mandible.

Pain was very seldom a presenting symptom, although swelling was sometimes encountered with the larger lesions. Usually the patient was unaware of the cementoid lesion's presence. Therefore, estimations of duration were considered unreliable. The tumors that were treated by surgery did not recur. The history in three cases indicated inadequate surgical removal at the first opera-

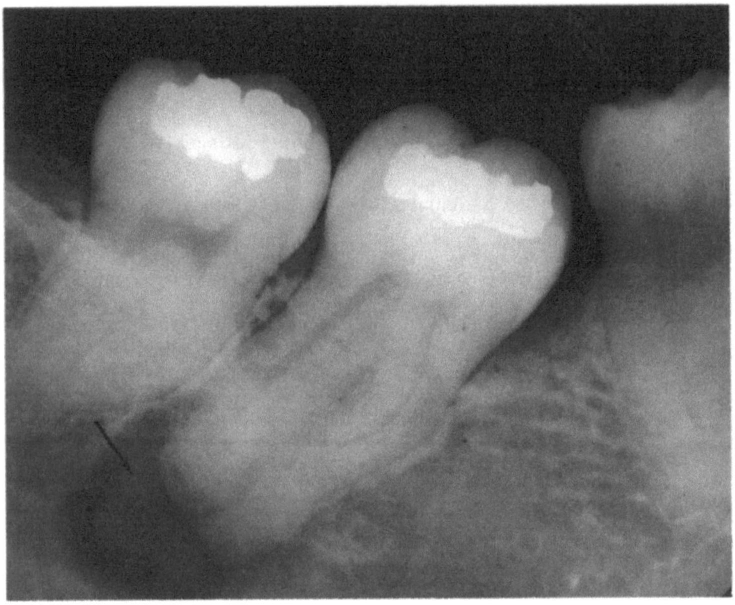

Fig. 3.45. Cementifying fibroma (*arrow*), right mandibular molar area. 38-year-old Caucasian female

tion, followed by later clinical appearance of the tumor. Follow-up information was obtained for 99/148 cases (66%).

The cementoid lesion begins as a small, painless periapical fibrous lesion, arising from the periodontal membrane, with limited local osteolysis. An enlarging periapical radiolucency is seen on periodic dental radiographs during the first stage. The initial radiolucency is sometimes mistakenly diagnosed as a dental cyst or granuloma. The pulp vitality in a tooth demonstrating a cementoid, osteoid, or mixed cemento-osteoid lesions is the important clinical differential diagnostic feature which rules out a dental granuloma or radicular cyst. Gradual mineralization usually occurs over the years, producing a small benign, calcified periapical radiopaque mass with a peripheral radiolucent halo (Fig. 3.45). The lesion may not pass beyond the cementifying stage, which appears radiographically as a radiolucent-radiopaque tumor. In other cases, the lesion progresses from this "donut" radiographic appearance to a more solid mineralized state, producing a more radio-opague tumor with a thin, well-defined radiolucent border at its periphery (Fig. 3.46).

Infrequently, a "true cementoma", which is a rare form of solid cementoma, possessing a direct cemental connection between tooth and tumor is seen. Cases have been reported by Kline et al. [154], Wertheimer et al. [155], and Gorlin et al. [125].

Microscopically, the cementifying fibroma consists of a mixture of cellular connective tissue and scattered round, ovoid masses or "droplets" of cementum.

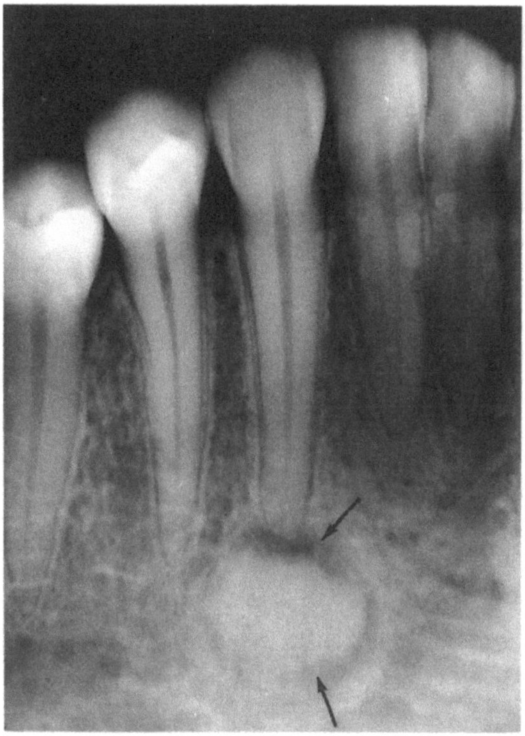

Fig. 3.46. Cementoma, solid-form appearing radiographically as a radiopaque mass with a thin radiolucent border (*arrows*)

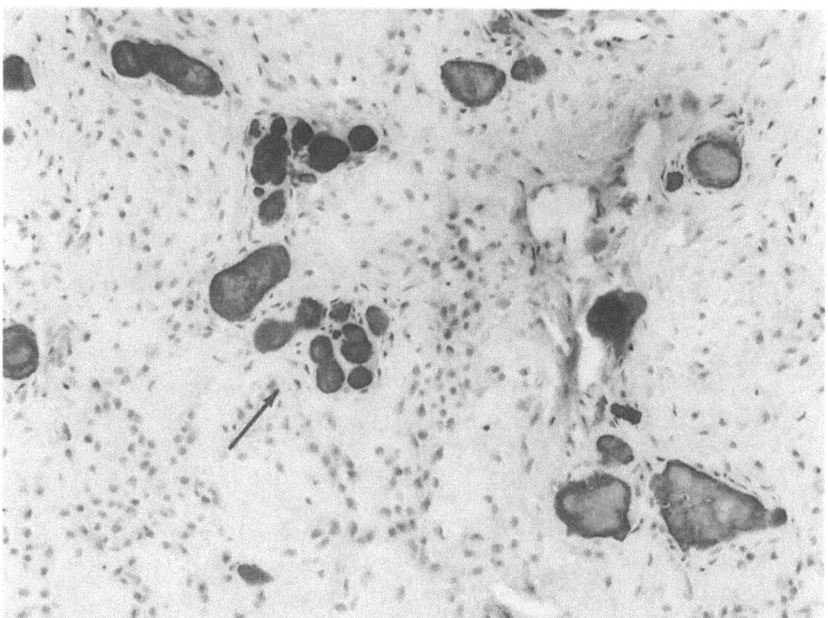

Fig. 3.47. Cementifying fibroma; note the spherical droplets of cementum (*arrow*). H. & E. stain, ×160

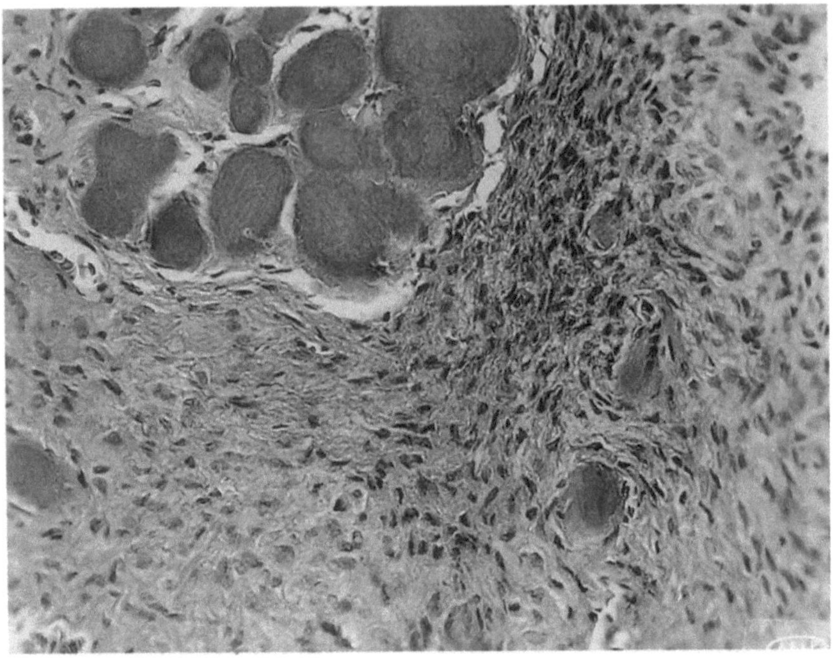

Fig. 3.48. Cementifying fibroma, H. & E. stain, ×300. (A.F.I.P. Accession #1129384)

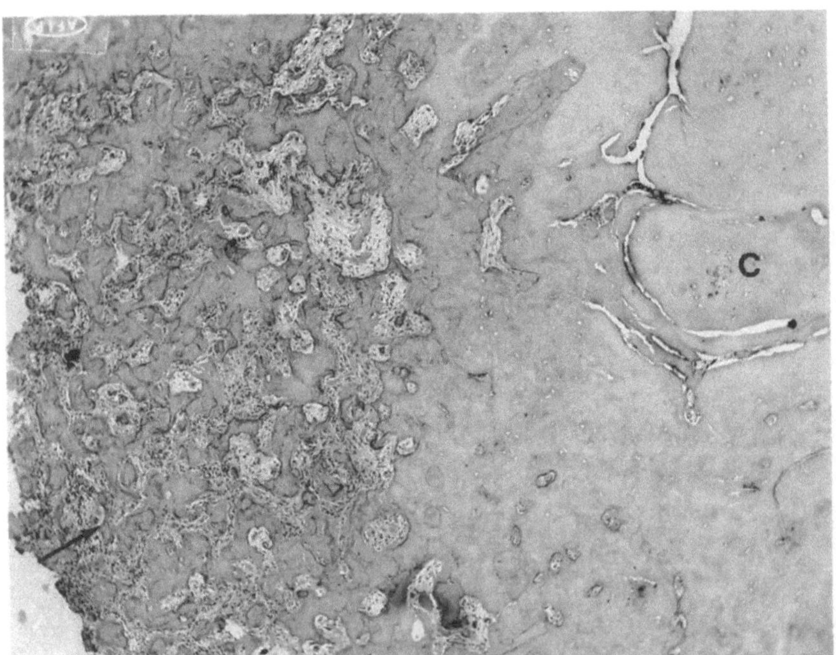

Fig. 3.49. Cementoma, solid center (*C*) with a mixed periphery (*arrow*). H. & E. stain, ×40. (A.F.I.P. Accession #665728)

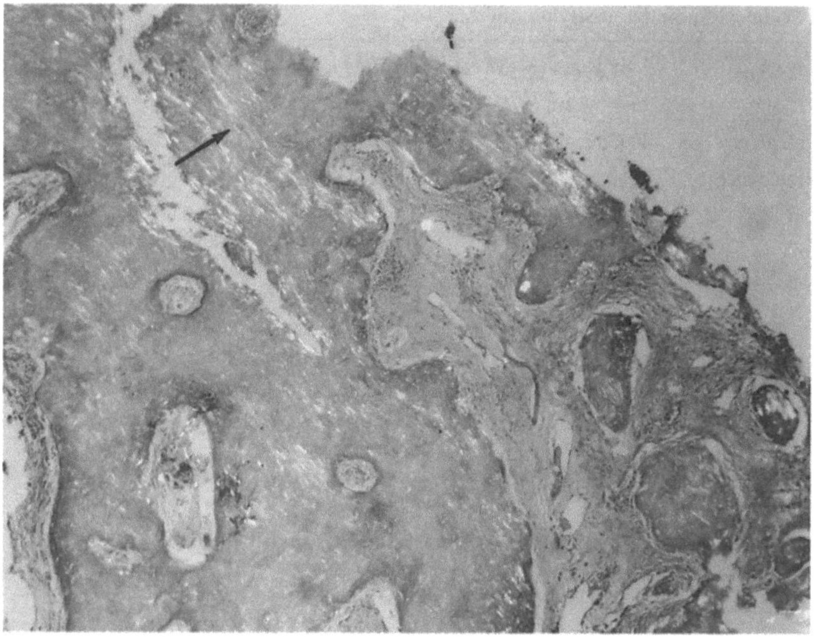

Fig. 3.50. Fine lines of parallel birefringence (*arrow*) in a cementoma under polarized light. H. & E. stain, × 160

The droplets vary in size and number, are acellular, and usually have a dark distinct periphery (Fig. 3.47). They may coalesce to form larger conglomerations of cementum. The stromal tissue consists of spindle shaped cells with flattened nuclei, resembling the fibrous tissue of the periodontal membrane. Cementoblasts may be prominent, appearing as plump cells with oval nuclei (Fig. 3.48). The cementoma is a more solid, calcified lesion than the cementifying fibroma, although some droplet cementum and fibrous tissue may be evident in the peripheral region (Fig. 3.49). One of the best means of distinguishing bone from cementum is by the use of polarized light. Although droplet cementum seldom polarized, it can be recognized by its distinct histologic appearance, i.e., acellularity and reddish purple staining quality with hematoxylin and eosin. However, the more solid or "mature" cementoma usually polarizes well in dark and light lines of parallel birefringence, similar to mature lamellar bone. Poor polarization quality is often due to improper decalcification in which the negative birefringence of the mineralized component cancels out the positive polarization of the collagen. The outstanding difference between bone and cementum in their polarization properties is the degree of fineness in the parallel lines of the latter. In a mature cementoma the parallel bireringent lines are finer and more delicate than the ones seen in lamellar bone (Fig. 3.50).

(B) Ossifying Fibroma

The ossifying fibroma, the second possible tumor of periodontal membrane origin, behaves and appears quite similar to the cementifying fibroma, except

Table 3.13. Clinical findings – ossifying fibroma [143]

1. Age range	7–58 years (57/57 cases recorded age)		
2. ($\bar{x}$) age	26.44 years (57/57 cases recorded age)		
3. Racial incidence	40 Caucasian (70%), 16 Negro (28%), 1 Mongol (2%)		
4. Sexual incidence	31 males (54%), 26 females (46%)		
5. Location	mandible – 39 cases (70%)	4 anterior area (15%) 22 posterior area (85%)	(13 not listed)
	maxilla – 17 cases (30%)	6 anterior area (60%) 4 posterior area (40%)	(7 not listed)
	One case did not list either jaw in location		
6. Multiple lesions	3/57 cases (5%) (2 mandible cases; 1 case in both jaws)		
	Caucasian – 1/3 cases	0 males 1 female	
	Negro – 2/3 cases	0 males 2 females	
7. Giant Lesions	3/57 cases (12%) (5 mandible cases; maxillary cases)		
	Caucasian – 3/7 cases	2 males 1 female	
	Negro – 3/7 cases	0 males 3 females	
	Mongol – 1/7 cases 0 females	1 males	

the mineralized component is mature, lamellar bone. Table 3.13 illustrates the clinical findings for this lesion. 57/249 A.F.I.P. cases of periodontal membrane lesions were classified as ossifying fibroma [143].

The age of patients at the time of discovery of their ossifying fibroma ranged from 7–58 years with a mean age ($\bar{x}$) of 26.44 years. This mean age represents a decrease of 10 years in comparison with the mean age of cementoid lesions. Caucasians were most prevalent in racial incidence (70%), although lesions occurred often in Negroes (28%) and in Mongols (2%). In contrast to the female sexual majority in the cementoid lesion group, more males (54%) presented with an ossifying fibroma. This figure is still small considering the male bias in the A.F.I.P. sample.

Again more lesions occurred in the mandible (70%) than in the maxilla (30%). Mandibular leisons were found more frequently in the posterior area of the jaw (85%), but maxillary ossifying fibromas occurred more often (60%) in the anterior region.

Multiple lesions were rarer (5%) as ossifying fibromas than as cementifying fibromas and occurred more often in Negroes. Also, giant lesions were more common (7/57 cases or 12%) in the osteoid group than the cementoid group. Large osteoid tumors were evenly divided racially; however, they were seen more frequently in females than males, whereas all the giant cementoid tumors occurred in males.

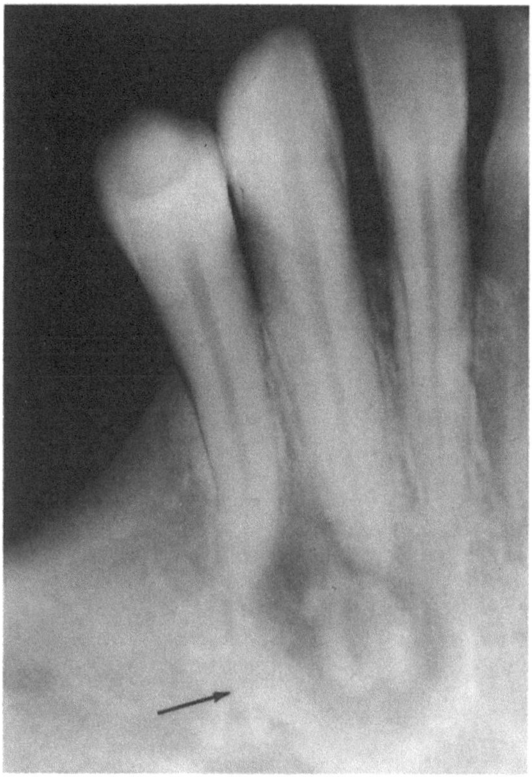

Fig. 3.51. Ossifying fibroma, a radiopaque central mass surrounded by a radiolucent periphery (*arrow*)

Clinically, in most instances, the ossifying fibroma is an innocuous lesion, similar to the other tumors of periodontal membrane origin. Pain, swelling, and paresthesia are seldom encountered except with the larger tumors. Discovery is usually based on routine dental radiographs. The ossifying fibroma responds well to thorough curettage and does not tend to recur.

Radiographically, the ossifying fibroma usually appears similar to the cementifying fibroma, i.e., a fairly well-circumscribed radiolucency with a varying amount of radio-opacity, depending upon the degree of mineralization located in the periapical region (Fig. 3.51).

Microscopically, the ossifying fibroma is composed of cellular fibrous connective tissue and numerous small trabeculae of lamellar bone. The trabeculae sometime join to form a larger solid mass and have smooth peripheries lined by osteoblasts (Fig. 3.52). Osteocytes are numerous within the trabeculae; osteoclasts occasionally may be present adjacent to the trabeculae. The stomal fibroblasts commonly have flat elongated nuclei, closely resembling the cells seen in the periodontal membrane.

Osteoblasts surrounding the bony trabeculae are oval shaped with dark prominent nuclei. Figure 3.53 quite clearly illustrates the periodontal membrane origin of the ossifying fibroma. The diagnosis may be enhanced by the use of polarized light. The trabeculae of bone in an ossifying fibroma polarize in dark and light lines of parallel birefringence that are more widely spaced

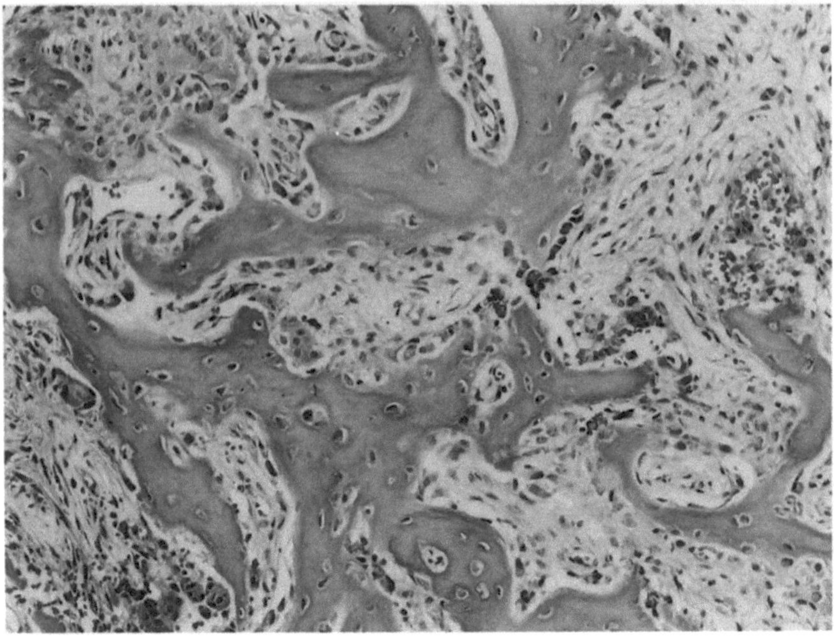

Fig. 3.52. Ossifying fibroma. H. & E. stain, × 160

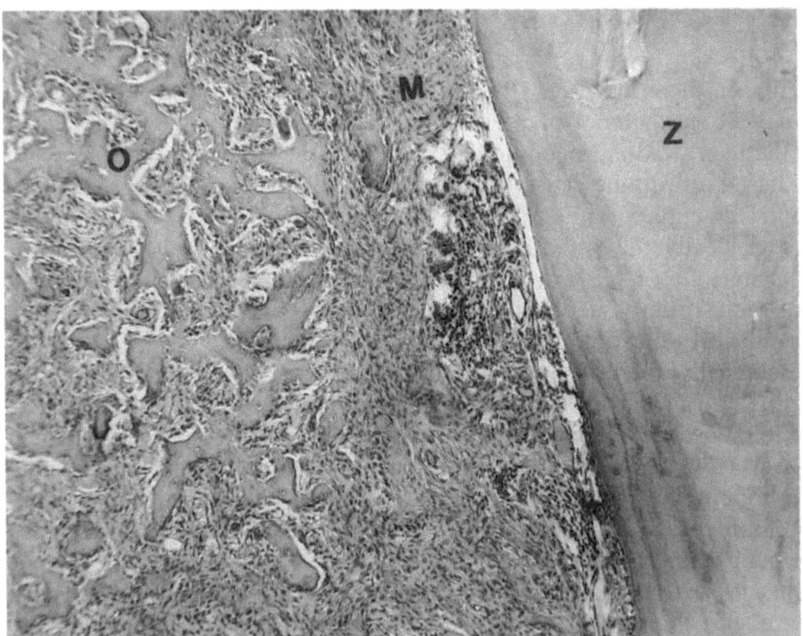

Fig. 3.53. Ossifying fibroma. *Z*, tooth; *M*, periodontal membrane; *O*, ossifying fibroma. H. & E. stain, × 80. (A.F.I.P. Accession #809964)

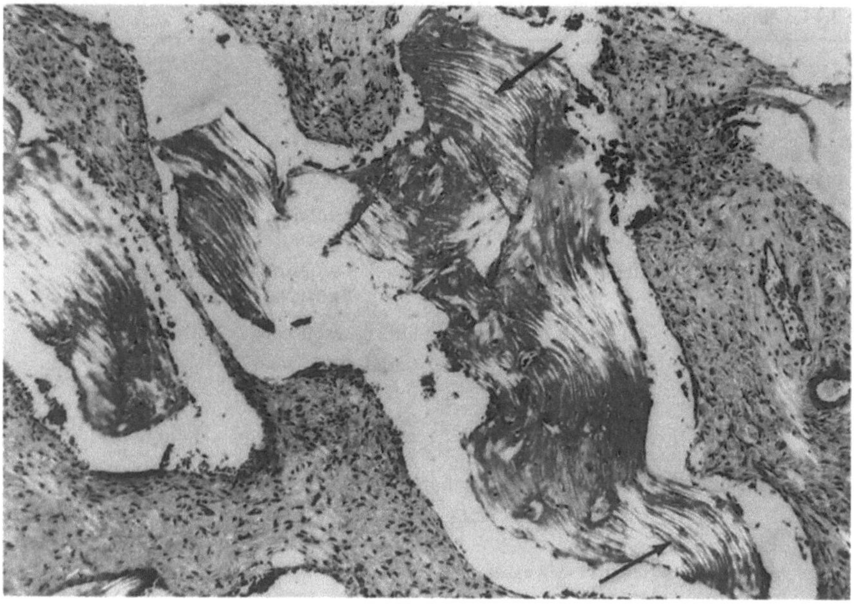

Fig. 3.54. Ossifying fibroma under polarized light. Parallel lines of birefringence are broader (*arrows*). H. & E. stain, ×100

than the parallel birefringent lines seen in a cementoid tumor under polarized light (Fig. 3.54).

(C) Cemento-Ossifying Fibroma

The third potential tumor of periodontal membrane origin is the cemento-ossifying fibroma. 42/249 A.F.I.P. surveyed cases fell into this category, and the clinical findings are depicted in Table 3.14.

Patients with cemento-ossifying fibromas ranged in age from 5–71 years with a mean ($\bar{x}$) age of 32.48 years [143]. Most of the patients were Caucasian (69%); however, 31% were Negroes. No Mongols were included in this sample population. Cemento-ossifying fibromas were seen most often in females (29/42 cases). The mandible again was more frequently involved (76%), especially the posterior area. Discovery of multiple tumors was fairly common (7/42 patients). All of the multiple tumors occurred in the mandible of female patients except for one cases that involved both jaws.

Seven giant tumors were noted, being fairly evenly divided between mandible and maxilla, male and female, Caucasian and Negro. The mixed form giant lesions tended to be larger and more aggressive than the giant forms of either the pure cementoid or osteoid lesions.

The mixed periodontal membrane tumors were indistinguishable radiographically from cementifying fibromas or ossifying fibromas. They appeared as painless fairly well-defined radiolucent/radiopaque lesions located in the periapical

Table 3.14. Clinical findings: Cemento-ossifying fibroma [143]

1. Age range	5–71 years (40/42 cases recorded age)		
2. ($\bar{x}$) age	32.48 years (40/42 cases recorded age)		
3. Racial incidence	29 Caucasian (69%), 13 Negro (31%), no Mongol		
4. Sexual incidence	13 males (13%), 29 females (68%)		
5. Location	mandible – 32 cases (76%)	8 anterior area (28%) 21 posterior area (72%)	(3 not listed)
	maxilla – 10 cases (24%)	3 anterior area (30%) 7 posterior area (70%)	
6. Multiple lesions	7/42 cases (17%) 6 mandible cases; 1 case in both jaws)		
	Caucasian – 5/7 cases	0 males 5 female	
	Negro – 2/7 cases	0 males 2 females	
7. Giant Lesions	7/42 cases (17%) (4 mandible cases; 3 maxillary cases)		
	Caucasian – 3/7 cases	1 males 2 females	
	Negro – 4/7 cases	3 males 1 females	

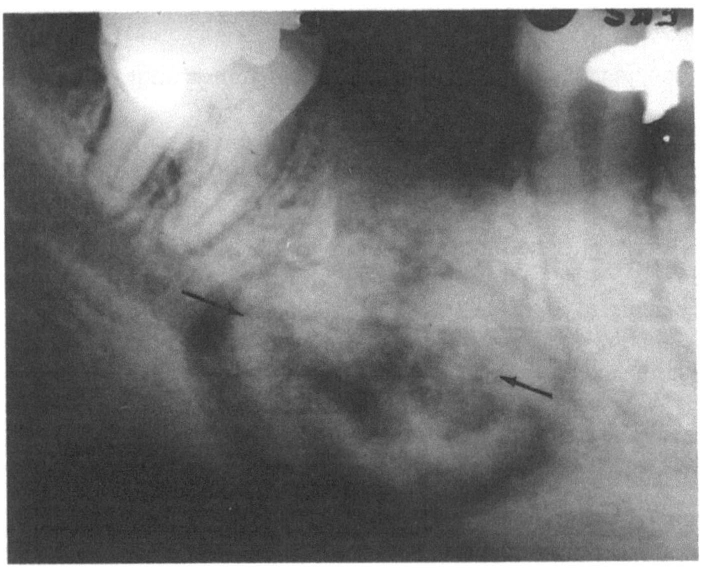

Fig. 3.55. Cemento-ossifying fibroma (*arrows*); radiographic appearance in a left mandibular missing tooth area

region (Fig. 3.55). Occasionally the tumors may be multiple, exhibiting all phases of radiolucency and radiopacity such as those seen in Fig. 3.56.

The microscopic picture shows a mixture of droplet cementum and lamellar bone trabeculae randomly scattered throughout a fibrous tissue stroma quite

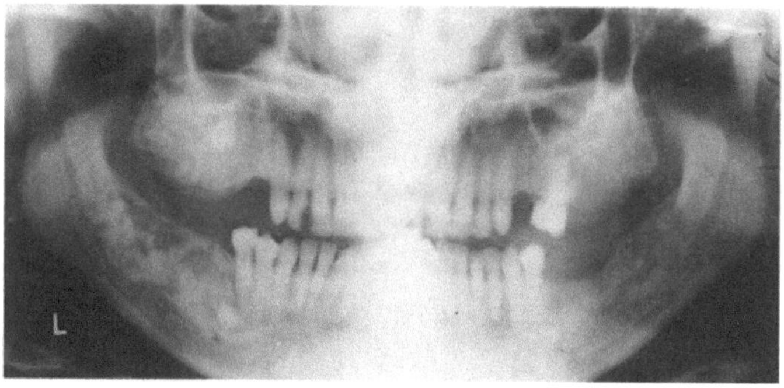

Fig. 3.56. Panorex radiograph illustrating multiple cemento-ossifying fibromas in the posterior regions of both the maxilla and mandible. (A.F.I.P. Accession #1218046)

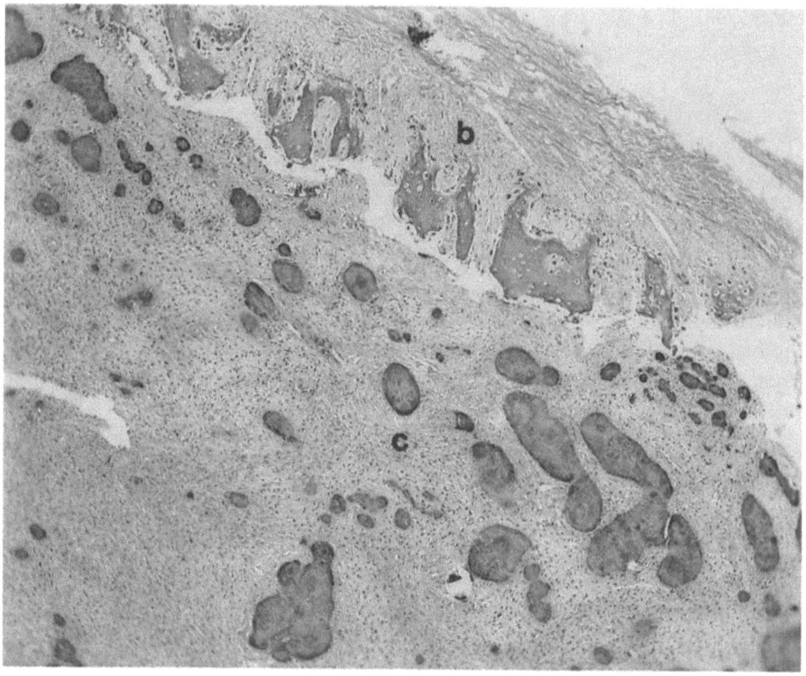

Fig. 3.57. Cemento-ossifying fibroma. *c*, cementum droplets; *b*, osteoid portion of tumor. H. & E. stain, × 50. (A.F.I.P. Accession #588894)

similar in cellular composition to that illustrated previously in cementifying fibroma and ossifying fibroma (Fig. 3.57). The cementum is usually in droplet form, acellular and darker staining than the bony trabeculae which are very cellular (Fig. 3.58).

In rare cases the cemento-ossifying fibroma can behave in an aggressive fashion and attain gigantic size. Two of the 7 giant lesions were discovered in the maxillae and maxillary antra of Negro children – a boy aged 5 and a girl aged 16 years. Both tumors acted in a very destructive manner. Both

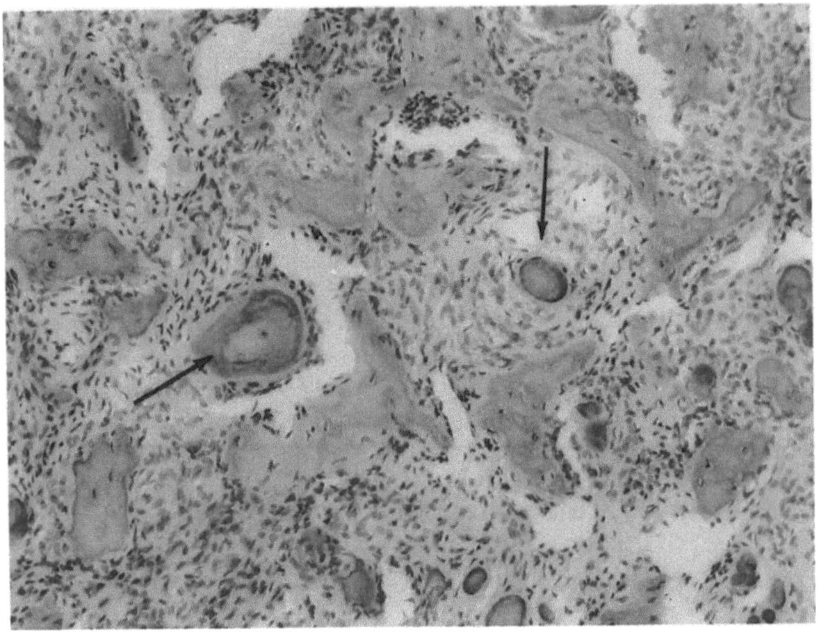

Fig. 3.58. Cemento-ossifying fibroma. *Arrows* point to cementum droplet portion of tumor. H. & E. stain, × 80

maintained a histologic picture of lamellar bone, cementum, and fibrous tissue without the criteria for malignancy, and both cases responded well to extensive initial surgery. The latter case will be shown in the final chapter's series of case examples.

(D) Central Fibroma

The fourth type of periodontal membrane origin lesion is the pure fibroma. Such lesions were extremely rare; only two out of the entire group of 249 A.F.I.P. cases were classified as central fibroma. Diagnosis was based on radiographic appearance (a well-defined radiolucency), intimate association with the periodontal membrane of the adjacent tooth, and histologic appearance.

One of the cases was a simple central fibroma, occurring in the right mandible premolar region of a 23 year-old Caucasian male. The other case was the desmoplastic variety of fibroma and was found in the left mandibular molar area of a 26 year-old Negro male. Growth was slow, swelling as slight, and pain was absent. Both tumors appeared on radiography and at surgery to be closely associated with the periodontal membrane of the involved teeth.

The central fibroma was a very cellular tumor with distinct prominent nuclei, a moderate amount of collagen, and a good blood supply (Fig. 3.59). Odontogenic epithelium and an embryonic dental papilla-like stroma were absent.

The desmoplastic fibroma contained few cells, a vast amount of collagen, and no odontogenic epithelium or mineralized tissues (Fig. 3.60).

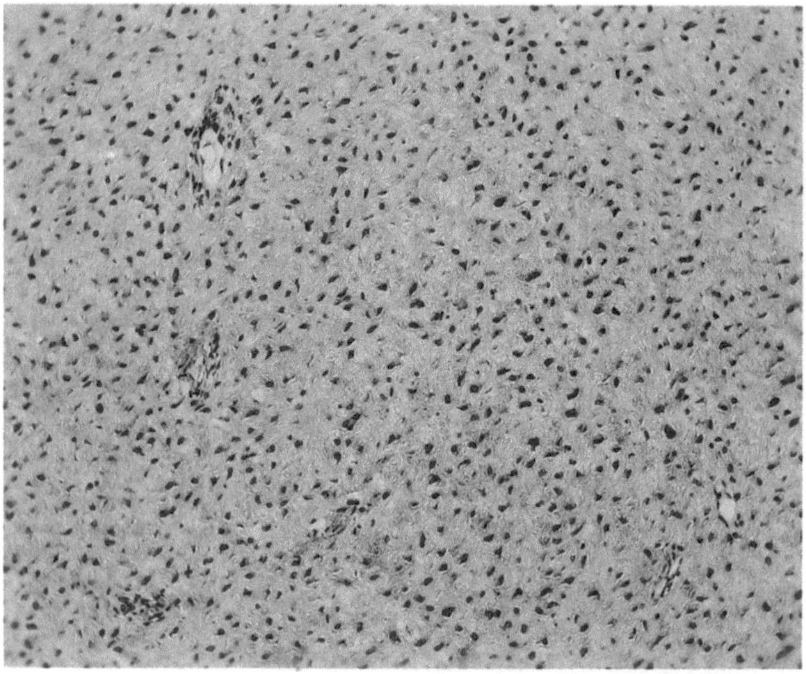

Fig. 3.59. Central fibroma. H. & E. stain, ×115. (A.F.I.P. Accession #778095)

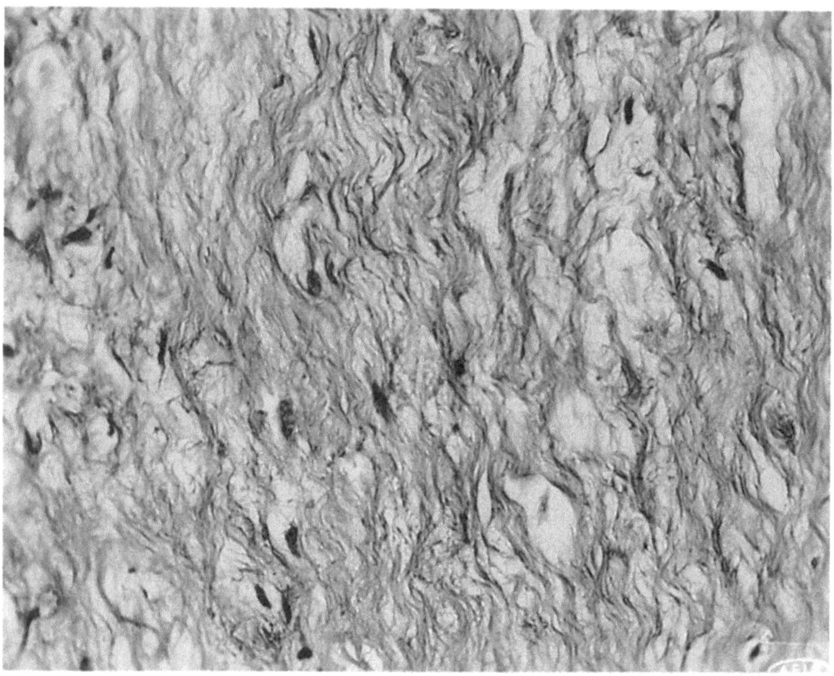

Fig. 3.60. Desmoplastic fibroma, H. & E. stain, ×300. (A.F.I.P. Accession #1057143)

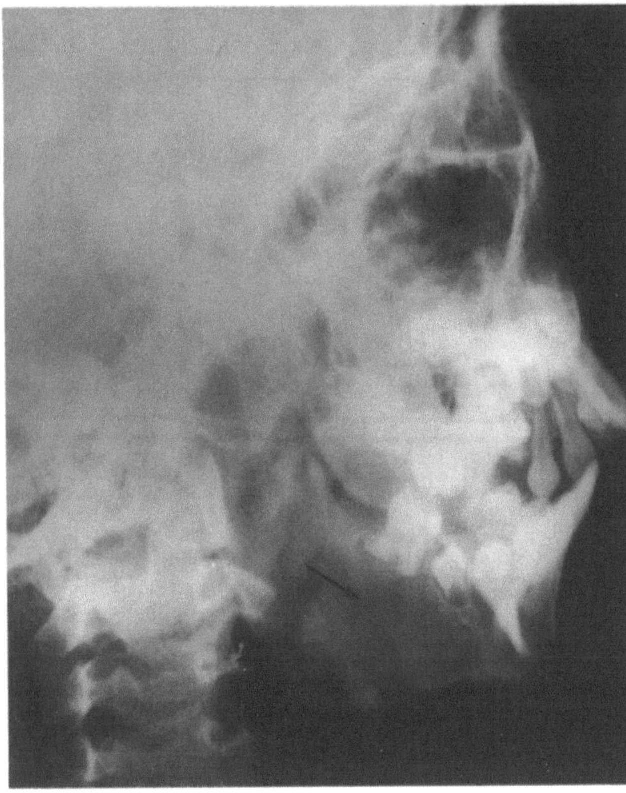

Fig. 3.61. Central fibroma (*arrow*), left body, angle, and ramus of the mandible, 9-year-old Caucasian female

Treatment consisted of extraction of the associated teeth and curettement of the tumor. Neither lesion recurred.

Even though the central fibroma is a rare tumor, controversy has arisen over it in regard to diagnosis and treatment. The central fibroma of periodontal membrane origin appears to behave in a benign fashion, although it can reach a large size as evidenced by the radiograph in Fig. 3.61. This reported case tumor was first noted at age 3 in a Caucasian girl. At the time of surgery at the National Institutes of Health, she was age 9, and the tumor then involved body, angle, and ramus of the left mandible extensively. The neoplasm was removed by thorough curettement, and again the histologic picture was innocuous (Fig. 3.62). Annual follow-up for three years showed no evidence of recurrence.

In 1958, Jaffe first presented a series of five cases of desmoplastic fibroma involving the tibia, scapula, and femor [156]. Whiteside and Ackerman described 3 cases in the head of the humerus, the neck of the humerus, and the ilium [157]. Scheer and Kuhlman later reported a similar tumor in the third lumbar vertebra of an 11-year-old child [158]. In 1965, Griffith and Irby described a desmoplastic fibroma in the left mandible of an 8-year-old girl [159]. To

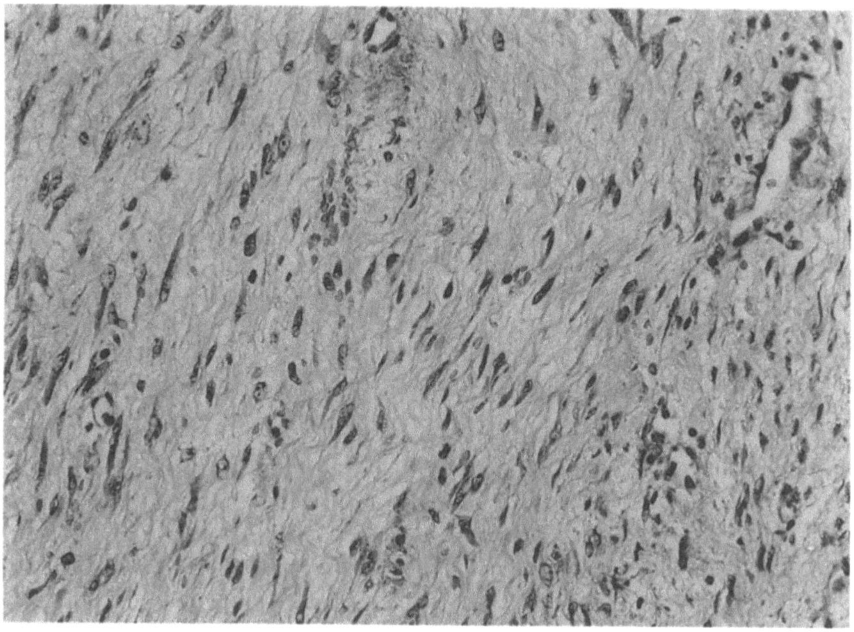

Fig. 3.62. Central fibroma, same case, H. & E. stain, ×250

Table 3.15. Facial bone desmoplastic fibromas reported in the literature

Author	Year	Age	Sex	Site	Treatment	Follow-up
1. Dahlin and Hoover [160]	1964	25	M	Mandible	Excision	No recurrence
2. Griffith and Irby [159]	1965	8	F	Mandible	Excision	No recurrence
3. Rabhan and Rosai [161]	1958	13	M	Mandible	Excision	Radiographs suggested relapse
4. Hamner et al. [143]	1968	26	M	Mandible	Curettage	No recurrence
5. Hinds et al. [162]	1969	15	F	Mandible	Excision	?
6. Hovingu and Ingenhoes [163]	1974	15	F	Mandible	Curettage	?
7. Wagner, et al. [164]	1977	25	M	Mandible	Curettage	?

date, six additional mandibular cases have been reported in the literature (see Table 3.15) [143].

The question is: Is the desmoplastic fibroma simply a variant of the central fibroma of periodontal membrane origin, or is it a separate entity? From its behavior, it seems to be a separate entity, yet it has been reported "cured" by thorough curettage as well as radical excision. The simple central fibroma of periodontal origin behaves in a totally benign fashion, is intimately involved with the adjacent periodontal membrane, and is successfully treated by curettement [143, 165].

2. Fibro-Osseous Jaw Lesions of Medullary Bone Origin

In the Armed Forces Institute of Pathology study, benign fibro-osseous lesions of periodontal membrane origin were found to be much more prevalent in the jaws (249 cases) than fibro-osseous lesions of medullary bone origin (154 cases). Medullary bone origin lesions may be differentiated by utilizing clinical, radiographic, hematologic, and histologic considerations. Differential diagnosis yielded the following number of cases for each medullary origin tumor: fibro-osteoma (40), active juvenile ossifying fibroma (14), cherubism (9), fibrous dyslasia (16), giant cell tumor (58), aneurysmal bone cyst (7), jaw lesion of hyperparathyröidism (3), and Paget's disease (3) [143].

(A) Fibro-Osteoma

The fibro-osteoma is usually a larger tumor than the ossifying fibroma of periodontal membrane origin, and thus, it frequently produces a painless clinical swelling. It is generally a slow-growing, solitary tumor that does not undergo malignant change. Blood calcium and phosphorus levels are typically within normal limits [5, 143, 166].

Radiographically, this tumor often involves an area encompassing several teeth, as illustrated in Fig. 3.63. Its radiopacity has been described as having a "ground-glass" appearance, and often this tumor is found in the maxillary antrum (Fig. 3.64) [167].

In microscopic appearance, the fibro-osteoma possesses larger trabeculae of mature lamellar bone than is customarily seen in the ossifying fibroma. These trabeculae are lined by osteoblasts, the fibrous stroma is more myxomatous, and the stromal cells also do not resemble the periodontal membrane tissues (Fig. 3.65). Under polarized light, broad parallel lines of alternating dark and light are clearly visable (Fig. 3.66).

Treatment is by curettage or conservative surgical excision, and the fibroosteoma does not tend to recur.

(B) Active Juvenile Ossifying Fibroma (A.J.O.F.)

The active juvenile ossifying fibroma (or osteoblastoma) is a very rare aggressive tumor most commonly seen in children and teenagers [143]. This tumor was first described as an "ostoblastoma" in the literature in 1956 in independent articles published by Lichtenstein and Jaffe [168, 169]. In 1954, Dahlin and Johnson had earlier published a report of 11 similar-type cases, but they had entitled the tumor a "giant osteoid osteoma" [170]. In this discussion, the term "active juvenile ossifying fibroma" (A.J.O.F.), coined by Lent C. Johnson at the Armed Forces Institute of Pathology, will be used because it is more accurate descriptively [171].

Lichtenstein reported that 75% of his 31 cases of osteoblastoma occurred between the ages of 7 and 20 years, with the eldest patient being 78 years old. He found the most common sites to be the limb bones, vertebral column,

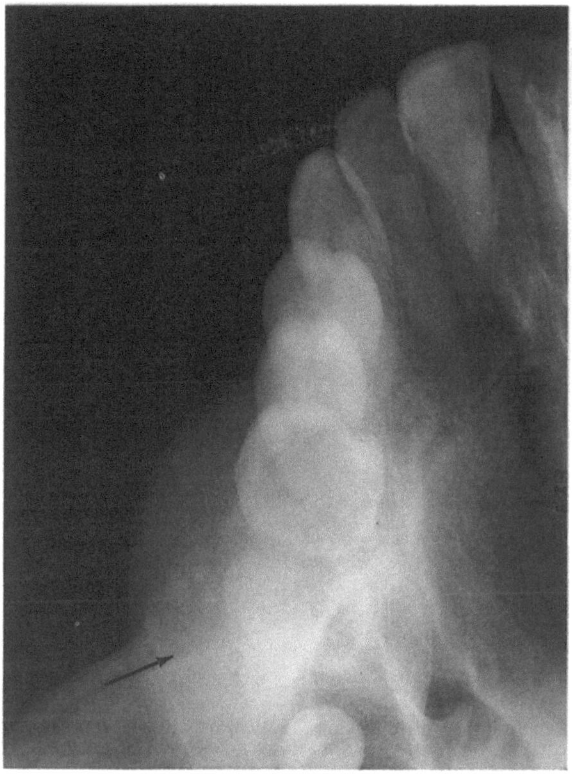

Fig. 3.63. Radiographic appearance of a fibro-osteoma (*arrow*), right maxillary molar and premolar areas

and the calvarium. Six of his 31 cases occurred in the calvarium (4 in the temporal bone, 1 in the occipital bone, and 1 in the frontal bone); no cases were found in the jaws [172].

Jaffe's findings in his 20 collected cases were essentially of the same view as Lichtenstein, however, he did not list specific tumor sites [169]. Clinical complaints obviously vary with the tumor's location. Tumors arising in the vertebral column may involve either the spinal cord or nerve roots, producing severe pain. In other bony locations, the pain has sometimes been described as dull or aching [168–170].

In 1967, Kramer reported a case of benign osteoblastoma arising in the left mandible of a 6-year old girl. Chief complaints were pain and swelling. Surgical treatment consisted of an intra-oral incision, reflection of a mucoperiosteal flap, and thorough curettement of the tumor tissue. Healing was uneventful, with no signs of recurrence 2 years later [173].

An analysis of 12 available Armed Forces Institute of Pathology cases of A.J.O.F. produced this clinical profile: age range = 7 to 20 years with an average age of 11.5 years; 8 males to 4 females; 6 Caucasians, 5 Negroes, and 1 Mongol; 8 mandibular cases to 4 maxillary cases – 2 of the latter also involved the

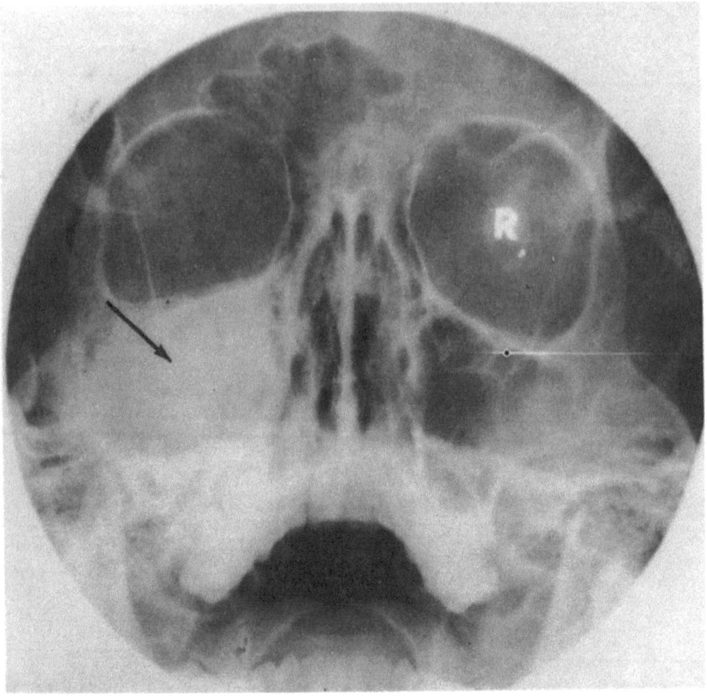

Fig. 3.64. Waters-view radiograph depicting the "ground-glass" appearance of a fibro-osteoma in the left maxillary antrum (*arrow*)

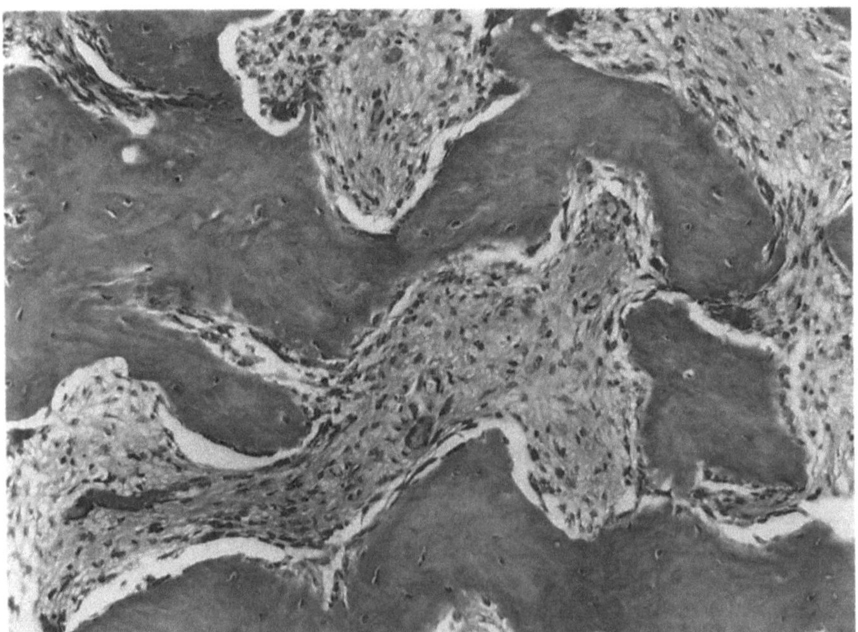

Fig. 3.65. Fibro-osteoma, 10-year-old Caucasian male. H. & E. stain, ×110

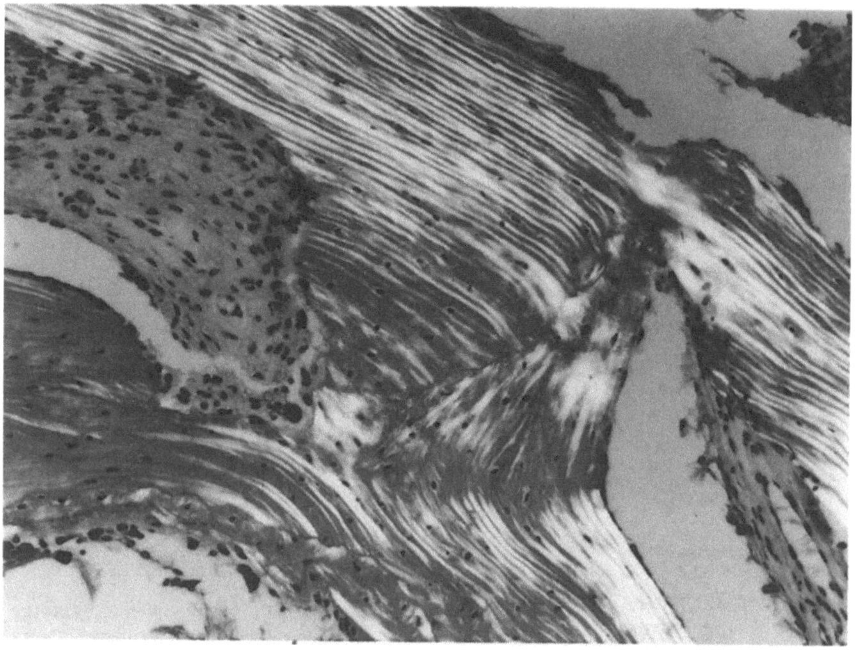

Fig. 3.66. Fibro-osteoma under polarized light. H. & E. stain, ×160

maxillary antrum; swelling was noted in all cases; and pain was absent in 6 cases and not listed in 6 cases [174].

The active juvenile ossifying fibroma often grows rapidly and may destroy adjacent anatomic structures, leading to death due to secondary infection or destruction of vital tissues. It has not been known to metastasize [171]. Figure 3.67 is a good example of a rapidly enlarging active juvenile ossifying fibroma in the right maxilla and right maxillary antrum of an 18-year-old Negro male.

Lichtenstein has described this tumor as being well-circumscribed on radiographic examination, and even though it may expand the bone quite markedly, it still is delineated by a thin shell of new cortical bone [172]. The tumor itself may be either radiolucent or mottled, depending upon the amount of ossification and calcification present. Figures 3.68 and 3.69 exhibit both of these two roentgenographic appearances.

The most outstanding histologic feature is that the stromal tissue is densely populated by osteoblasts, which often appear to be arranged in a primitive trabecular pattern with osteomucin being laid down (Fig. 3.70). The numerous osteoblasts, which give the tumor its name, are surrounded by osteomucin, as they attempt to form trabeculae – hence, it appears quite cellular (Fig. 3.71). Mature bone may be present in areas, and if so, its periphery is packed with osteoblasts – another diagnostic feature. The most important factor to consider is the differentiation of this tumor from the osteosarcoma. Close scrutiny will reveal that the active juvenile ossifying fibroma does not have numerous or

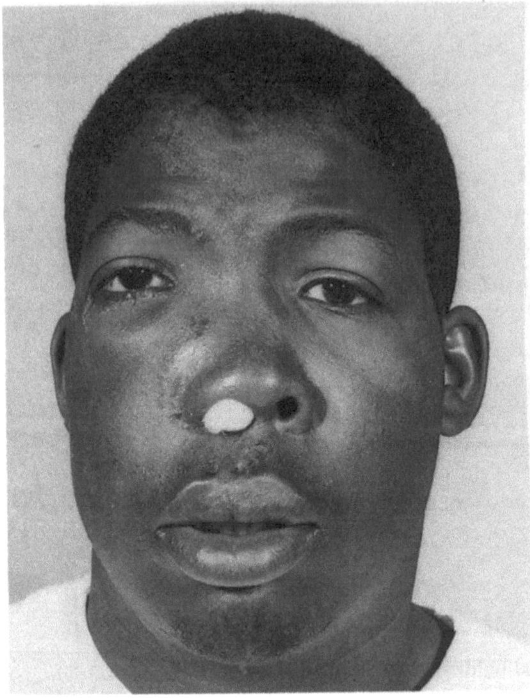

Fig. 3.67. Active juvenile ossifying fibroma in the right maxilla and right maxillary autrum of an 18-year-old Negro male

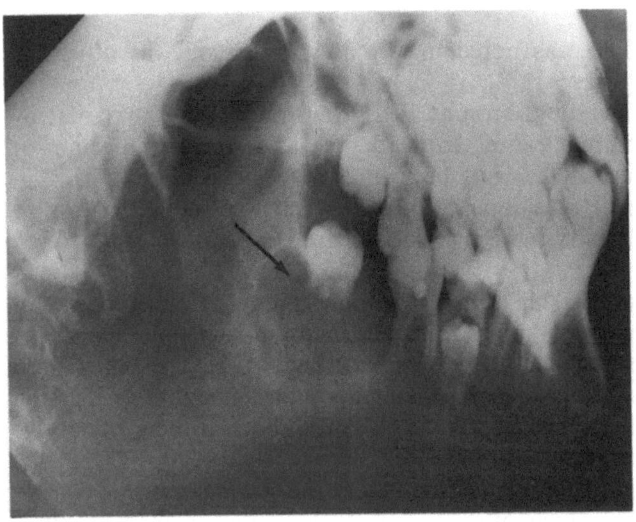

Fig. 3.68. Lateral head film of an active juvenile ossifying fibroma, appearing as a posterior mandibular radiolucency (*arrow*) in an 11-year-old Caucasian female

atypical mitoses, sarcoma giant cells, tumor cartilage, or other hallmarks of sarcoma malignancy.

Lichtenstein and Jaffee have recommended conservative surgical excision in treating this specific tumor [169, 172]. Kramer achieved good healing and

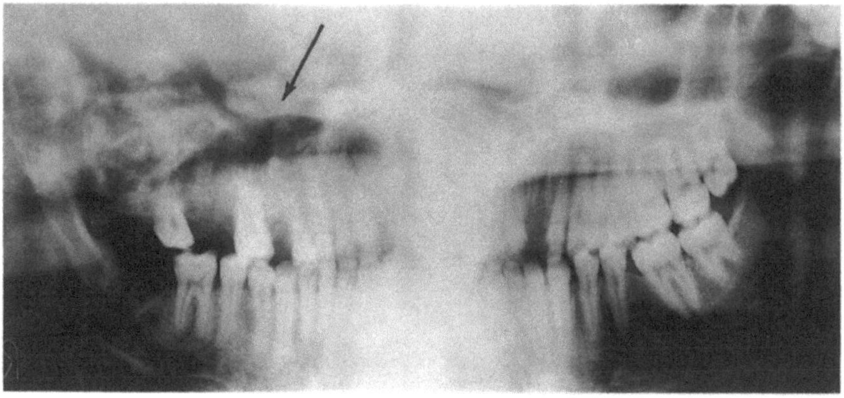

Fig. 3.69. Panorex film demonstrating an extensive active juvenile ossifying fibroma (*arrow*) in the right maxilla and maxillary antrum of an 18-year-old Negro male

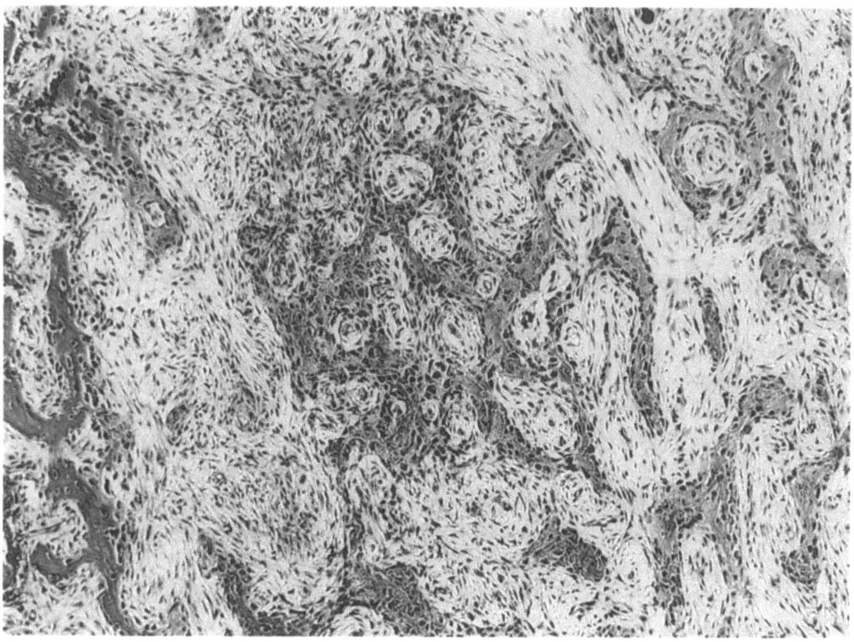

Fig. 3.70. Active juvenile ossifying fibroma with numerous osteoblasts forming primitive trabeculae. H. & E. stain, ×85

a positive surgical result using thorough curettage for an A.J.O.F. in the left mandible of his reported patient. However, 6 out of 12 jaw-involved cases in the Armed Forces Institute of Pathology study required surgical removal more than one time. One case required five surgical procedures, but eventually all 12 cases were cured except for one who died during surgery. None of these cases had metastatic lesions or transformed to malignancy [174].

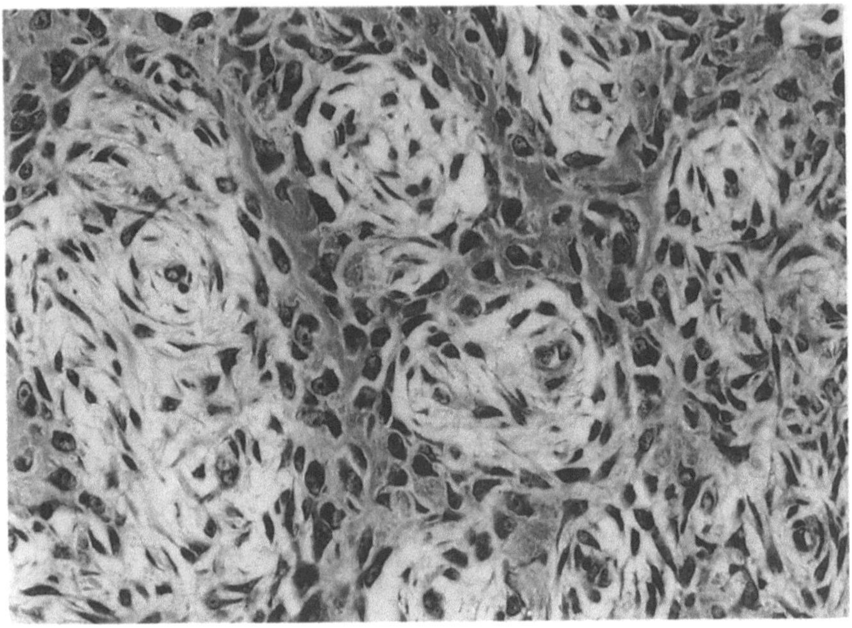

Fig. 3.71. Active juvenile ossifying fibroma. H. & E. stain, × 370

(C) Cherubism

In 1933, cherubism was first reported by Jones as a clinical entity in three young Jewish siblings [175]. Cherubism is a tumorous lesion of the jaws affecting children and is characterized by bilateral, painless mandibular (and often corresponding maxillary) swellings that cause fullness of the cheeks, firm protuberant intra-oral alveolar masses, and missing or displaced teeth [175, 176]. Submaxillary lymphadenopathy is described as an early, fairly constant feature that tends to subside after age 5 years and usually has regressed by age 12 years [177, 178]. Maxillary involvement can often produce a slight upward turning of the child's eyes, revealing an abnormal amount of sclera beneath them. It was the upward "looking toward heaven" cast of the eyes, combined with the characteristic facial chubbiness of the children, that prompted Jones to coin the term "cherubism" [175].

Since its original description, numerous patients with cherubism have reportedly given rise to a group of synonyms, such as "familial multilocular cystic disease" [175], bilateral giant cell tumors [179], "familial fibrous swelling" [176], "familial intraosseous fibrous swellings" [180], "familial fibrous dysplasia" [181], "disseminated juvenile fibrous dysplasia" [182], "familial osseous dysplasia" [183], and "hereditary fibrous dysplasia" [184].

Anderson, et al., first considered the genetic aspects of cherubism in their review of 65 cherubism patients in 21 families. They concluded that cherubism was related to a dominant gene with a pentrace of nearly 100% in males and between 50–75% in females [184]. Their analysis and conclusion were based on information gleaned from the 65 cherubism cases in the literature by 1962 that were acceptable for statistical analysis. The main problem in any valid genetical analysis is having accurate clinical and radiographic information on all family members for at least three successive generations.

Caffey and Williams recorded a hereditary history in one family in which cherubism was passed from the maternal grandmother to the mother to two of four children in one family. In another of the families that they surveyed they reported cherubism as being transmitted from the father to one of three children [176]. The family reported by Burland showed a similar familial pattern. He concluded that cherubism arises as a result of a spontaneous mutation, resulting in the formation of a nonsex-linked dominant gene [185].

Recently in 1979, Peters reported an extensive study of twenty cases of cherubism occurring in one family, covering five successive generations. His genetic findings confirmed that cherubism does follow an autosomal dominance pattern of inheritance that is nonsex-linked. Of the ten individuals who transmitted this condition, eight themselves were affected, thus demonstrating an 80% penetrance [186]. Therefore, from the viewpoint of genetic counseling, it can be estimated that there is a 40% chance of an affected member of the family producing an affected offspring [186].

Cherubism has a very early clinical onset, the youngest previously reported affected child being 18 months old [187]. Rapid progression of the disorder can occur during the next several years, encompassing all of the areas that will become affected and causing clinical features which vary according to the anatomy involved and the severity of the genetic disorder. The typical initial painless, bilateral, symmetrical enlargement of the posterior mandible and rami has been described in all of the reported cases. However, the maxillae are often affected simultaneously, giving rise to the upward cast of the eyes by tumor encroachment on the orbital floor and often causing partial obliteration of the palatal vault with a resulting "V"-shaped cleft [177, 185, 187, 188]. The clinical appearance may vary from barely discernible posterior swellings of a single jaw to marked anterior and posterior grotesque expansion of both jaws with concomitant difficulties in mastication, speech, swallowing, and respiration [175, 182, 187, 189]. Figure 3.72 illustrates the typical "cherubism" look in a 3-year-old Negro boy.

The early rapid rate of size increase usually declines with advancing age, so that a period ensures that is characterized by minimal clinical change [178]. As the child reaches puberty, the facial appearance may begin to improve as the normal bony growth pattern evolves toward adulthood facial features. The maxillary lesions often tend to regress, although the mandibular lesions may continue to progress until age 15 years. Reshaping of the bone has been described between age 20 and 30 years with regression of the mandibular lesions, resulting in a mandible that is only a bit larger than normal [187, 190, 191].

Radiographically, the lesions of cherubism appear as multiple, well-defined, multilocular radiolucencies in the mandible and maxillae (see Fig. 3.73). These rarefactions begin in the posterior avelolar and rami regions and can spread anteriorly. They are irregular in size and usually cause marked destruction of the alveolar bone. Numerous displaced and unerupted teeth appear to be float-

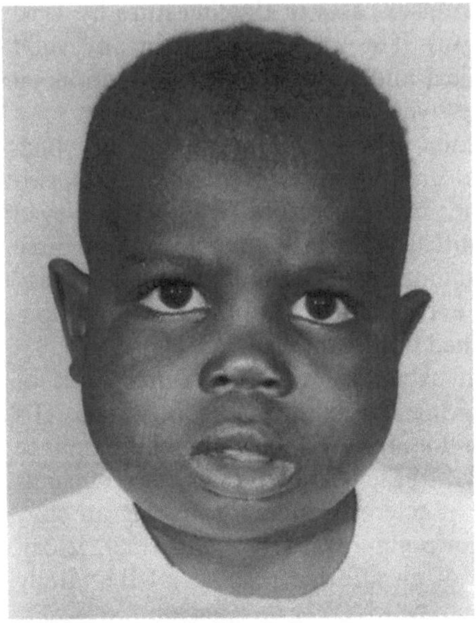

Fig. 3.72. A 3-year-old Negro male with cherubism. Note the chubby facial contours and a slight amount of sclera apparent under his pupils

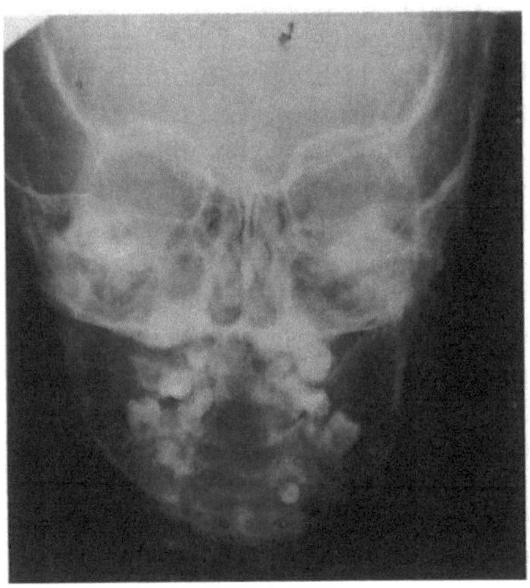

Fig. 3.73. Waters-view radiograph demonstrating the bilateral multilocular mandibular radiolucent lesions typical of cherubism in a 4-year-old Caucasion female

ing in the multiple radiolucent spaces. As the child reaches adulthood, the multilocular rarefactions of cherubism become replaced by bone, described radiologically as having a dense granular or "ground-glass" appearance. Some radiolucent areas have been reported to persist for years [185, 187, 188].

Blood chemistry values, such as serum calcium and serum phosphorus, are within normal limits for cherubism patients, while the serum alkaline phosphatase level may be elevated [10, 185].

Histologically, the cherubism jaw lesion can bear a close resemblance to the benign giant cell tumor (giant cell reparative granuloma), having a loose

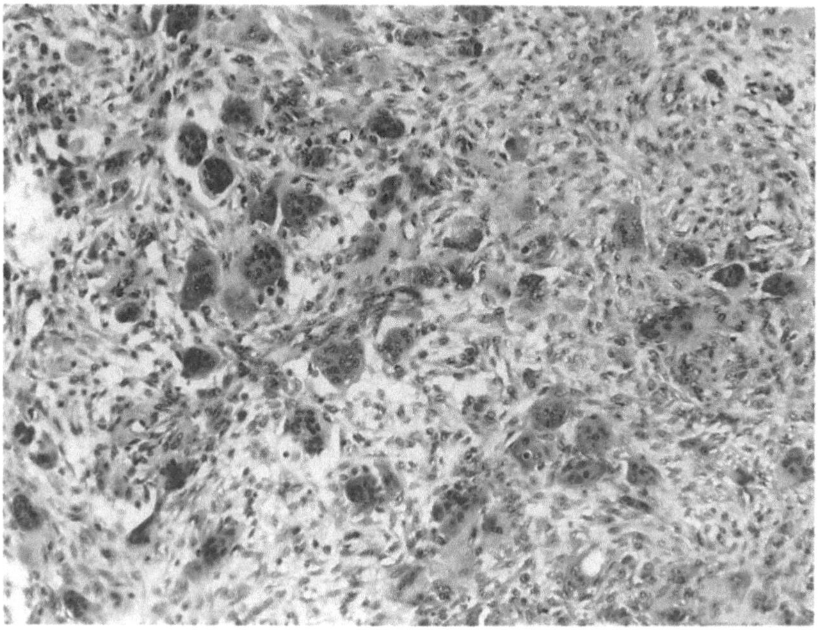

Fig. 3.74. Cherubism lesion with a plump cellular stroma and numerous giant cells. H. & E. stain, ×160

fibrillar stroma with numerous multinucleated giant cells featuring prominent nuclei and nucleoli, spindle-shaped fibroblasts, red blood cells, and hemosiderin deposits (see Fig. 3.74). Other cherubism tissue specimens have been described as being more mature with a greater amount of fibrous tissue and collagen and fewer giant cells. Figure 3.75 exhibits a cherubism lesion with a very loose myxomatous stroma with no giant cells. The prominent eosinophilic perivascular cuffing material noted around capillaries in these lesions has been shown by special stains to be collagen, which is very a important differential diagnostic feature (see Fig. 3.76 and 3.77) [192]. The Masson Trichrome and Rinehart stains are especially useful for this purpose.

The clinical features of bilateral, firm, painless, mandibular swellings beginning in the posterior alveolar body angle and ramus area with or without corresponding maxillary swelling and possible orbital encroachment causing the "cherubic look", coupled with submaxillary lymphadenopathy in a very young child, strongly suggest cherubism. Multilocular radiolucencies in the jaw radiographs render even more support for this diagnosis, and histopathologic demonstration of a loose fibrillar stroma with varying numbers of multinucleated giant cells and perivascular deposition of collagen confirm cherubism.

The problem of clinical management and surgical treatment is a more arduous one because each child must be evaluated individually according to the degree of tumor manifestation.

The reported treatment of cherbuism has varied considerably with advocates for each of the following methods: (a) no active treatment, (b) extraction of

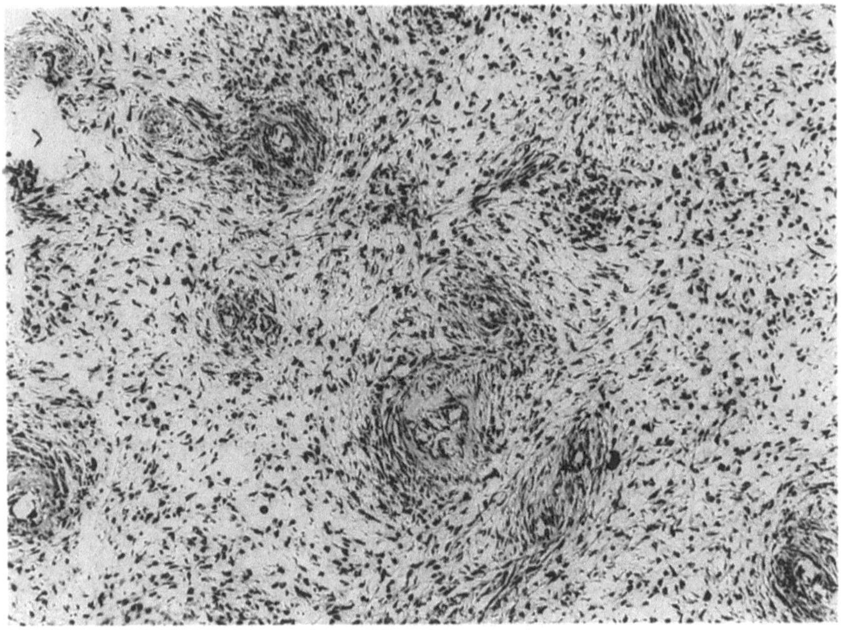

Fig. 3.75. Cherubism lesion with a more loose, myxomatous stroma and no giant cells. H. & E. stain, ×80

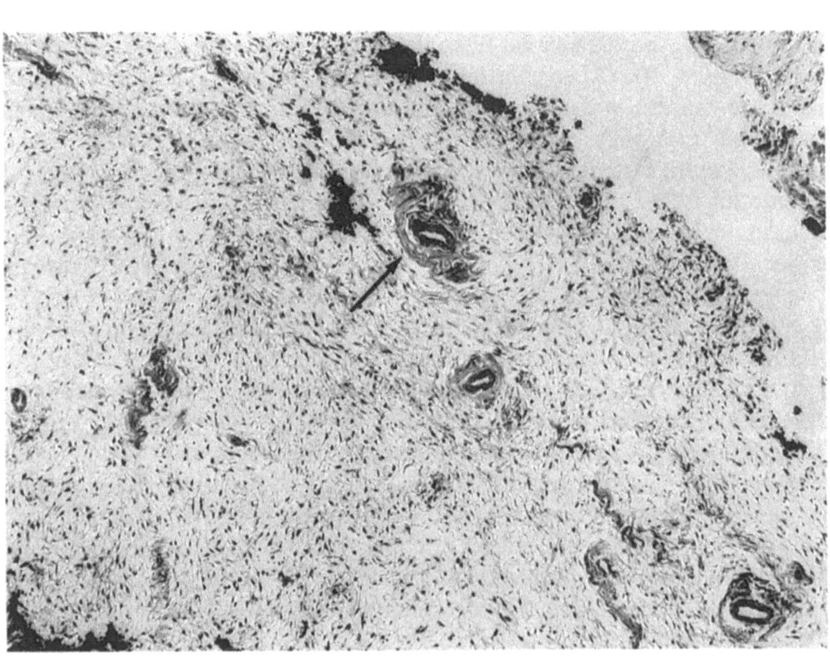

Fig. 3.76. Cherubism lesion with perivascular cuffing of collagen (*arrow*). Masson trichrome stain, ×65

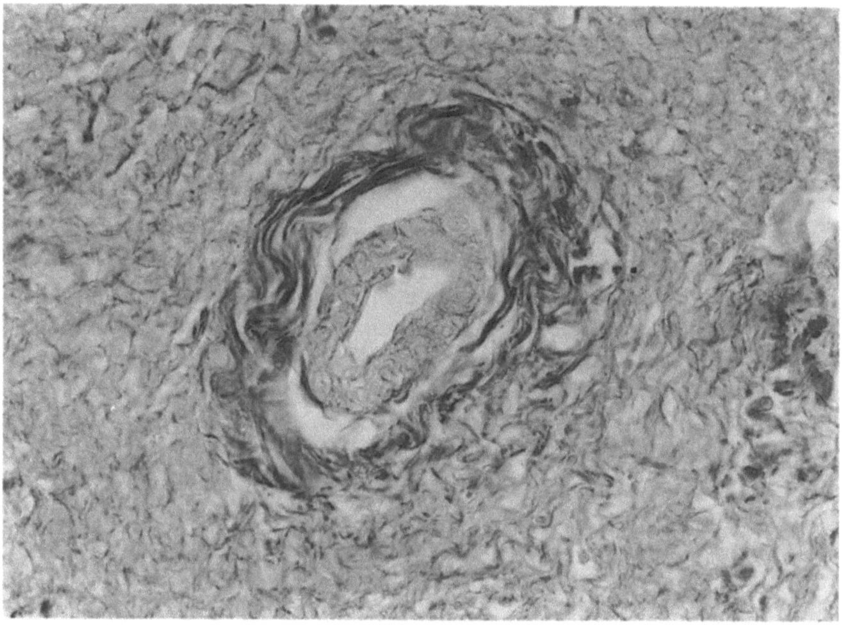

Fig. 3.77. Perivascular cuffing of collagen, diagnostic for cherubism. Rinehart stain, ×450

teeth in the involved areas, (c) surgical contouring of expanded lesions, and (d) complete curettage.

The statement has been repeated in the literature that many occrurrences of cherubism have resolved spontaneously when there was no treatment instigated, yet no one documented such a philosophy of "watch and wait" with any long term follow-up of actual case results [193].

The belief that a policy of non-surgical interference will eventually result in an adult with a symmetrical facial appearance obviously has been based on casual familial histories of a parent having vague jaw swellings as a child that eventually did "regress", so that the typical manifestation of cherubism was not present in adulthood. No child with early typical cherubism has been carefully follow to adulthood without some form of treatment. The children in Jones' original report refused treatment initially, then were later operated by curettement as teenagers with gratifying cosmetic results. Their jaw lesions did uniformly progress to reach grotesque proportions without treatment, yet continuous postoperative follow-up revealed no further extension of the lesions after curettement, but rather a gradual remodeling of bone toward normal facial symmetry by age 30 [177, 178, 190].

What may be ideal in theory, such as the policy of watching and waiting, is not always possible in practice concerning treatment of these children. The continued progress of the tumor lesions in both of the cases reported by Hamner and Ketcham bears out this fact [187].

Jones had steadfastly maintained that the permanent teeth are somehow associated with the bone disturbances of cherubism. His observations on the first and second generations of the cherubic family he originally reported in 1933 led him to the conclusion that the tumor lesions seem to recede about the time the permanent teeth in the affected area are either shed or extracted [190]. Hence, he concluded that extraction of the teeth in the involved area would be a conservative therapeutic approach to surgical management.

In our estimation, extraction of teeth in the involved cherubism sites is not a good policy. Cherubism lesions can usually be controlled by thorough curettement, so the permanent teeth especially should be preserved whenever possible in order to insure the best possible future masticatory function. If curettement provides the same end result as extraction, as cited by Jones, then it would be preferable to employ curettage and save as many teeth as possible, so as not to end up with an edentulous child with all the attendant prosthetic and psychologic problems that would entail.

Recontouring of the involved cherubism jaw swellings has been used with satisfactory results by many surgeons. As tumor growth continues to reach a point of clinical or cosmetic intolerability, the expanding lesion is merely trimmed down again to a more normal contour. This act may alleviate the immediate problem and control the swellings over the years of their continued progression, however, occasionally recontouring will elicit a rapid, fulminating enlargement of the lesions. Most supporters of the recontouring philosophy believe results are better, using the trimming method, when all growth of the lesion has ceased [185, 188–190]. In practice, it is seldom possible to wait until "all growth of the lesion has ceased". Also, determination of growth terminis is a difficult state to pinpoint in a child's jaw development.

Complete curettement of cherubism has also produced its share of good and bad results [176, 190, 194, 195]. One interesting report concerned the use of autogeneous bone chips from the patient's iliac crest to fill the surgical curettement defects caused by enucleation of bilateral mandibular cherubism lesions in a 10-year-old boy. The benefit obtained by the use of bone chips in a surgical defect has always been debatable. It could be that the same good results would have evolved without the use of bone chips [196]. Such statements as, "no untoward reactions to surgery in either childhood or adolescence have occurred" [191], and "recurrence or activation of the condition following surgical intervention has never been recorded" [185], are poorly substantiated in extolling the efficiency of surgery. Whenever the decision is made to extensively curette these lesions, or to merely recontour them, it should be borne in mind that the possibility exists that such surgery can cause aggravation to the tumor which can "recur" with rapid devastation of the jaws. Several investigators have reported cases which have shown a recurrent, more aggressive course following surgery [180, 181, 195].

The use of radiation in any form of therapy for cherubism is now universally condemned because of the dangers of sarcoma induction, osteoradionecrosis, and interference in bone growth and facial development in these children [186, 187, 190, 191, 196].

It is our experience that cherubism is a relentless process in the early stages, and if the jaws are extensively involved or even moderately so, thorough curettement of all possible tumor, taking pains to spare as many of the teeth as possible, is the treatment of choice. Both of the children in the National Institutes of Health Study exhibited steady progression of the tumor lesions whether the initial surgery was extensive or more conservative [187].

If the lesions are mild on initial manifestation with minimal bone involvement and are noticed only on radiographs, they can be observed and followed closely in relationship to the corresponding jaw growth. A surge in tumor growth can occur quickly, necessitating surgery. Lesions causing initial expansion of the rami appear to steadily enlarge, if left untreated. Curettement and recontouring must usually be combined to obtain the best esthetic result. Merely trimming a large lesion is not satisfactory.

The prognosis is enhanced if cherubism occurs in only one jaw, preferably the mandible. Anterior as well as posterior lesions in both jaws present a grave situation. Cherubism lesions in the maxillae act in a more agressive manner than their mandibular counterparts, and due to the anatomical considerations pose the more serious problem.

(D) Fibrous Dysplasia

Polyostotic fibrous dysplasia of bone was first described as a pathological entity in the late 1930's by Albright and Lichtenstein [197, 198]. Later, solitary lesions of bone that were indistinguishable from the lesions of polyostotic fibrous were recognized as the localized, or "monostotic", form of this same disease [199]. Patients with the monostotic form of fibrous dysplasia generally do not exhibit the marked disturbances in skeletal growth, sexual maturation, and cutaneous pigmentation that are associated with polyostotic fibrous dysplasia. Many authors began to follow a trend to use the label of "fibrous dysplasia" as a general term to encompass lesions that were formerly delineated as fibro-osteomas, ossifying fibromas, cherubism, periapical cementomas, etc. As a result of being thus carelessly employed, "fibrous dysplasia" became a meaningless wastebasket term for a whole group of largely unrelated and often clinically dissimilar lesions. Reed and others have clearly described the basic histologic differences that serve to differentiate fibrous dysplasia from the other fibro-osseous lesions, so therefore, we shall discuss fibrous dysplasia as a separate, distinct entity [143, 200, 201].

Fibrous dysplasia can occur in either the maxilla or the mandible in both the monostotic and polyostotic forms, but it is rarer than the literature would lead one to believe [171, 202, 203]. Using the strict histopathologic criteria of having a fibrous stroma with loose myxomatous areas, a good blood supply, and feathery, irregular-shaped trabeculae of immature bone that lack a well-defined periphery and an osteoblastic lining and polarize in a random birefringent pattern, 16 cases of fibrous dysplasia were included in the Armed Forces Institute of Pathology study. Of these 16, 11 were the monostotic form, and 5 were the polyostotic form. The clinical findings from this survey are shown in Table 3.16. The monostotic form was more prevalent – 11/16 cases. The patients' ages ranged from 6 to 43 years with an average age of 22 years. Yet, 10/16 cases were in the 20 years and younger group, thus casting this lesion in the role as one that affects a younger population. The sex distribution

Table 3.16. Clinical findings in fibrous dysplasia

Case no.	Form	Age	Sex	Race	Location	Swelling	Pain	Parasthesia	No. surgical treatments
1	monostotic	37	M	Caucasian	Mandibular molar	yes	no	no	1
2	monostotic	23	M	Caucasian	Maxilla and antrum	yes	no	yes	1
3	monostotic	20	M	Caucasian	Maxilla	yes	?	?	2
4	monostotic	20	M	Caucasian	Mandibular molar	yes	no	no	3
5	monostotic	8	F	Caucasian	Maxilla; antrum; ethmoids	yes	?	?	1 (pt. died)
6	monostotic	12	F	Eskimo	Maxilla, palate; zygoma	yes	no	no	2
7	monostotic	23	M	Negro	Maxillary antrum	yes	yes	no	1
8	monostotic	8	F	Negro	Maxillary anterior palate	yes	no	no	1
9	monostotic	40	M	Caucasian	Maxillary molar	yes	no	no	4
10	monostotic	17	M	Caucasian	Maxilla and antrum	yes	?	?	2
11	monostotic	11	F	Caucasian	Mandibular molar	yes	?	?	2
12	polyostotic	45	F	Caucasian	Max. antrum; skull mandible; tibia	yes	?	?	1
13	polyostotic	19	F	Caucasian	Maxilla; malar; sphenoid	yes	no	no	1
14	polyostotic	6	F	Caucasian	Maxilla; humerus; vertebrae	yes	yes	no	1
15	polyostotic	20	F	Caucasian	Maxilla; mandible; frontal; malar	yes	?	no	1
16	polyostotic	43	M	Negro	Mandible; facial sinuses	yes	no	no	1

was equal; however, it is interesting to note that 4/5 of the polyostotic form cases were females. Racially, it occurred predominantly in Caucasians (12 cases) with 3 cases found in Negroes and 1 case in a 12 year old Eskimo female. More cases were discovered in the maxilla (12) than the mandible (4). Swelling was a universal symptom, but pain and parasthesia varied where these entities were even recorded in the patient histories. The number of surgical treatments is misleading, since the follow-up information for most of these patients was rather sketchy. This A.F.I.P. sample size is a very small one, so these statistics must be viewed with that fact in mind.

It appears that fibrous dysplasia can have a sudden onset and can progress quite rapidly, often coinciding with bodily growth spurts. Or, it can progress in a slower, steady fashion. It often can be destructive locally and tends to recur if not adequately removed surgically. Elevation of the serum alkaline phosphatase level is common in cases of fibrous dysplasia that have large lesions [171].

Figures 3.78, 3.79, and 3.80 demonstrate the radiographic appearance of fibrous dysplasia as a left mandibular lesion, an anterior maxillary/palatal lesion, and a maxillary antral lesion, respectively. These tumors appear radiolucent or radiopaque, depending upon the amount of immature bone present. Fibrous dysplasia can be very destructive of bone and cause marked displacement of teeth.

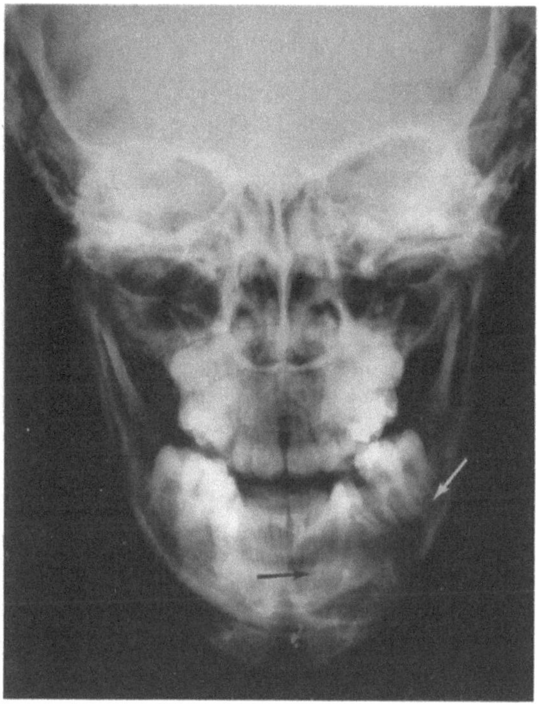

Fig. 3.78. Waters-view radiograph of fibrous dysplasia in the left mandible (*arrows*) of an 11-year-old female

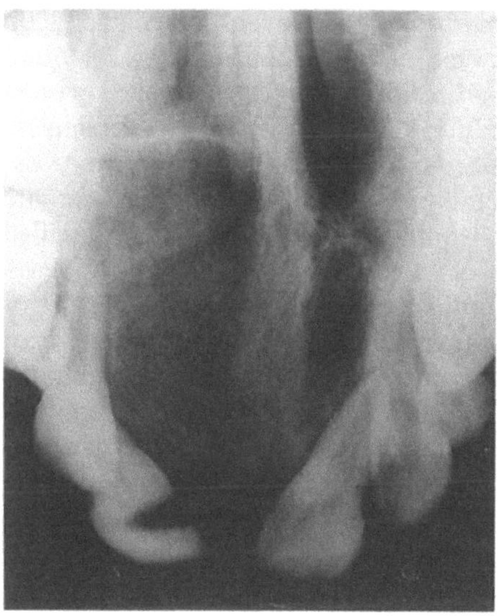

Fig. 3.79

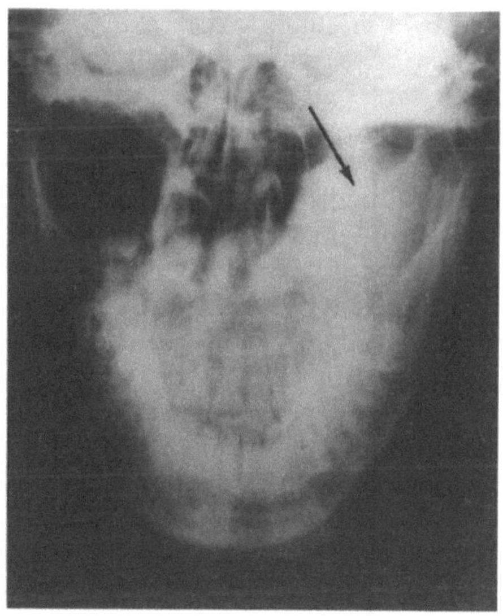

Fig. 3.80

Fig. 3.79. Occlusal film of a rapidly expanding, destructive fibrous dysplasia lesion in the anterior maxilla/palatal area of an 8-year-old female

Fig. 3.80. Fibrous dysplasia (*arrow*) appearing as a large radiopaque lesion in the left maxilla, palate, and zygoma of a 12-year-old female

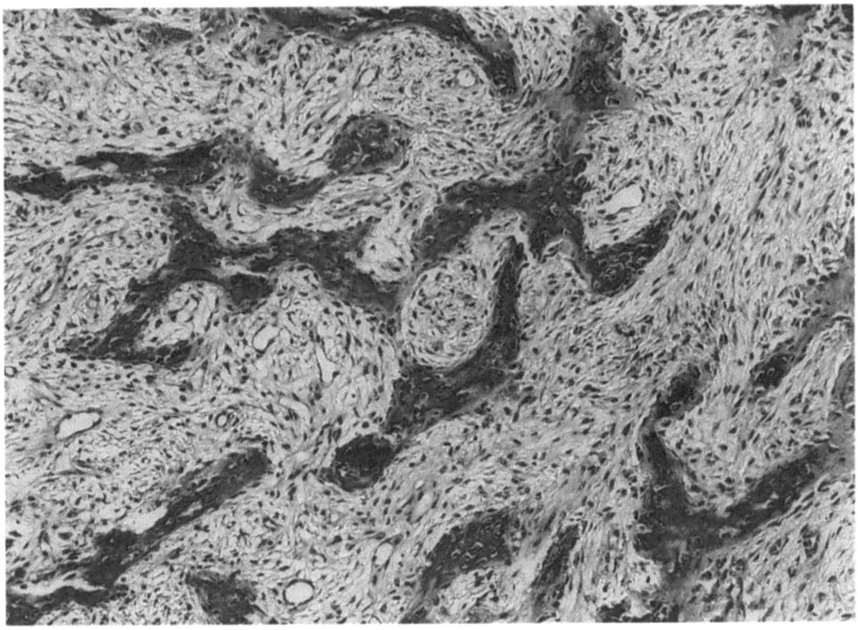

Fig. 3.81. Fibrous dysplasia. H. & E. stain, ×100

Microscopically, fibrous dysplasia is a specific fibro-osseous lesion characterized by a maturation arrest of bone formation at the woven bone stage [200]. Woven bone is a structurally inefficient type of bone that is normally found in the early stages of intramembranous ossification and in the periosteal growth of bone formed by endochondral ossification [204, 205]. There is a complete absence of lamellar bone formation in fibrous dysplasia. Therefore, since osteoma, fibroosteoma, ossifying fibroma, and osteoid osteoma all show varying degrees of lamellar bone formation, they should not be erroneously classified as variants of "fibrous dysplasia".

Fibrous dysplasia has a delicate, acidophilic myxomatous stroma. The stromal cells exhibit round or oval nuclei with inconspicuous nucleoli and scant cytoplasm (Fig. 3.81). The trabeculae are composed of woven, immature bone that often resemble "Chinese characters" (Fig. 3.81). Under higher magnification one can see a distinct lack of osteoblastic rimming of the trabeculae, and the peripheries of the trabeculae are irregular, feathery, and not defined (Fig. 3.82). Whorling of the fibrous stromal tissue may be present with isolated spicules of woven bone, as see in Fig. 3.83. Another very important differential diagnostic feature for fibrous dysplasia is the appearance of woven bone under polarized light. Unlike the even parallel dark and light lines of birefringence typical of lamellar bone, woven bone polarizes with a totally different random birefringence pattern (Fig. 3.84).

Treatment of fibrous dysplasia should be complete surgical removal, taking care to preserve as much normal tissue as possible. Tillman, et al., obtained a good surgical result and absence of recurrence with thorough surgical curettage

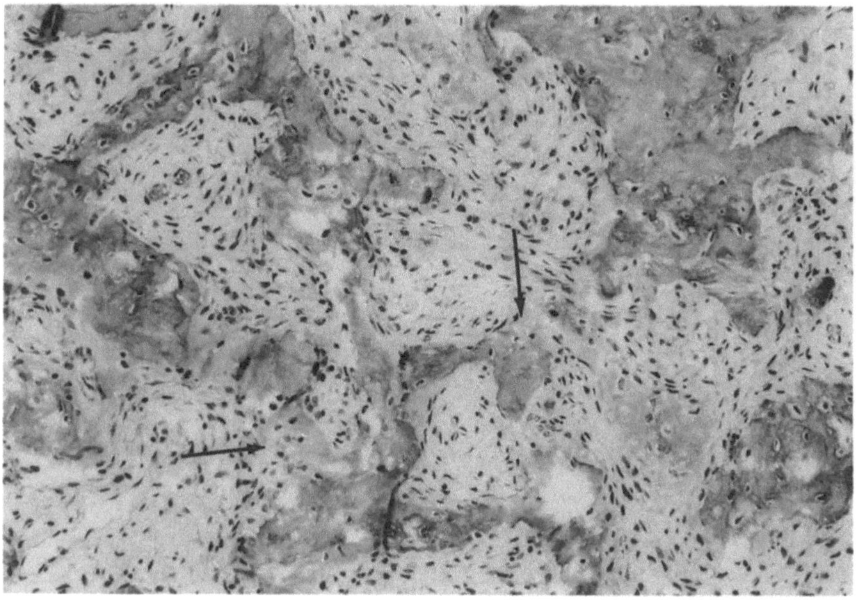

Fig. 3.82. Fibrous dysplasia. Note the irregular, feathery trabeculae borders with no osteoblastic rimming. H. & E. stain, ×160

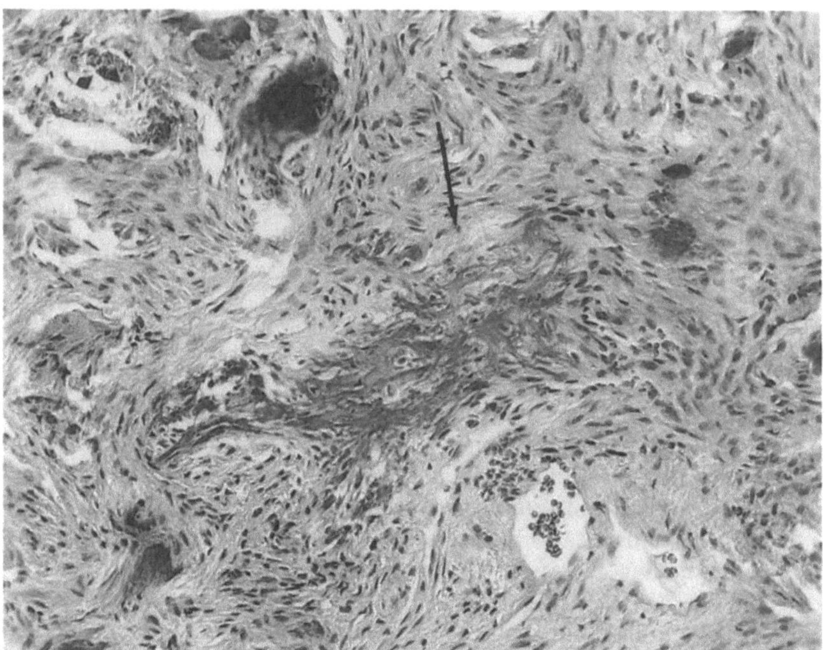

Fig. 3.83. Whorling of fibrous stroma, sometimes seen in fibrous dysplasia. Isolated spicule of woven bone (*arrow*). H.&E. stain, ×180

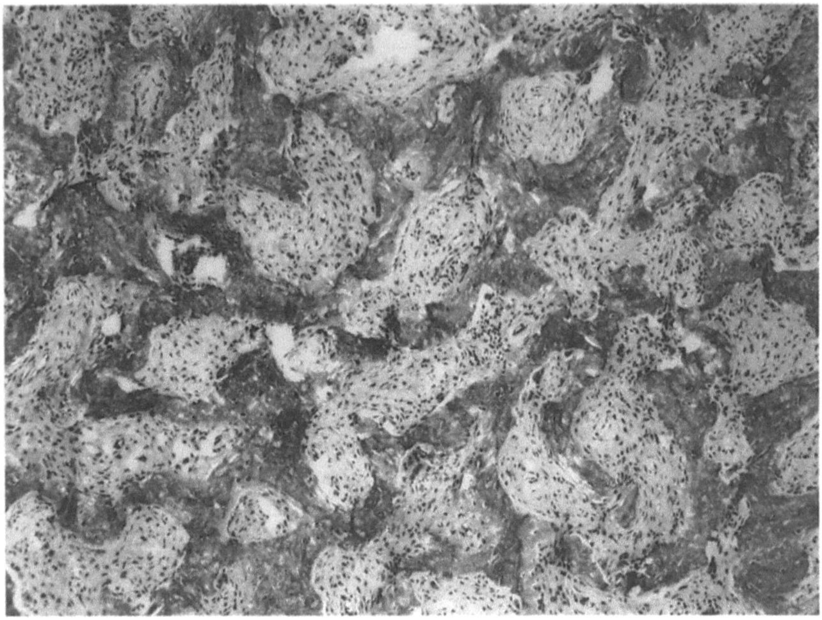

Fig. 3.84. Randon birefringence of woven bone in fibrous dysplasia under polarized light. H. & E. stain, × 80

of fibrous dysplasia in a 7-year-old boy [202]. Most of the 16 A.F.I.P. cases responded well to conservative surgery, however, 6/16 did require more than one operation. In contrast, Ramsey, et al., encountered a difficult progressive fibrous dysplasia lesion in the maxilla of a 3-year-old boy, causing grotesque deformity during a period of 13 years of treatment by radiation and surgery, ending in this patient's death at age 16 after an unsuccessful attempt at surgical resection [206]. Again, this example points out that each case must be evaluated on an individualistic basis in regard to proper treatment.

(E) Giant-Cell-Tumor

The benign giant-cell tumor of the jaws is the same lesion that Jaffe designated as the "giant-cell reparative granuloma" [207]. It is Johnson's contention that the term giant-cell tumor should be retained, and the lesions should be classified as benign or active giant-cell tumor [171]. The vast majority are benign. Only 5/58 of the A.F.I.P. study cases were the active variety, and two of these had a history of therapeutic radiation. In his thesis on the subject, Jacoby [208] concluded that the name giant-cell reparative granuloma is an unsuitable one, and we agree. These tumors are neither reparative nor granulomatous. An excellent analysis of 38 similar cases by Waldron and Shafer supports the view that central "giant-cell reparative granuloma" of the jaws and "benign giant-cell" tumor of other bones are identical lesions [209].

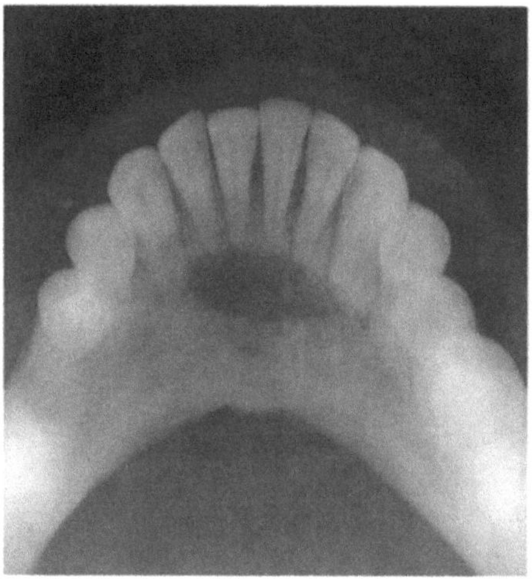

Fig. 3.85

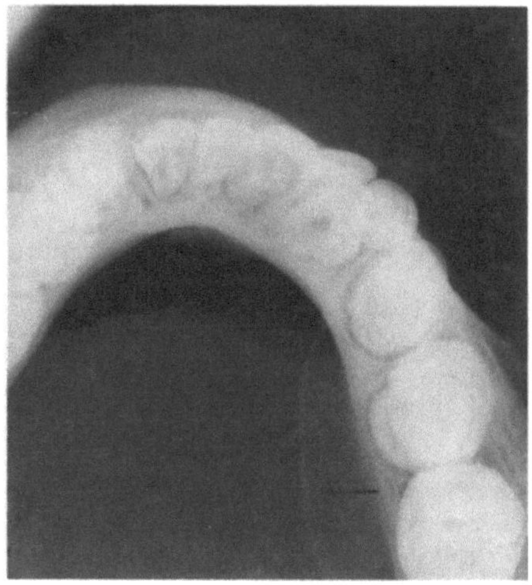

Fig. 3.86

Fig. 3.85. Benign giant-cell tumor in the mandibular anterior area

Fig. 3.86. Benign giant-cell tumor demonstrating expansion and thinning of the cortical plates of bone (*arrow*), right mandible

This tumor occurs more often in children and young adults according to Jaffe and Austin [207, 210]. The sex distribution in Waldron and Shafer's study was approximately 2:1 of females over males [209]. Two-thirds of their 38 cases occurred in the mandible, while 1/3 were found in the maxilla – the lesions were also more frequent in the anterior segment of the jaws [209]. In the A.F.I.P. cases, 28 were seen in men, 26 in females for benign giant-cell tumor, but it must be remembered that there is male sex distribution bias in such a military population. 38/58 of the benign giant-cell tumors were detected in the mandible. Pain is uncommon with this tumor, but bony expansion of the cortical plates usually is noted in the involved region.

The benign giant-cell tumor presents radiographically as a destructive radiolucent lesion with either a smooth or jagged border, sometimes demonstrating faint trabaulae (Fig. 3.85). The cortical plates of bone may be thinned and expanded by the enlarging tumor as shown in Fig. 3.86.

Histologically, the benign giant cell tumor is composed of a loose, fibrillar connective tissue stroma featuring interspersed proliferating fibroblasts, small capillaries, reactive osteiod and bone in the periphery, and a variable distribution of multinucleated giant-cells with numerous nuclei containing prominent nucleoli (Fig. 3.87 and 3.88).

Treatment of the benign giant cell tumor consists of either curettement or surgical excision. The tumor space usually fills in with new bone, and healing is uneventful [209, 211, 212].

The active giant cell tumor behaves in a much more aggressive fashion, as demonstrated in the clinical findings for the five A.F.I.P. cases (Table 3.17). One patient was 70 years old, one was 52, one was 24, and two children were

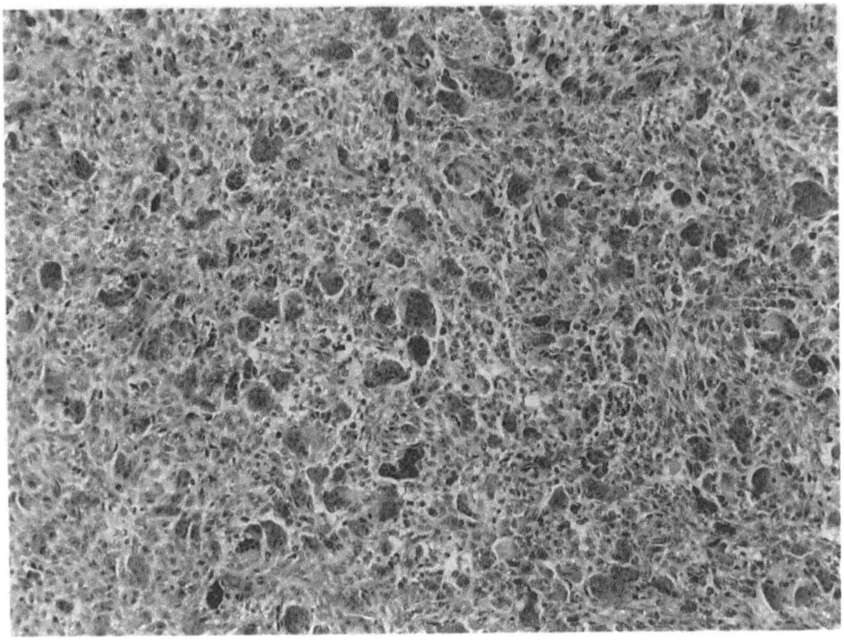

Fig. 3.87. Benign giant-cell tumor. H. & E. stain, ×100

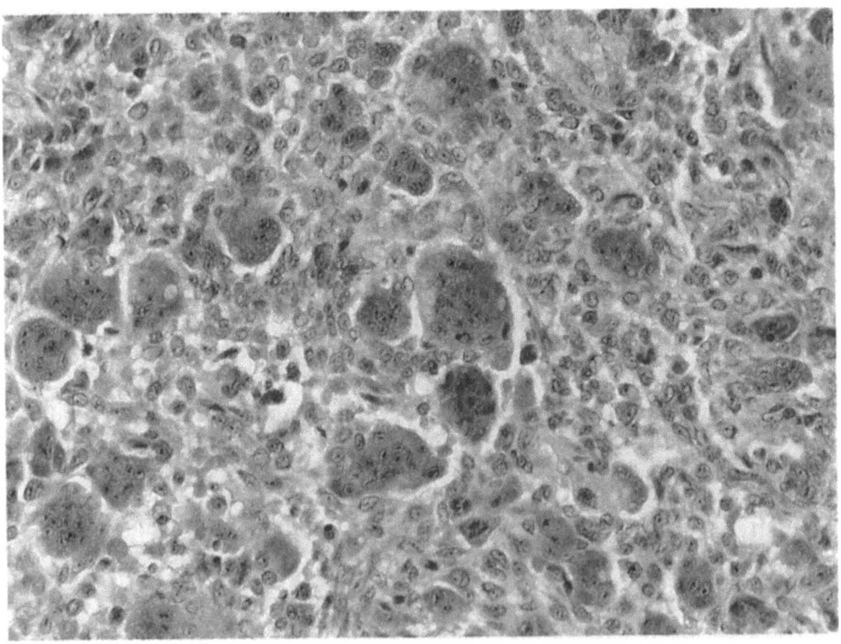

Fig. 3.88. Benign giant-cell under higher magnification. H. & E. stain, ×250

Table 3.17. Giant cell jaw tumor – active type clinical findings

Case no.	Age	Sex	Race	Site	Treatment	Prognosis
1	70	Male	Caucasian	Maxillary molars region	Surgical curettement; plus 11,300 R in 4 radiation treatments	Tumor recurred; patient died 9 years later
2	52	Male	Caucasian	Maxillary sinus and ethmoids	Surgery 3 times, plus >2,000 R in radiation therapy	3 Recurrences, patient died 10 years later
3	6	Male	Caucasian	Maxillary central incisors to molar area and palate	Curettement, followed later by total hemimaxillary excision	Recurred twice. No recurrence for 10 years after resection
4	24	Male	Caucasian	Mandibular right cuspid to left third molar region	Surgical excision of half of mandible	No recurrence
5	5	Male	Caucasian	Mandibular right 2nd premolar to left cuspid	Surgical excision 2 times	Recurred initially after 4 years

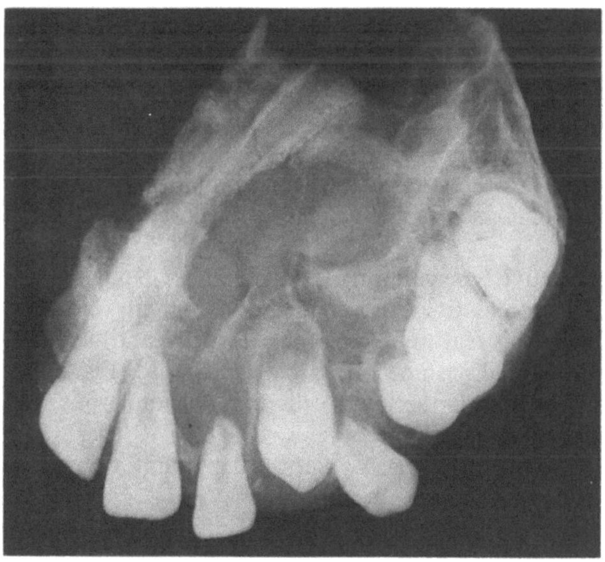

Fig. 3.89. Radiograph of the maxillary surgical specimen of an active type giant-cell tumor in a 6-year-old Caucasian male. (A.F.I.P. Accession #741190)

6 and 5, respectively. All of them were male Caucasians. A larger area of the jaws and/or maxillary sinis was involved as a tumor site for the active type of giant-cell tumor, and each tumor grew in a rapid, aggressive, destructive fashion. Treatment on the two older patients combined various doses of radiation (from 2,000 to 11,300 R) with surgery after the inital surgical effort. Again,

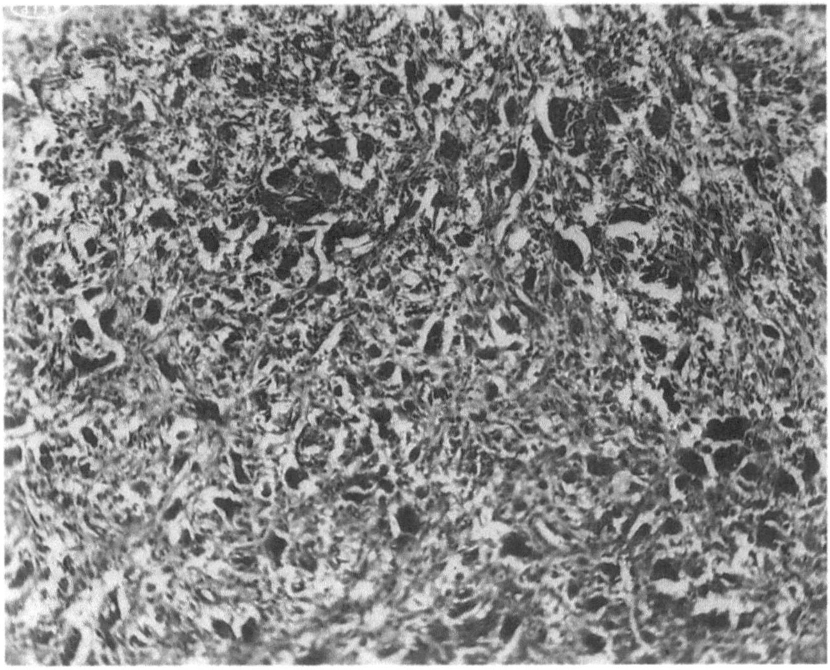

Fig. 3.90. Giant-cell tumor, active type. H. & E. stain, ×90. (A.F.I.P. Accession #529424)

radiation therapy proved to be ineffective against a fibro-osseous lesion, possibly produced a harmful effect, and thus, it should not be used. Radical surgery proved to be the most effective procedure in preventing recurrence. Figure 3.89 is a radiographic representation of the surgical excision specimen of an active giant-cell tumor in a 6-year-old Caucasian male. Note the large, destructive radiolucent tumor.

The histopathology of the active type varies markedly from the benign giant-cell tumor of the jaws. The stromal tissue is much looser and myxomatous (Fig. 3.90). Under higher power this feature is even more evident, and the giant cells tend to be more numerous and assume rather bizarre shapes (Fig. 3.91), whereas in the benign giant-cell tumor the giant cells may be numerous, but they are much more uniform in size and shape.

The treatment of choice for the active form of giant-cell jaw tumor is radical excision.

(F) Aneurysmal Bone Cyst

The term, "aneurysmal bone cyst", was coined by Jaffe and Lichtenstein to describe this separate fibro-osseous clinicopathologic entity [213]. The "aneurysmal" portion describes the "blown-out" appearance of the bony contour of the affected area, whereas the "bone cyst" portion designates that the lesion is located in a blood-filled cavity. In their first report of 35 cases, most patients

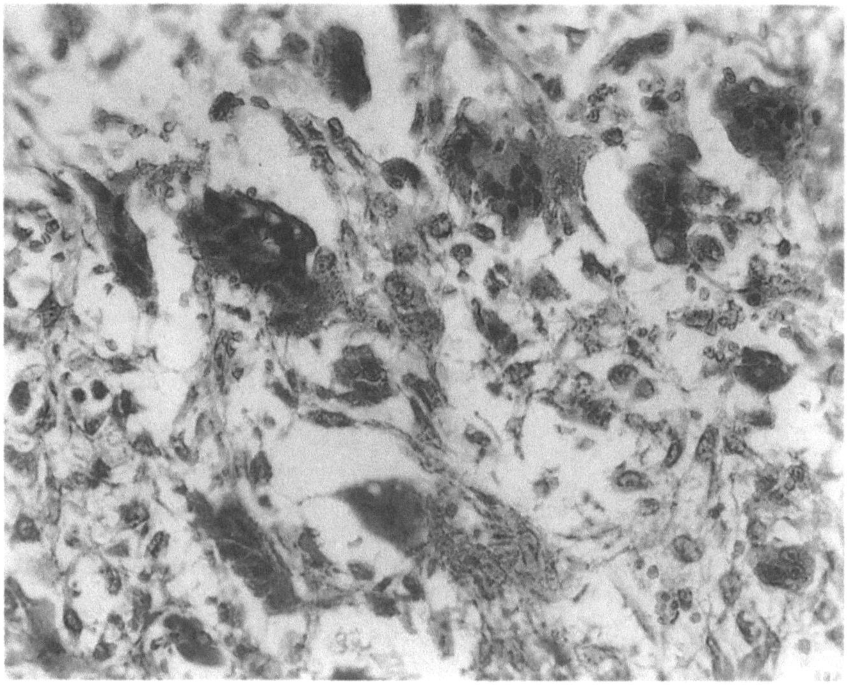

Fig. 3.91. A higher magnified view of the same tumor; note the bizarre giant-cells. H. & E. stain, ×350

were older children or young adults with a preponderance of females. This lesion has been observed in nearly all skeletal parts, however, over 50% of them occur in the long bones and vertebral column [214].

Bernier and Bhaskar reported the first two cases of an aneurysmal bone cyst occurring in the jaws. One was found in the mandible of an 11-year-old female, and the other one was detected in the mandible of a 59-year-old female [215]. They believed that this lesion resembles the central benign giant-cell tumor of the jaws (reparative granuloma) in patient age, clinical features, and prognosis. They suggested that both lesions represented "overzealous attempts of connective tissue to replace a hematoma in bone marrow". Provided the hematoma maintained a circulatory connection with its damaged vessel, an aneurysmal bone cyst would develop, but if this connection were lost, a giant cell reparative granuloma would result [215]. This theory remains unproven.

Daugherty and Eversole's review of the literature in 1971 yielded 17 reported cases of aneurysmal bone cyst in the jaws [216]. They missed the 7 A.F.I.P. cases reported by Hamner in 1968 [143]. Since then, other single cases have been described by Ellis and Walters in 1972 [217], by Oliver in 1973 [218], and by Reyneke in 1978 [219]. This total figure of only 27 literature cases indicates the rarity of this particular fibro-osseous lesion.

The aneurysmal bone cyst is a solitary, expansile, non-neoplastic lesion. Typically, the patient's chief complaint is mild pain and swelling in the affected bony part. It is not a true cyst in the sense of being an epithelial lined cystic

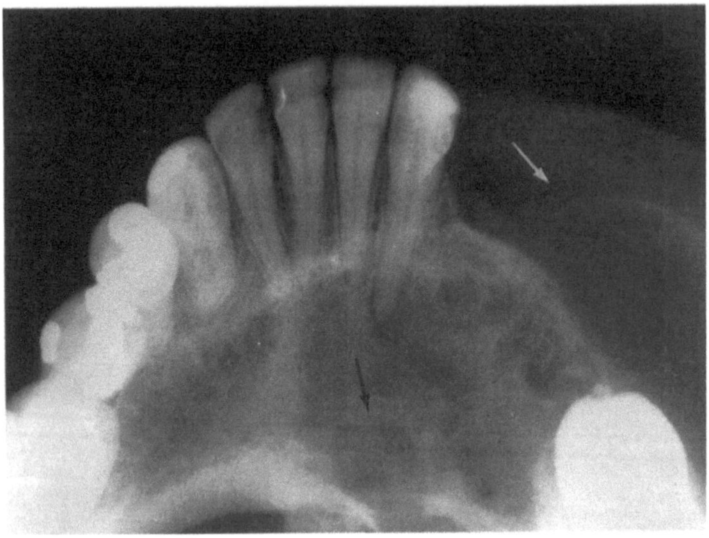

Fig. 3.92. Mandibular aneurysmal bone cyst with the radiolucent "soap bubble" aspect; mandibular lesion in a 29-year-old Caucasian female. (A.F.I.P. Accession #931546)

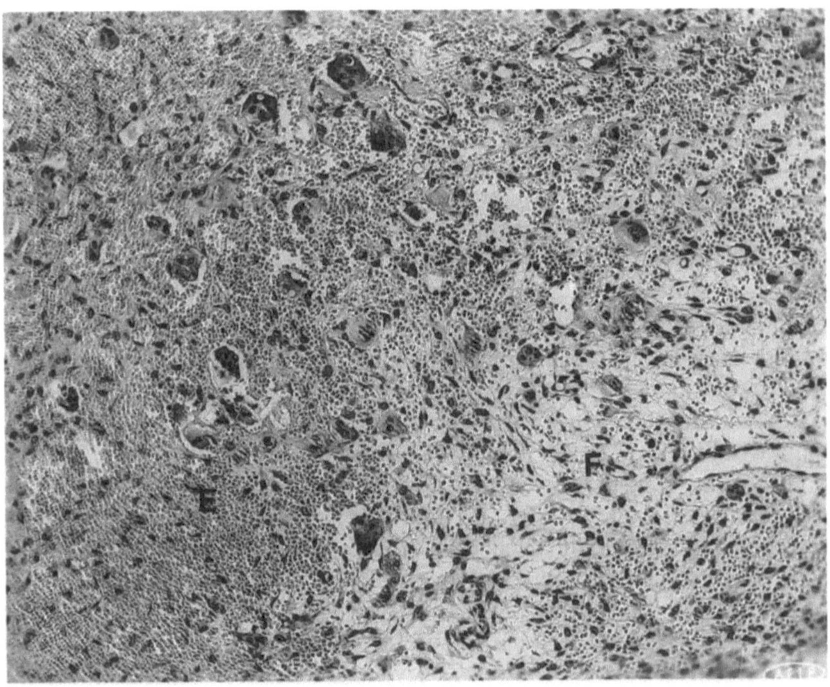

Fig. 3.93. Aneurysmal bone cyst with young fibroblasts (*F*); scattered giant-cells, and numerous erythrocytes (*E*). H. & E. stain, ×65

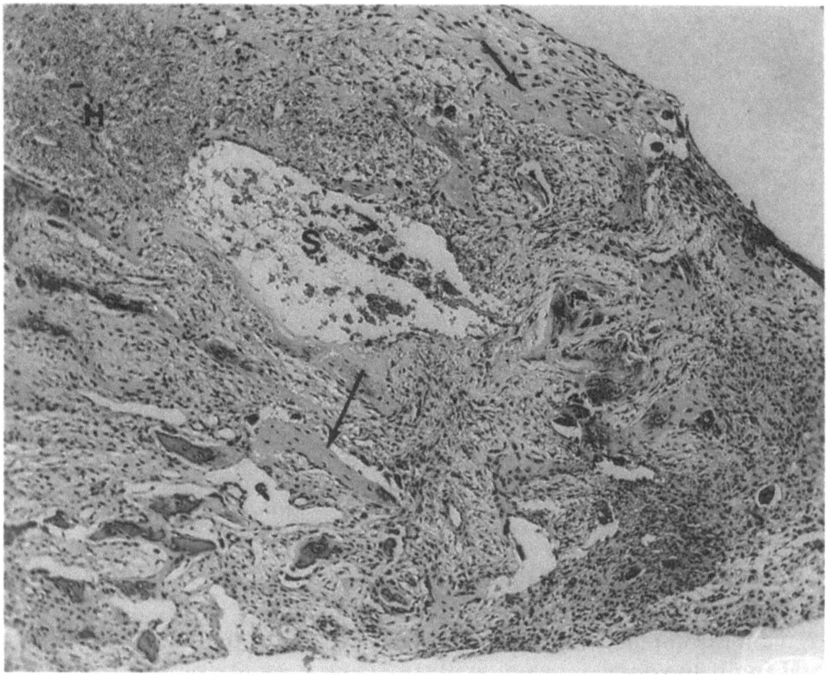

Fig. 3.94. Aneurysmal bone cyst; *S*, sinusoidal space; *H*, blood; new peripheral osteoid formation (*arrows*). H. & E. stain, ×65

space. It is found more often in patients younger than 25 years of age. The average age for the seven Armed Forces Institute of Pathology cases was 22.4 years. Five of these seven patients were women, and 5/7 of the aneurysmal bone cysts were discovered in the mandible.

X-rays of this lesion in other bones characteristically demonstrate a "blown-out tire" appearance that is typical for the aneurysmal bone cyst. Due to angulation and anatomic considerations during technique, dental radiographs of the jaws, especially periapical films, are not normally taken in a manner that will reveal this feature. Figure 3.92 is an occlusal x-ray film that does show the "honeycomb" or "soap bubble" aspect of this lesion [10].

Histologically, the aneurysmal bone cyst is quite similar to the benign giant-cell tumors of the jaws. The fibrous connective tissue stroma contains many young fibroblasts and a patchy distribution of multinucleated giant cells (Fig. 3.93). The most helpful diagnostic feature is the pooling or laking of blood (Fig. 3.94), which give it the cystic portion of its name. The stromal connective tissue is richly vascularized with numerous cavernous or sinusoidal spaces filled with blood.

Surgical curettage is the treatment of choice for aneurysmal bone cyst. Because of the spongy texture of the lesion, it is not easily removed in toto. Excessive bleeding often is encountered in the central part of the tumor mass. Blood tends to "well-up" from the tissue due to the slow flow of blood through the lesion, however, it can be controlled with careful surgical manipulation.

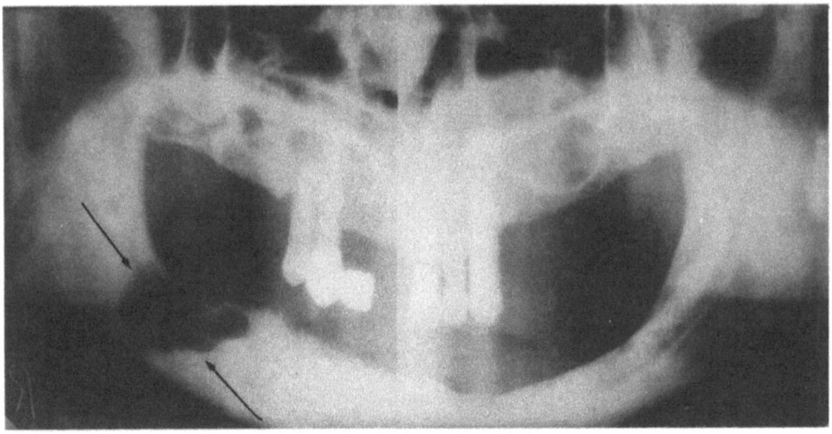

Fig. 3.95. Hyperparathyroid jaw lesion (*arrows*) in the right mandible of a 48-year-old Caucasian male

(G) Jaw Lesion of Hyperparathyroidism

In 1891, von Recklinghausen first described hyperparathyroidism as a bone disease, giving it the name – osteoitis fibrosa cystica generalisata [10]. Because this disease affects both calcium and phosphorus metabolism, it is associated with genitourinary disorders, gastrointestinal disease, muscular function, the central nervous system, and dental disorders. A patient suffering from primary hyperparathyroidism has an excessive quantity of parathyroid hormone, caused most often by a parathyroid adenoma (80–90% of cases), or less frequently carcinoma, or hyperplasia of the parathyroids.

Hypercalcemia, resulting from hyperparathyroidism, can produce the following signs and symptoms: decreased neuromuscular excitability with weakness, fatigue, abdominal distension, constipation, and anorexia. Some patients may exhibit shortening of the Q–T interval on an electrocardiogram. The diuretic effect of parathyroid hormone produces polyuria, and hypercalciuria can result in urinary stones, depending upon the concentration of salts in the urine, while nephrocalcinosis may result in other patients [220].

Von Recklinghausen's disease of bone (hyperparathyroidism) is a chronic progressive disorder affecting the entire skeleton. Generalized osteoporosis is evident on radiographs, and compact bone is replaced by spongy bone. Advanced cases reveal osteoclastic bone resorption of the marrow spaces, and benign giant-cell lesions may be found throughout the skeleton. Hematology provides the key for diagnosis, since the patient has increased serum calcium and decreased serum phosphorus levels [220, 221]. The total serum protein level should also be checked because a normal serum calcium level associated with a low serum protein may reflect an actual high serum calcium level, since 60–70% of the serum calcium is protein bound [221].

On x-ray, these jaw lesions of hyperparathyroidism frequently appear as either sharply defined round, or punched-out oval, radiolucencies that may

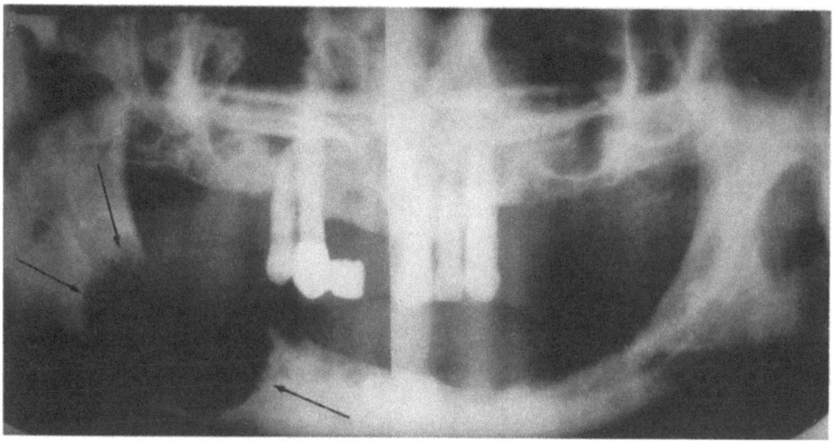

Fig. 3.96. Marked increase in the size of the hyperparathyroid jaw lesion in the same patient after only 4 months

or may not be lobulated. Figure 3.95 illustrates such a punched-out radiolucent jaw lesion of hyperparathroidism, located in the right mandibular molar and angle of the jaw region. Because of its location at the angle of the mandible, this lesion was suspected to be a metastasis from the patient's primary parathroid carcinoma, since he did have proven rib metastases. Four months later, a follow-up panorex film showed that the lesion had undergone extremely rapid growth and bony destruction of the mandible, now involving even more of the ramus (Fig. 3.96). However, excisional biopsy revealed that the tumor was a giant-cell lesion of hyperparathyroidism.

Loss of the lamina dura on dental periapical x-rays has long been cited in the past literature as diagnostic evidence of hyperparathyroidism [10]. Of the 220 hyperparathyroid patients included in Rosenberg and Guralnick's study, 62 were not examined in regard to the lamina dura, and 42 were edentulous. Of the 116 patients who were checked by dental x-rays, 47 (40%) exhibited absence of the lamina dura, while 69 (60%) demonstrated an intact lamina dura [221]. Thus, the absence of the lamina dura is better considered as an aid to differential diagnosis, but its absence is not necessary for a positive diagnosis of hyperparathyroidism.

Upon surgical exposure, this tumor has a reddish-brown clinical appearance giving it the name "brown tumor of hyperparathyroidism". Microscopically, it also closely resembles the benign giant-cell tumor of the jaws with an increase in red blood cells and hemosiderin deposits. The giant cells are benign, plentiful, and uniform in appearance (Fig. 3.97).

(H) Paget's Disease

Paget's disease of bone (osteitis deformans) was first defined by Sir James Paget in 1877 as a localized destructive lesion of bone [222].

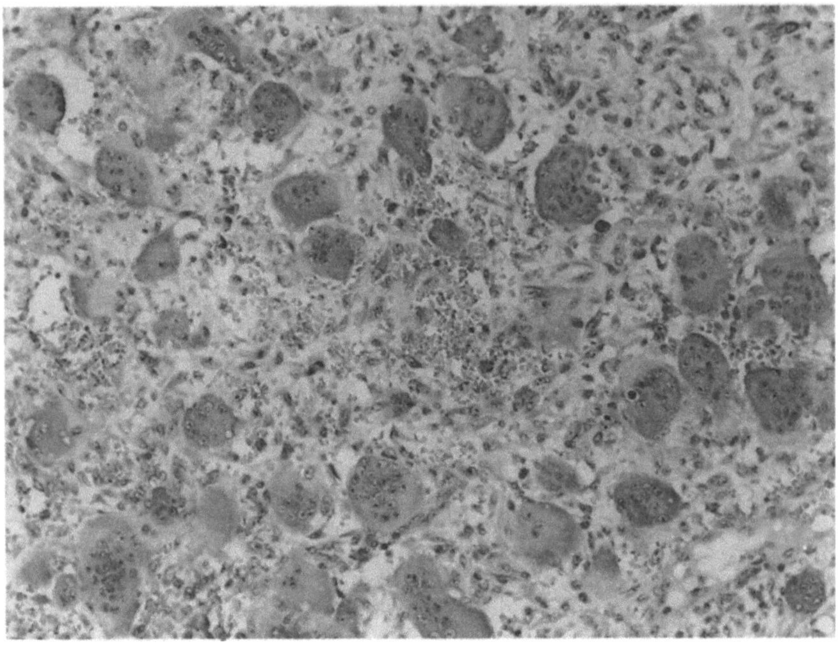

Fig. 3.97. Giant-cell jaw lesion of hyperparathyroidism. H. & E. stain, ×160

The exact etiology of this malady remains unknown. Paget's disease is a condition of middle and old age, occurring twice as common in men as women [223]. Some evidence suggests a familial aspect, and the condition has been seen in identical twins [224, 225]. An advanced case of Paget's disease presents as a patient with an enlarged head, sunken chest, curved back, bowed legs, and disproportionaltcly long arms. The onset is insidious, and the course of the disease is slowly progressive. Later, the patient usually becomes aware of a bone deformity. Another symptom that may cause the sufferer to seek medical attention is a deep, dull constant ache in the bones. Headache and deafness can also ensue, if the skull is involved [223].

One laboratory characteristic of patients with Paget's disease is an elevated serum alkaline phosphatase. In Woodward's study of 144 patients with uncomplicated Paget's disease, 25 with osteogenic sarcoma, and 2 with giant-cell tumor complicating Paget's disease, the median level of serum alkaline phosphatase was 23 Bodansky Units (normal) for an adult is 1.5–5 B.U.) with a range of 4 to 267. Patients who had only minor elevation or no change in their serum alkaline phosphatase levels had either very small lesions or else inactive bone lesions [226].

The radiographic picture depends upon the stage of progression of Paget's disease. During the early osteolytic phase, bone density is decreased, and a "ground-glass" appearance is common. Teeth in the affected jaw may show hypercementosis (Fig. 3.98). As the disease progresses, osteoblastic activity increases, and irregular osteosclerosis becomes a prominent feature. The combined

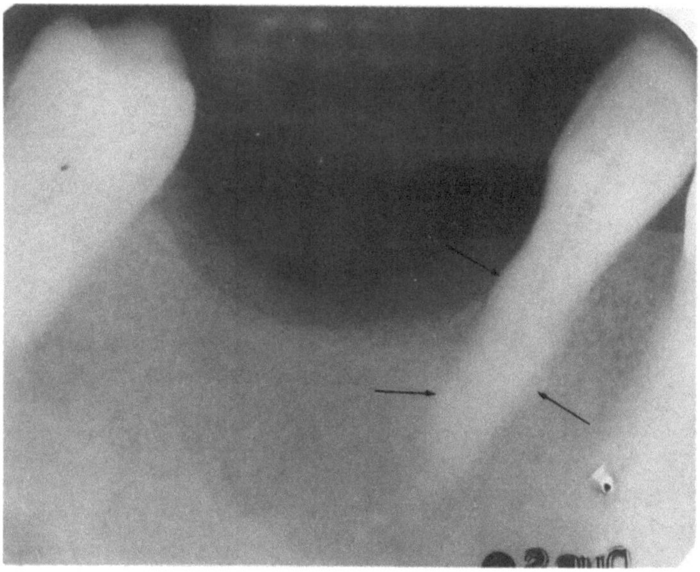

Fig. 3.98. Hypercementosis (*arrows*) in a patient with Paget's disease of bone

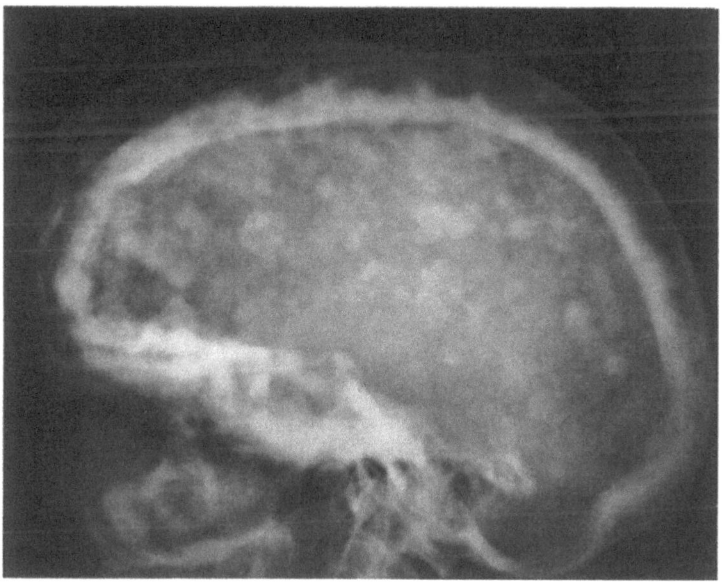

Fig. 3.99. "Cotton-wool" appearance of the skull in a radiograph during a combined phase of Paget's disease. (Courtesy of Drs. D. Wilner and R.S. Sherman)

phase of both bone absorption and production can produce the "cottonwool" appearance of the skull and separation of bony tables (Fig. 3.99) [227].

Microscopically, the initial lesions are characterized by vascularity, fibrosis, and multinucleated giant cells that resorb bone in an expanding fashion. The

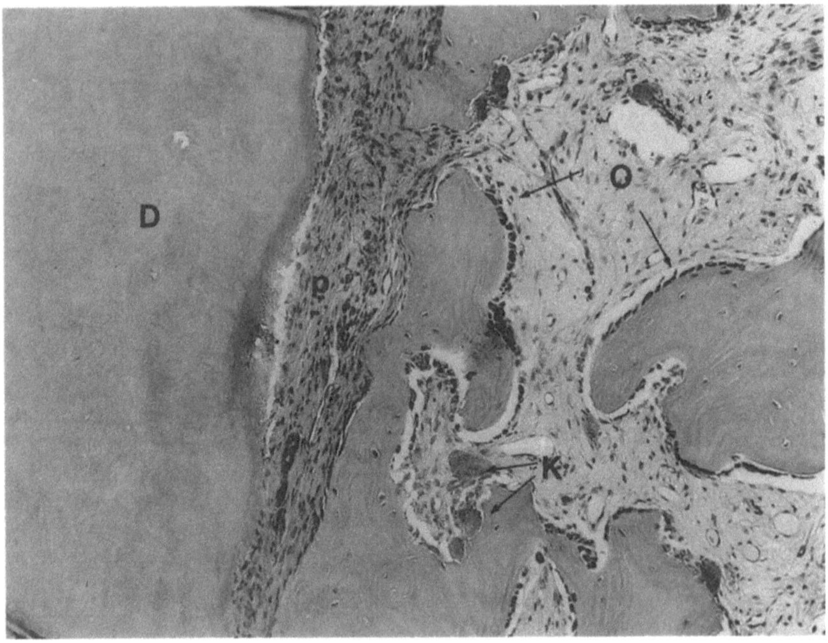

Fig. 3.100. Paget's disease of bone. *D*, tooth; *P*, periodontal membrane; *O*, osteoblastic activity; *K*, osteoclastic activity. H. & E. stain, ×100

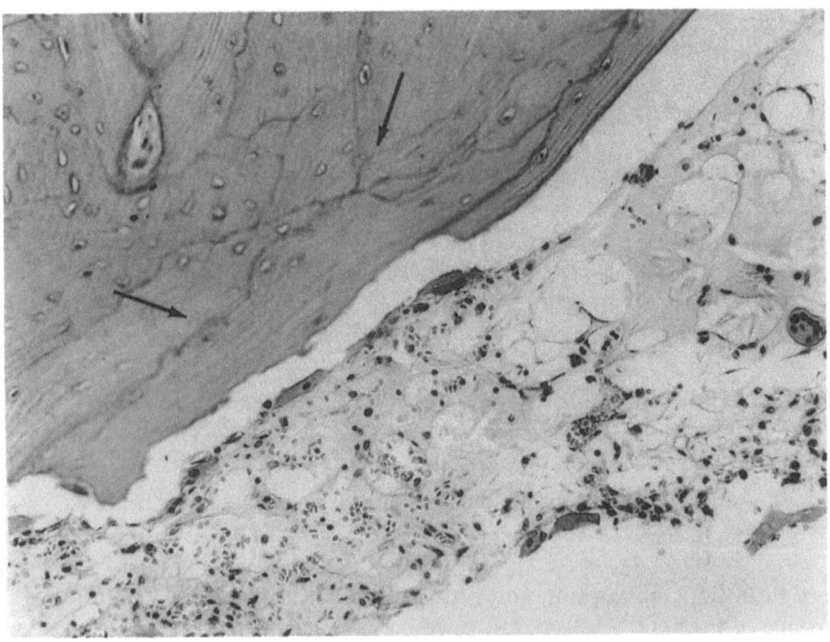

Fig. 3.101. "Mosaic pattern" of cement lines in bone (*arrows*) in Paget's disease. H. & E. stain, ×160

osteoblastic and osteoclastic phases can occur simultaneously, as shown in Fig. 3.100. Because both destruction and repair of bone tend to repeat themselves in the same area, there is a bizarre, patternless arrangement of the cement lines, which has been described as the "mosaic pattern" of Paget's disease (Fig. 3.101).

3. Malignant Fibro-Osseous Lesions of the Jaws

The three malignant fibro-osseous tumors of the jaws are fibrosarcoma, osteosarcoma, and chondrosarcoma.

(A) Fibrosarcoma

In their 1972 article, Richardson, Fine, and Goldman reported a maxillary case of fibrosarcoma and presented a review of the literature on this malignancy [229]. They found eight histologically documented cases of fibrosarcoma and added one of their own. Hamilton's case was missed [230], Saw reported a case in 1978 [231], and the 13 cases from Dahlin and Ivin's Mayo Clinic study were not included [136]. Even so, a total of only 24 cases indicates the rarity of fibrosarcoma occurring in the jawbones.

From this paucity of case information the following picture emerges. It has been estimated that less than 20% of body fibrosarcomas occur centrally in the bone, and it is often difficult to determine whether the tumor arose in soft tissue or intraosseously [232]. Of the 24 intra-oral fibrosarcomas of the jaws, 20 have been found in the mandible. It customarily appears as a bulky, slow-growing, locally invasive neoplasm. Teeth in the affected area become loosened and mobile, and ulceration of the overlying mucosa can occur. Asymmetric swelling is a common finding; pain and parasthesia are later symptoms, indicating nerve involvement [229].

Metastasis of fibrosarcoma occurs late, is predominantly hemotagenous, and usually goes to the lungs. Twelve of the 13 patients in Dahlin and Ivin's survey were available for followup. Eight of the 12 died within 5 years, one was a terminal case with widespread metastases in the fifth year, and three were alive with no evidence of disease [136].

X-rays of the central fibrosarcoma reveal an osteolytic, radiolucent tumor with poorly defined, irregular margins [229], Histologically, this tumor is composed of pleomorphic spindle-shaped cells arranged in bands or interweaving patterns with variable amounts of collagen interspersed between them (Fig. 3.102). The nuclei are hyperchromatic, elongated, and have a "combed" appearance. Mitoses may be sparse or plentiful and assume bizarre forms [10]. Saw reported strong alkaline phosphatase activity in these tumor cells in her histochemical study [231]. Radical surgery is the most commonly accepted method of treatment [136].

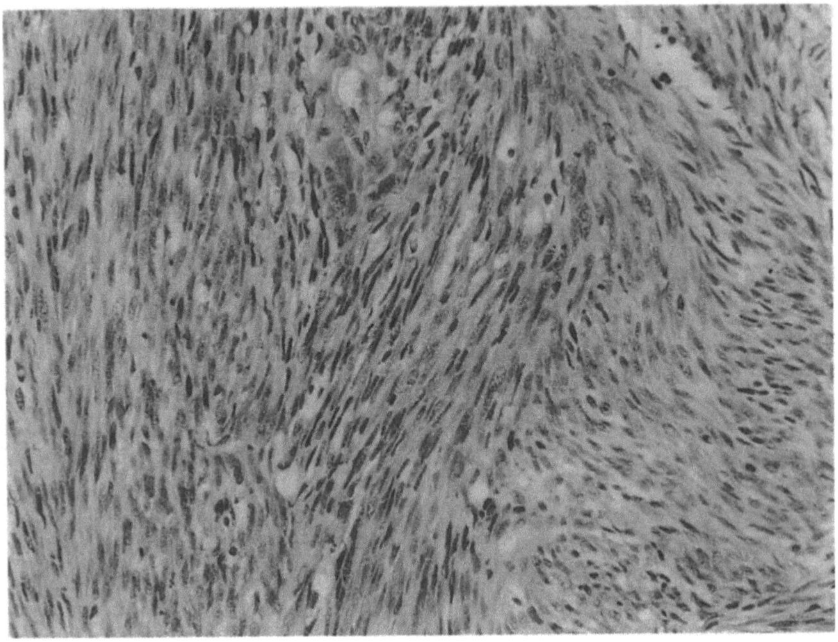

Fig. 3.102. Fibrosarcoma. H. & E. stain, ×250

(B) Osteosarcoma

The best summation of osteogenic sarcoma of the jaws is afforded by Garrington, et al.'s Armed Forces Institute of Pathology analysis of 56 osteosarcomas and 36 chondrosarcomas [223].

The age range for these 56 osteosarcomas of the jaws was 4 to 64 years. The median age for osteosarcoma of the maxilla was 28 years, while the median age for patients with mandibular osteosarcoma was 25 years. Maxillary tumors peaked (41%) in the 20–29 year old group, whereas mandibular tumors followed a more normal distribution, occurring in both the young and the elderly. The mean age for osteosarcoma of the jaws is about 10 years later than for osteosarcoma in other bony locations [233]. Of the 55 patients in which sex was specified in the available history, 31 were males and 24 were females. In regard to site of origin, 38 osteosarcomas were located in the mandible and 18 in the maxilla. 22/24 of the female patients presented with mandibular tumors [233].

The etiology of most osteosarcomas remains unknown. Some have arisen in pre-existing lesions, and others have been iatrogenically produced by radiation [234–236]. Trauma has been mentioned as a possible cause, however, most investigators now generally believe that the traumatic episode probably only draws attention to a pre-existing lesion, rather than being instrumental in its pathogenesis [167]. In Garrington's survey of jaw sarcoma, only 9/56 had a history of possible trauma to the affected site [233]. Kragh, Dahlin and Erich found only 2/44 of the Mayo Clinic patients with osteosarcoma of the jaws

Table 3.18. Frequency of presenting symptoms for jaw osteosarcomas

	Kragh et al. [237] (no. of cases)			Garrington et al. [233] (no. of cases)		
Symptom comparison	Maxilla	Mandible	Total	Maxilla	Mandible	Total
1. Swelling or tumor mass	12/14	18/19	30/33	16/16	34/38	50/54
2. Pain	4/14	8/19	12/33	5/16	18/38	23/54
3. Parasthesia	0/14	5/19	5/33	0/16	7/38	7/54
4. Loosening of teeth	1/14	1/19	2/33	3/16	6/38	9/54

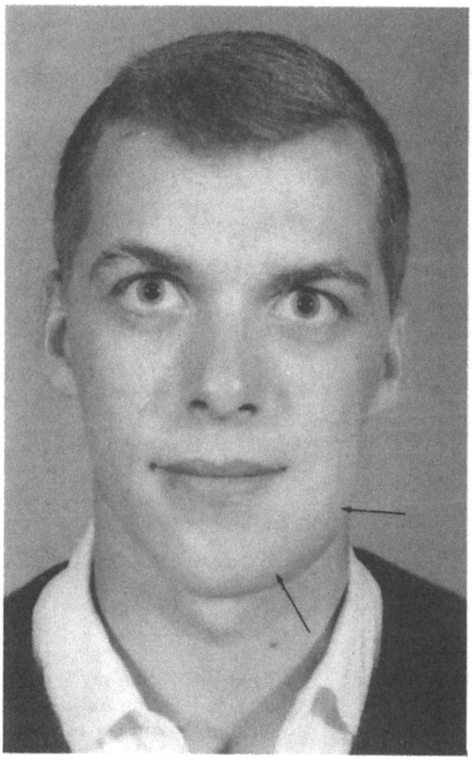

Fig. 3.103. Osteosarcoma in a 24-year-old Caucasian male, producing left mandibular swelling (*arrows*)

and facial bones who described a history of trauma, and the traumatic episode had transpired many years prior to the onset of osteosarcoma in both cases [237].

Presenting symptoms may include swelling, pain, parasthesia, loosened teeth, bleeding, headache, toothache, etc. Table 3.18 compares the frequency of presenting symptoms for osteosarcoma in either the maxilla or mandible in the Garrington and Kragh surveys. Similar to osteosarcoma's symptoms in other bones, swelling and pain were most prominent. An example of such neoplastic swelling is seen in Fig. 3.103, obvious asymmetric clinical enlargement of the left mandible in a 24-year-old Caucasian male with osteosarcoma. Figure 3.104

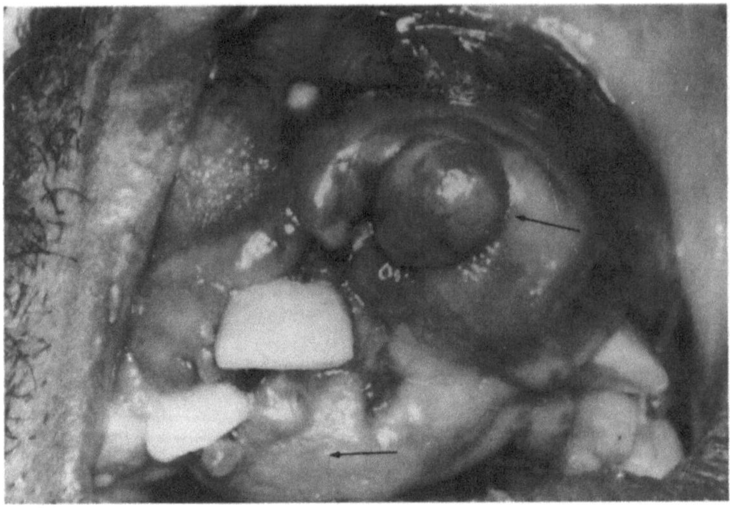

Fig. 3.104. Maxillary midline osteosarcoma (*arrow*) extending into the palate (*arrow*) in a 34-year-old Negro male

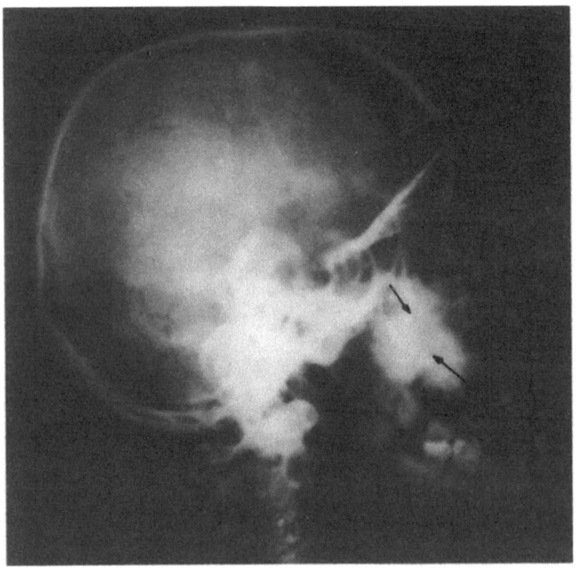

Fig. 3.105. "Sun-ray" effect in a radiograph of a right maxillary antral osteosarcoma (*arrows*), sclerotic type, in a 20-year-old Caucasian male. (A.F.I.P. Accesion #328118)

illustrates a bulky, expansile osteosarcoma that has extended from the maxillary midline into the palate, causing both loss and displacement of the remaining teeth.

The radiographic appearance of osteosarcoma can vary from radiolucent to radiopaque, depending on whether it is a lytic, sclerotic, or mixed type. Certain of the osteosarcomas exhibit the "sun-ray" effect with ossific laminae radiating out in a sunburst pattern about the periphery of the tumor (Fig. 3.105).

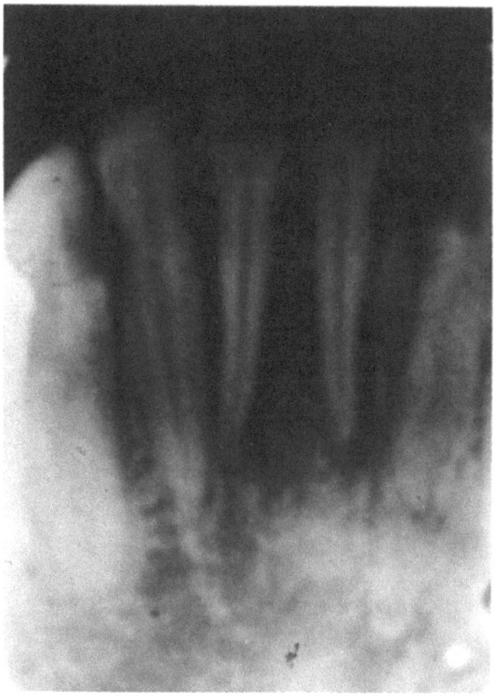

Fig. 3.106. Dental periapical x-rays demonstrating marked symmetrical widening of the periodontal membrane by a mandibular symphysis osteosarcoma in a 26-year-old Caucasian male

This pattern was seen in 25% of the A.F.I.P. survey cases [223], and while it is helpful in adding to the diagnostic value of the x-ray, it isn't essential for diagnosis. The "sun-ray" pattern has been noted in other bone conditions.

Symmetrical widening of the periodontal membrane, seen on dental periapical films of teeth in the tumor-affected area, has been described as prominent radiographic evidence of osteosarcoma [233, 238]. This finding is important because this early feature is often quite striking before the tumor shows other definite radiographic characteristies to indicate its presence. This same feature was noted by Garrington in some of his chondrosarcoma cases [233]. Figure 3.106 shows such marked periodontal thickening. Scleroderma is the only other known disease which shows periodontal membrane thickening [10].

Osteosarcoma is characterized histologically by tumor osteoid and/or osseous tissue arising directly from a sarcomatous stroma without passing through a cartilagenous phase [167, 237]. The stromal tissue is composed of malignant spindle cells or polyhedral cells. Therefore, the stromal cells may be predominately osteoblastic (Fig. 3.107), chondroblastic (Fig. 3.108), or fibroblastic (Fig. 3.109). The osteoid and bone portions can vary from small, randomly scattered foci to densely packed interlacing, irregularly calcified malignant bone [167].

The therapy of choice, in terms of survival, is radical surgery [167, 233, 237]. If palpable positive lymph nodes are present, neck dissection does improve survival [233]. In Garrington's follow-up on 56 jaw osteosarcoma cases, the 5-year survival rate was 35%, the 10-year survival rate was 30%, and the 15-year survival rate was 22% [233]. The prognosis for mandibular osteosarcomas is

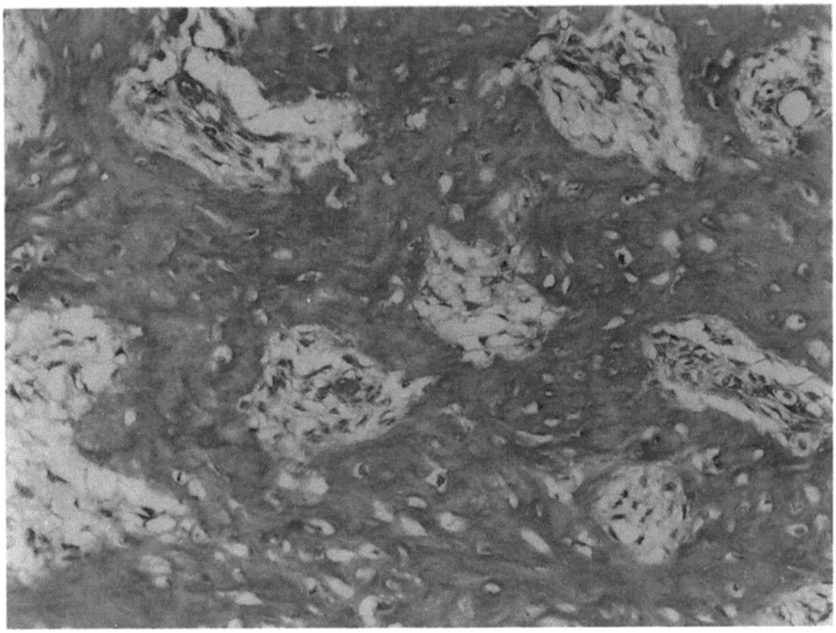

Fig. 3.107. Osteogenic osteosarcoma. H. & E. stain, ×250

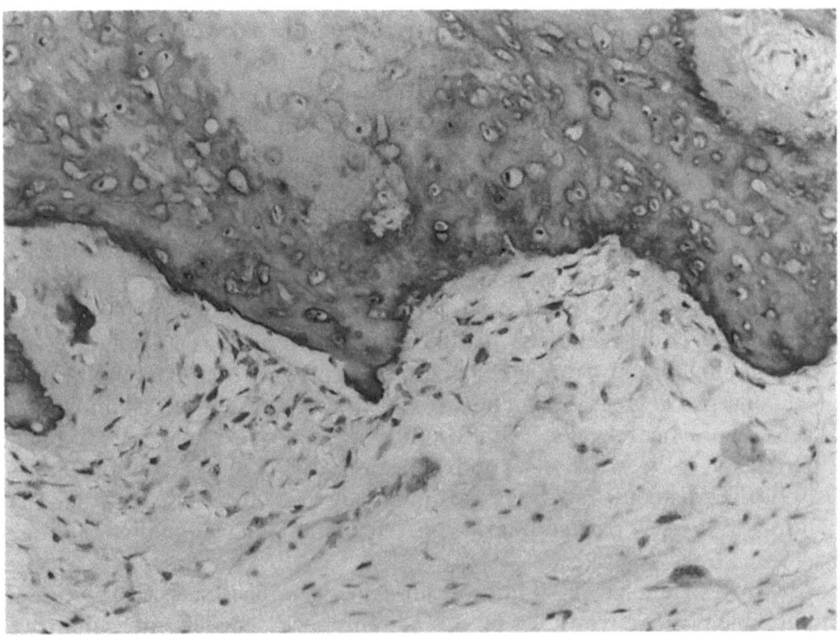

Fig. 3.108. Chondroblastic osteosarcoma; transition form cartilage to malignant bone. H. & E. stain, ×250

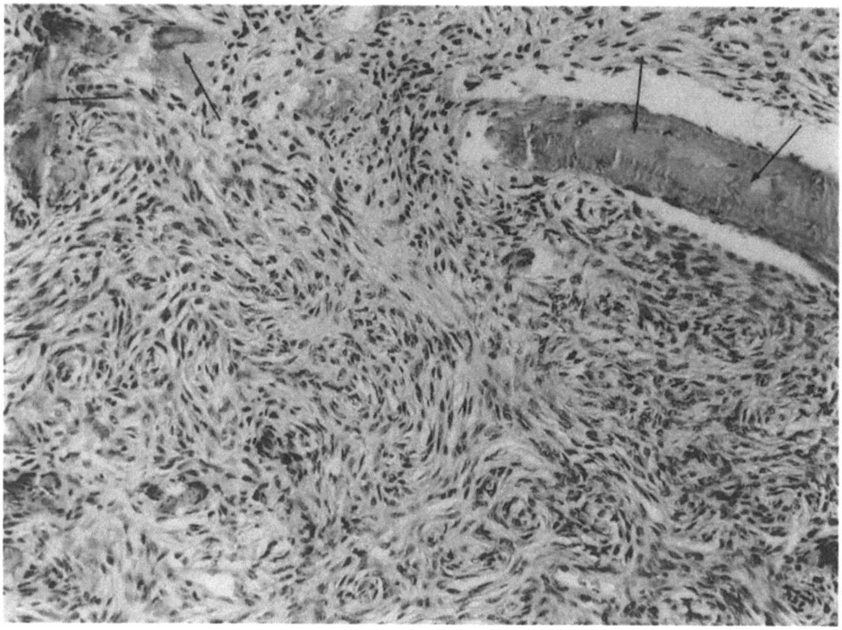

Fig. 3.109. Fibroblastic osteosarcoma; malignant bone and osteoid portion (*arrows*). H. & E. stain, ×160

better than that for the maxillary counterpart. The worst survival rate in the A.F.I.P. study was seen in the maxillary antral tumors.

Parosteal osteosarcoma is a very rare bone-forming neoplasm that represents less than 4% of all osteosarcomas [239]. Newland and Ayala reported a maxillary parosteal osteosarcoma in 1977 and reviewed the other 4 literature cases involving the jaws [240].

This tumor is a slow-growing variant of osteosarcoma. It usually is associated with the distal end of the femur and arises in either the periosteum or adjacent parosteal connective tissue, merging with the subjacent cortex along part of its sessile base [167, 241]. The lesions thus present as hard masses attached to the affected bone. Microscopically, the tumor consists of a sparse, malignant fibrous stroma with abundant, irregular bony trabeculae attached to the underlying cortex along the tumor base [167, 240]. Three of the 4 previously reported parosteal osteosarcomas of the jaws were free of local recurrence or metastases after 5 years [240].

(C) Chondrosarcoma

Chondrosarcomas are the second most common primary malignant tumor of the bone. It is a malignant cartilaginous tumor, arising de novo in bone or superimposed upon a pre-existing benign cartilaginous tumor. These neoplasms grow slowly, often extending along pathways of least resistance. However, it is capable of vascular invasion with metastases being most commonly seen

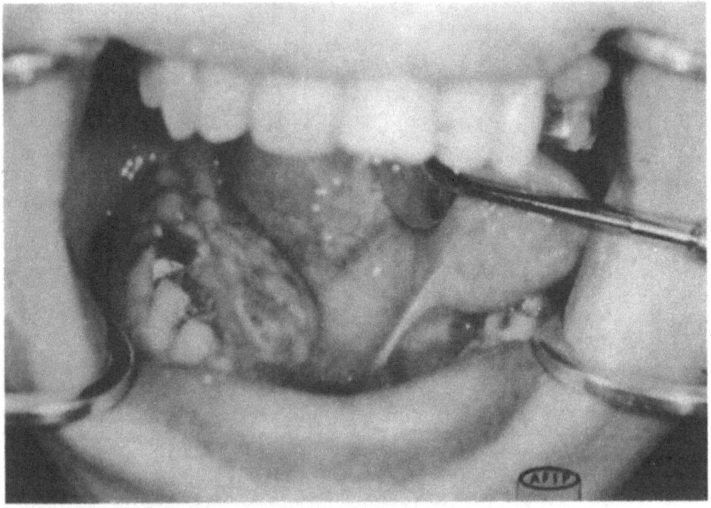

Fig. 3.110. Chondrosarcoma with lingual expansion of the right posterior mandible by the tumor in a 20-year-old Caucasian male. (A.F.I.P. Accession #930763)

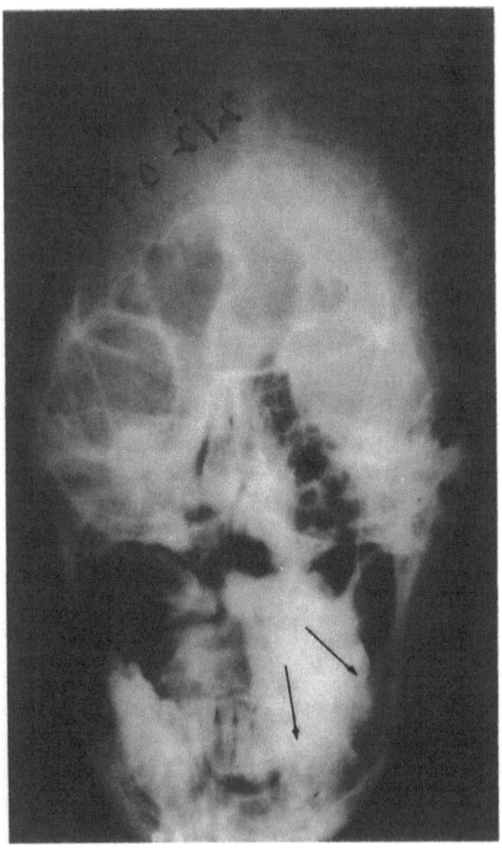

Fig. 3.111. Chondrosarcoma, left maxilla of a 29-year-old Caucasian male; note the partial "sun-ray" effect on the lower periphery of the x-ray (*arrows*)

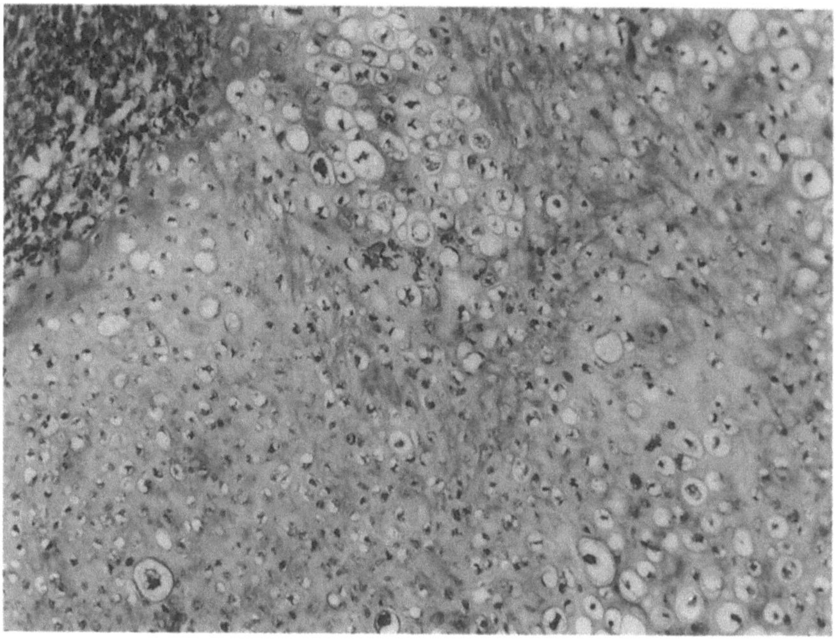

Fig. 3.112. Chrondrosarcoma. H. & E. stain, ×100

in the lungs and occasionally in liver, kidney, and brain. Metastasis via lymph nodes are quite rare.

Through 1974, the Armed Forces Institute of Pathology had collected 60 cases of chondrosarcomas of the jaws (compared to 141 accessioned cases of osteosarcoma). The age range of these patients was from 12 to 80 years [242]. Swelling and some degree of pain are the chief clinical features. Figure 3.110 illustrates tumor swelling and surface ulceration on the lingual side of the right mandible of a 20 year-old Caucasian male with chondrosarcoma. The patient died 2 years later with lung metastases.

The radiographic appearance of the chondrosarcoma varies from a radiolucent lytic lesion to one with radiopaque calcifications, such as Fig. 3.111, which has a partial "sun-ray" effect on the lower periphery.

The histologic diagnosis of chondrosarcoma can pose problems since many of the well-differentiated tumors are easily confused and erroneously diagnosed as benign cartilaginous neoplasms. Therefore, several blocks of tissue should be examined. The malignant cartilaginous cells appear in hypercellular fashion (Fig. 3.112) and contain nuclei that may be plump, bizarre, grotesquely enlarged, and bipolar or tripolar (Fig. 3.113). In addition to changes in the cartilage cells, foci of bone formation, myxoid zones, and calcification may be seen. Calcification is more common in the moderate to well-differentiated chondrosarcomas [167].

Slootweg reported the only case of clear-cell chondrosarcoma occurring in the maxillary left cuspid area of a 50 year-old Caucasian woman in 1980 [243].

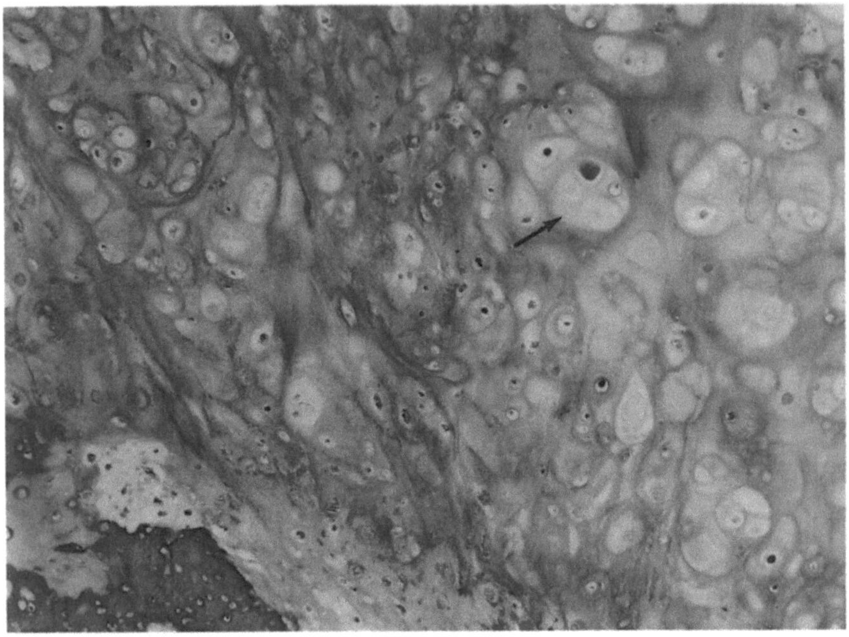

Fig. 3.113. Chondrosarcoma with bizarre, tripolar nuclei (*arrow*). H. & E. stain, ×160

This tumor is a slowly growing variant of chondrosarcoma, and it is characterized by the present of giant cells, clear cells, and pleomorphic cells in a cartilaginous matrix [243].

In 1981, Caravolas, et al. described a case of mesenchymal chondrosarcoma, occurring in the left posterior mandible of a 12-year-old Caucasian boy [244]. It is a highly malignant variant of chondrosarcoma which has a strong tendency to recur and metastasize. Fifteen of the previously reported cases in a review of 81 cases by Joshi were located in either the maxilla or mandible [245].

Treatment for chondrosarcoma is radical block resection of the affected portion. Five-year survival rates vary form 48% to 76%, and 10-year survival rates vary from 35% to 69% [167].

VII. Salivary Gland Tumors

One classification of salivary gland tumors is depicted in Table 3.19. The listed percentage of occurrence is the incidence rate in the United States for salivary gland tumors. These neoplasms are rare, comprising only 1–4% of all head- and neck tumors. The malignant varieties account for 35% of all salivary gland tumors [5, 10].

Diagnosis of salivary gland tumors is based upon patient history, palpation, clinical signs and symptoms, sialography, radioisotope scans, and surgical biopsy.

Table 3.19. Classification of salivary gland tumors with percentage of occurrence

	%[a]
I. *Benign*	
(1) Pleomorphic adenoma (mixed tumor)	58
(2) Papillary cystadenoma lymphomatosum (Warthin's tumor)	6
(3) Oxyphilic adenoma (oncocytoma)	1
II. *Malignant*	
(1) Malignant mixed tumor	7
(2) Mucoepidermoid carcinoma	12
(3) Adenocarcinoma	11
(A) Adenoid cystic carcinoma (cylindroma)	
(B) Acinic cell adenocarcinoma	
(4) Epidermoid carcinoma	5

[a] The listed percentage of occurrence is the incidence rate for major salivary gland tumors in the United States

Table 3.20. Survival rates for malignant salivary gland tumors

Type	Five-year survival rate (%)	Twenty-year survival rate (%)
1. Malignant mixed tumor	50	20
2. Mucoepidermoid carcinoma		
A) Low-grade tumor	95	
B) High-grade tumor	50	
3. Adenoid cystic carcinoma	75	15
4. Acinic cell adenocarcinoma	90	56
5. Epidermoid carcinoma	25	5

The malignant salivary gland tumors exhibit no sex predominance and tend to be more prevalent after 50 year of age. Clinical signs and symptoms typically include pain, sudden growth, facial nerve paralysis, a firm consistency, poor demarcation with infiltration into the surrounding tissues, and metastatic spread by either lymphatic or hematogenous routes [5, 10, 246].

In terms of anatomic site, approximately 80% of salivary gland tumors occur in the parotid gland, 10% in the submandibular gland, 1% in the sublingual gland, and 9% in minor salivary glands [5, 10, 246].

Treatment is most often surgical resection or surgery used in conjunction with radiation therapy. The latter regimen is more effective for epidermoid carcinoma than for the adenocarcinomas. Survival rates are listed in Table 3.20. Unfortunately, salivary gland tumors tend to recur because of the difficulty of complete surgical eradication and a tendency to distant metastases. In spite of fairly good 5-year survival rates, these cancers often pursue a relentless course over the years, resulting in a much lower 20-year survival rate [5, 10].

For the purpose of diagnostic clarification, we shall limit the discussion of salivary glands tumors to a brief resume of pertinent clinical features and the histopathological differentiation of each, with appropriate examples.

1. Benign Tumors

(A) Pleomorphic Adenoma (Mixed Tumor)

This tumor is not truly teratomatous – only the epithelial element is neoplastic; the other tissues represent metaplastic stroma. It comprises the majority (58%) of all salivary gland tumors and 90% of all benign salivary gland tumors. Most investigators believe that this tumor originates through neoplastic transformation of glandular ductal epithelium. The parotid gland is the most common site. It occurs chiefly in the age group 30–60-years old. It presents as a painless, slowly enlarging nodule without fixation to skin or deeper tissues. The skin seldom ulcerates, although the tumors can grow to huge sizes. Histologically, it is the most diverse salivary gland tumor. Cuboidal cells may be arranged in tubes or duct-like structures which contain an eosinophilic coagulum. In other areas tumor cells can assume stellate, polyhedral, or spindle form [247]. Loose myxoid material, foci of hyalinized connective tissue, cartilage, or even bone may be present (see Fig. 3.114). Recurrence is a tedious problem because the tumor cells frequently infiltrate the fibrous capsule (Fig. 3.115).

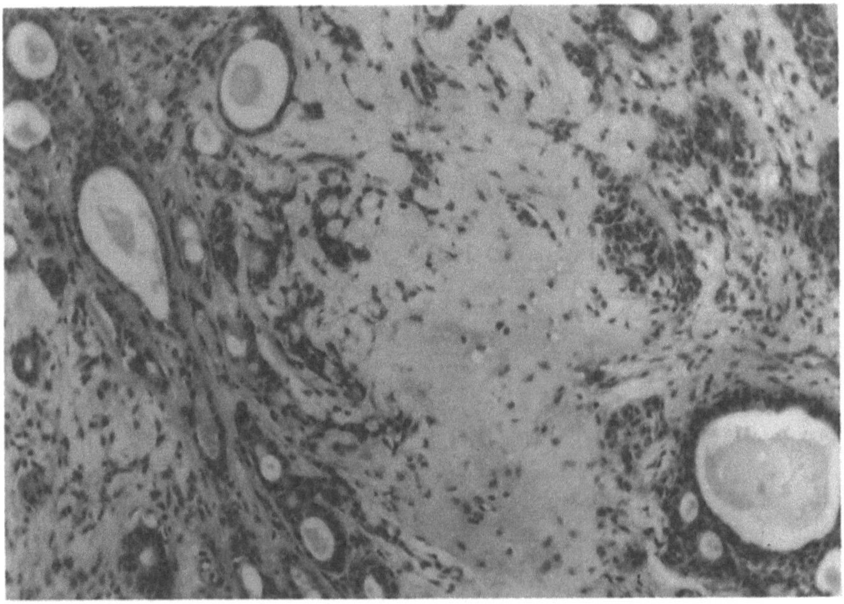

Fig. 3.114. Mixed tumor, parotid. H. & E. stain, ×65

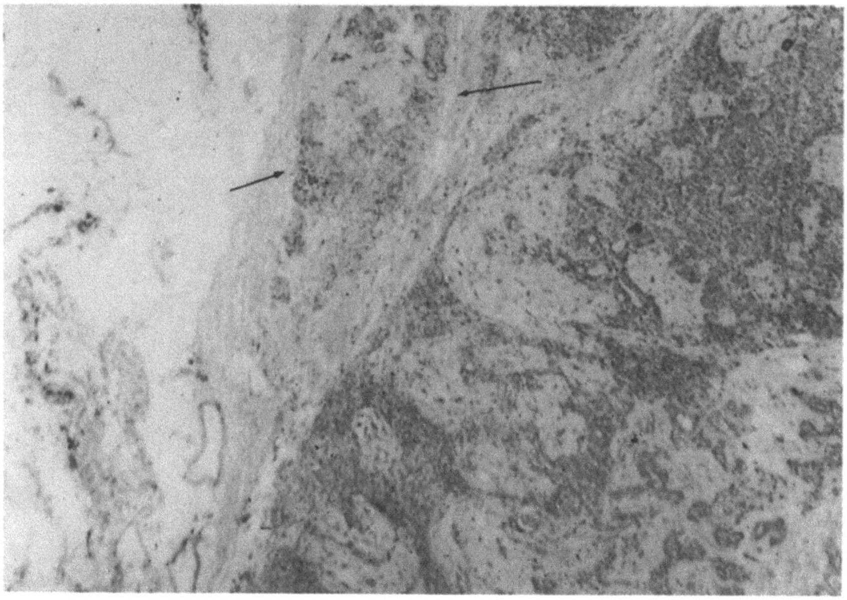

Fig. 3.115. Mixed tumor, parotid; note the tumor cells (*arrows*) infiltrating the fibrous capsule. H. &E. stain, ×90

(B) Papillary Cystadenoma Lymphomatosum (Warthin's Tumor)

This benign tumor occurs almost exclusively in the parotid gland. The most accepted theory of histogenesis is that this tumor originates from heterotropic salivary gland tissue entraped or included within lymph nodes during embryogenesis. It occurs chiefly in men in a 5:1 ratio within the 41–70 year age bracket, is generally a superficial tumor, and seldom exceeds 4 cm in diamter [5, 10, 44].

Histologically, Warthin's tumor is an adenoma exhibiting cystic spaces and a lymphoid matrix with germinal centers. The epithelial cells covering the papillary projections are columnar or cuboidal cells arranged in two rows (Fig. 3.116).

(C) Oxyphilic Adenoma (Oncocytoma)

This is an extremely rare, benign salivary gland tumor found most often in the parotid gland. The name "oncocytoma" is derived from the resemblance of these tumor cells to normal cells which have been called "oncocytes" and which are found in numerous locations, e.g., salivary glands, respiratory tract, breast, thyroid, pancreas, parathyroid, pituitary, testicle, fallopian tube, liver, and stomach. The cytoplasm is choked with mitochondria [5, 10, 44, 247].

It is seen chiefly in women among elderly persons. The oncocytoma occurs as a discrete 3–5 cm, encapsulated mass, and pain is usually absent. The characteristic tumor cells are large with eosinophilic cytoplasm, have distinct cell membranes, and are arranged in rows or cords. They can occur in sheets and exhibit an alveolar or lobular pattern (Fig. 3.117).

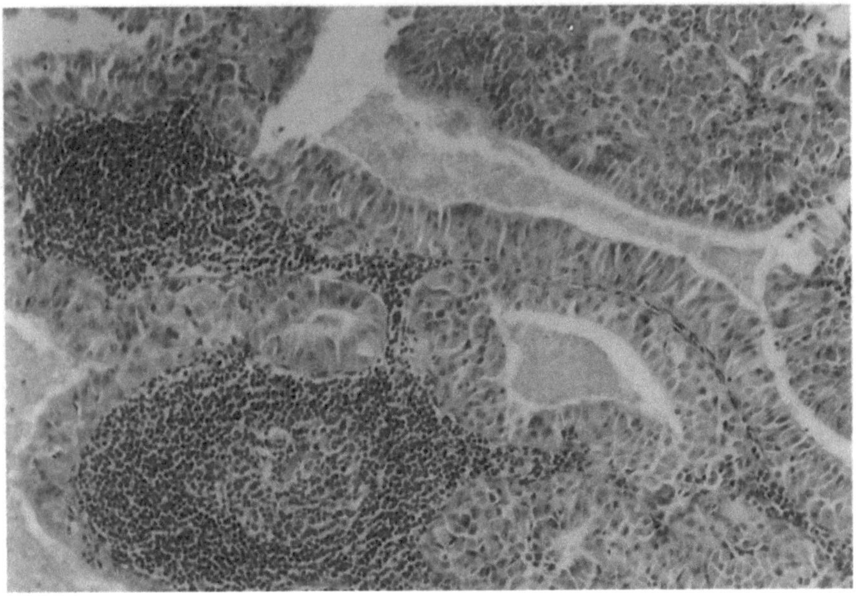

Fig. 3.116. Papillary cystadenoma lymphomatosum, parotid. H. & E. stain, ×115

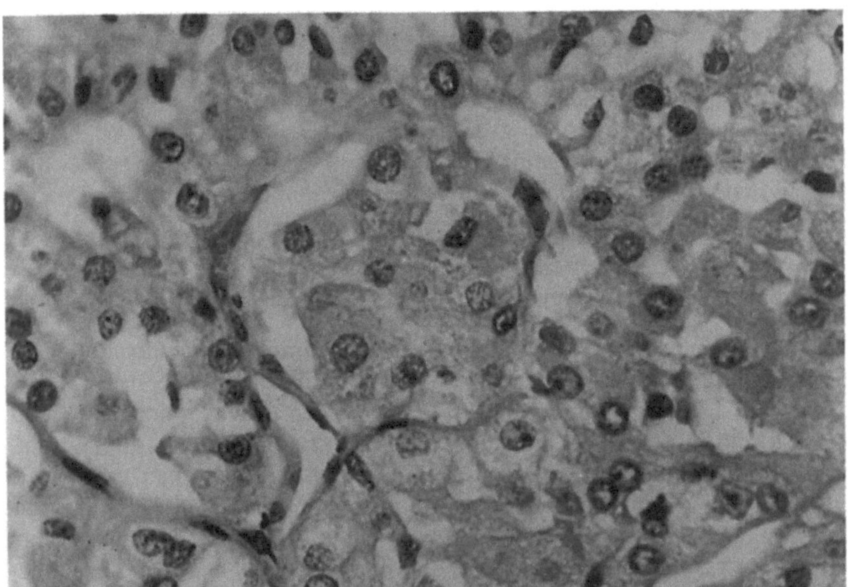

Fig. 3.117. Oxyphilic adenoma with its characteristic oncocyte cells, parotid. H. & E. stain, ×250

2. Malignant Tumors

(A) Malignant Mixed Tumor

This tumor is rare and has no obvious clinical differences from the benign mixed tumor except for deeper tissue fixation, possible pain, and the likelihood of metastatic lesions. Often, it is metastasis that establishes the diagnosis. Careful histologic study is needed to demonstrate the malignant areas in certain cases, while in others the malignant cells overgrow the benign areas. Specific histologic changes are those criteria indicative of malignancy elsewhere, e.g., nuclear hyperchromatism, abnormal mitotic figures, a disproportionate nuclear/cytoplasm ratio, etc. Figure 3.118 is an example of malignant mixed tumor. Distant metastases are common as well as regional lymph nodal involvement, and unfortunately, the recurrence rate is high [5, 10, 247].

(B) Mucoepidermoid Carcinoma

This pleomorphic tumor occurs in the 20–60 year age bracket equally in both men and women [15]. It may grow slowly or rapidly depending on the degree of malignancy.

The mucoepidermoid carcinoma is composed of three main cell types: mucus-secreting cells, epidermoid-type cells, and intermediate cells. Mucus-secreting cells and epidermoid-type cells predominate in the low-grade carcinoma (Fig. 3.119). The intermediate cells appear to give rise to the other two types, are smaller in size, and occur in solid epithelial sheets. Mucin is easily demon-

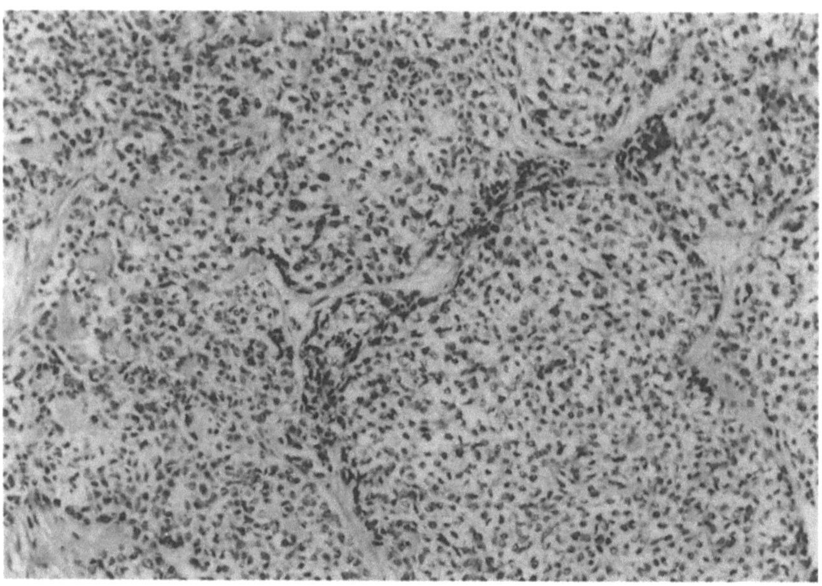

Fig. 3.118. Malignant mixed tumor, parotid. H. & E. stain, ×65

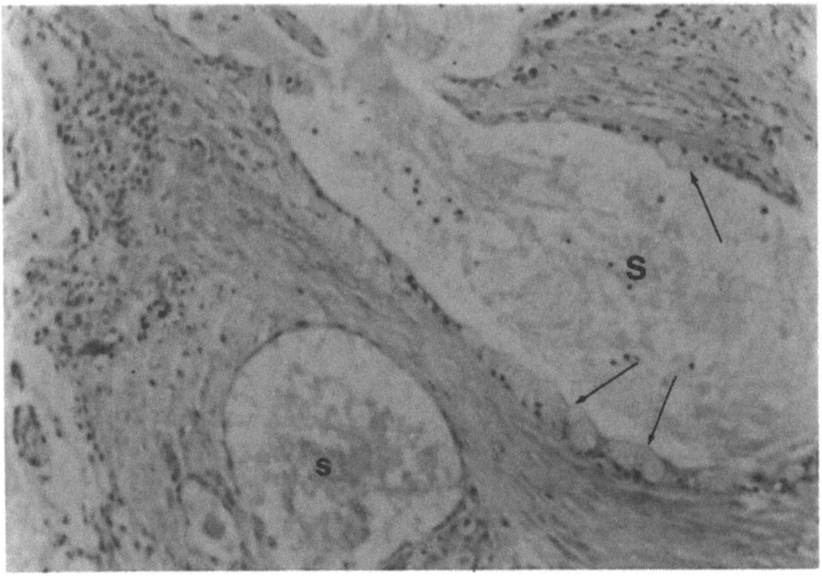

Fig. 3.119. Mucoepidermoid carcinoma (low-grade variety), parotid; note the mucus-secreting cells (*arrows*) and cystic spaces (*S*). H. & E. stain, ×160

strated in the columnar cells of the more highly-differentiated tumors by the mucicarmine stain. These cells can present an arrangement of glandlike structures with microcyst formation [5, 10, 247].

Ultrastructural studies have identified three forms of the intermediate cells: mitochondria-rich cells, glycogen-rich cells, and ribosome-rich cells. The cells which are rich in glycogen appear as the "clear cells" under light microscopy. Ribosome-rich cells appear basophilic, and mitochondria-rich cells appear lightly eosinophilic under normal light microscopy [248, 249].

(C) Adenocarcinoma

This malignant salivery gland tumor can occur in two types.

(a) Adenoid Cystic Carcinoma (Cylindroma)

This tumor is often found in the parotid, the submandibular, and accessory glands in the tongue and palate. It occurs usually in the 40–60 year age group. In Nochomovitz and Kahn's review of 384 salivary gland tumors in South Africa, 30/384, or 8%, were adenoid cystic carcinomas. The 30 tumors were divided 16 to 14 among women and men. The age range was 20 to 90 years with a mean age at diagnosis of 57.3 years. Eleven cases were detected in the parotid, 9 in the palate, 5 in the submandibular gland, and 5 in other locations [250].

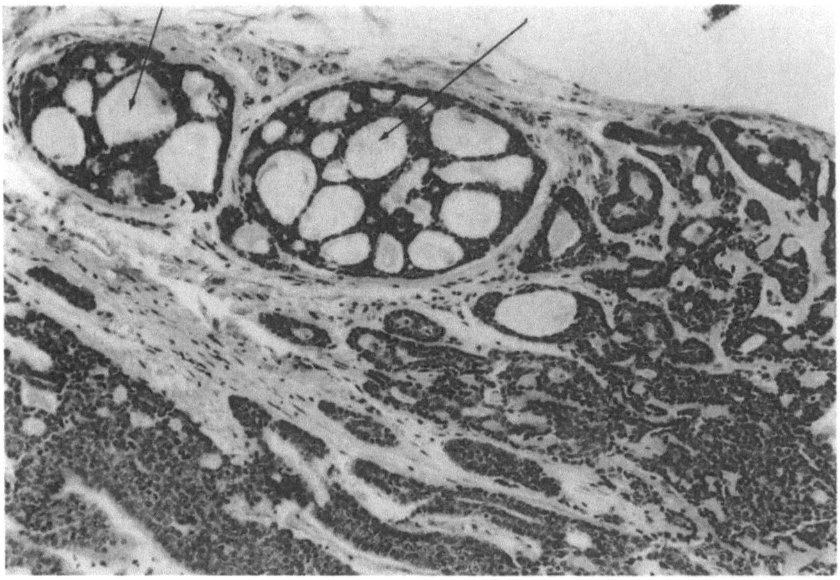

Fig. 3.120. Adenoid cystic carcinoma, parotid; note the cylindromatous, "Swiss-cheese" appearance (*arrows*). H. & E. stain, ×100

Clinical features include: early local pain, facial nerve paralysis, deeper tissue fixation, and local invasion. Prognosis is not favorable. In the South African study 25/30 cases were available for follow-up. Ten of the 25 patients had died between five months and 10 years following diagnosis; four of them had distant metastases. About half of the remaining 15 had evidence of persistant malignancy with a mean follow-up time of 81 months [250].

The adenoid cystic carcinoma (cylindroma) is composed of small, darkly staining uniform cells closely arranged in anastomosing cords or ductlike patterns, the central portion of which may contain mucoid or hyaline material (Fig. 3.120). The end result is a honeycomb or "Swiss cheese" appearance. The stromal tissue often becomes hyalinized, and because it surrounds the tumor cells, a cylindromatous pattern evolves. This tumor is extremely malignant, yet the histological appearance is deceptively benign [5, 247, 250].

(b) Acinic Cell Adenocarcinoma

Abrams, et al's fine clinico-pathologic analysis of 77 cases of acinic cell adenocarcinoma at the A.F.I.P. serves as the benchmark for this malignancy. In his study, the parotid gland was the most common site of tumor occurrence; the 20–30 year age group was the most frequently affected; these tumors were more common in females than males; and pain and fixation were ominous clinical features in terms of prognosis [251]. Abrams' review of 9 new cases and 20 literature cases of acinic cell adenocarcinomas in minor salivary glands presented a similar picture [252].

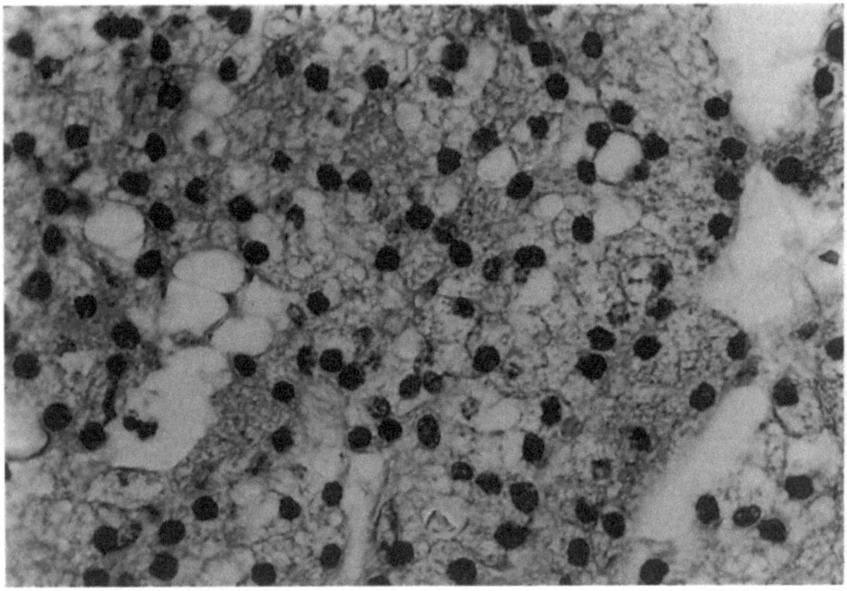

Fig. 3.121. Acinic cell type acinic cell adenocarcinoma in a solid parenchymatous growth pattern. H. & E. stain, ×250

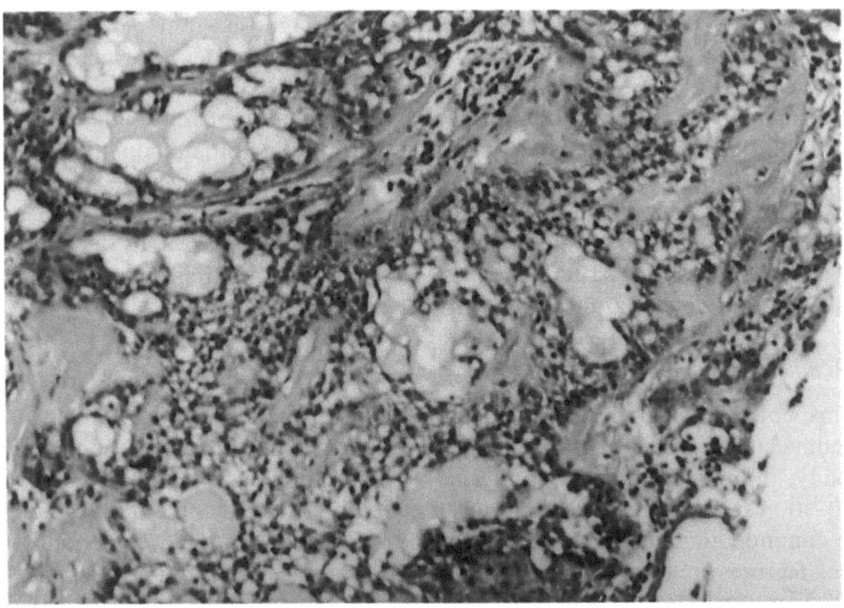

Fig. 3.122. Acinic cell adenocarcinoma, vacuolated cell type. H. & E. stain, ×110

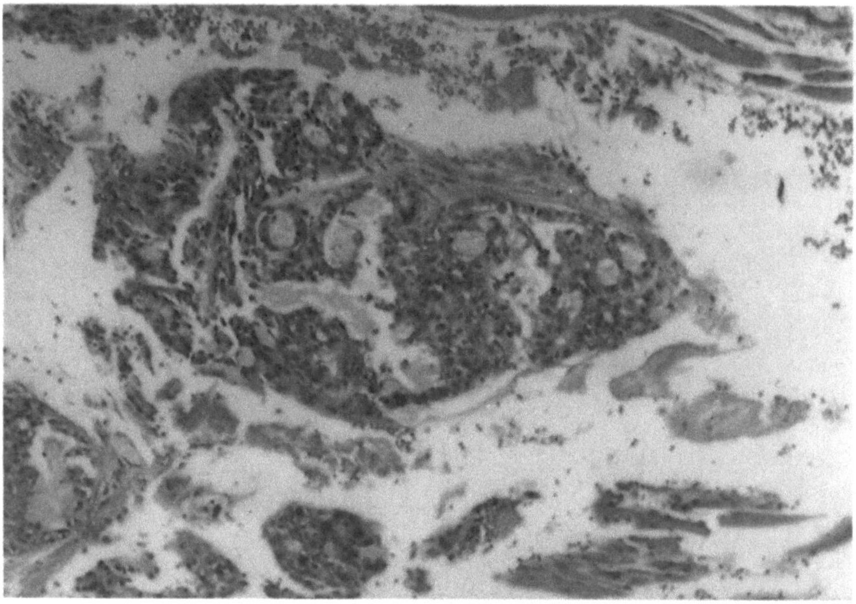

Fig. 3.123. Acinic cell adenocarcinoma, intercalated-duct cell type. H. & E. stain, ×120

The acinic cell adenocarcinoma arises from intercalated-duct cells rather than serous acinar cells. Abrams reported five variations of tumor cells for this neoplasm: acinic, intercalated-duct, vacuolated, clear, and nonspecific glandular cells [251]. Transitions between acinic, vacuolated, and intercalated-duct cells, and between vacuolated and nonspecific glandular cells were frequently seen. This adenocarcinoma can also assume four various growth patterns: solid parenchymatous mass, microcystic configuration, papillary cystic configuration, or follicular [251].

Figure 3.121 illustrates the acinic cell type of the acinic cell adenocarcinoma in a solid parenchymatous mass growth pattern. The nuclei are round, uniformly small, and hyperchromatic. The cytoplasm is basophilic and granular. Figures 3.122 and 3.123 demonstrate the vacuolated cell type and interculated-duct cell type, respectively.

(D) Epidermoid Carcinoma

Although the epidermoid carcinoma is an exceedingly rare malignant salivary gland tumor, its presence implies a grave prognosis because this tumor tends to infiltrate aggressively, metastasizes early, and commonly recurs [5, 247]. It is most frequently discovered in either the parotid or the submandibular gland [10, 44].

It probably arises from ductal epithelium which has undergone squamous metaplasia. The histopathologic picture resembles epidermoid carcinoma seen elsewhere (see Fig. 3.124).

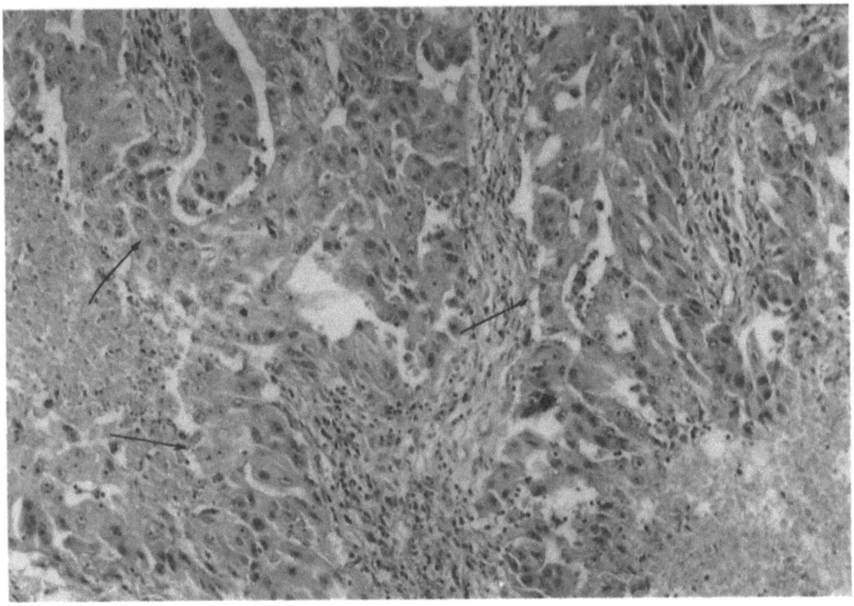

Fig. 3.124. Epidermoid carcinoma (*arrows*), parotid. H. & E. stain, ×120

VIII. Biopsy

A correctly taken biopsy is the heart of any accurate histopathologic diagnosis. It is considered to be the *only* confirmative method for properly evaluating the cancerous or precancerous nature of a lesion. Three techniques may be employed when taking biopsies of the oral mucosa.

1. Incision Biopsy Procedure

An incision biopsy is used when the suspicious lesion is large. It should always include the tumor tissue, border zone, and adjacent normal mucosa.

1) Anesthetize the lesion area with 2% lidocane hydrochloride anesthetic solution with or without a vasoconstrictor. Give the injection by local infiltration around the lesion and not directly into it.

2) Make parallel incisions 2 to 3 mm apart in the lesion area. Make another incision at each end, joining the two ends of the parallel incisions.

3) Now lift this end of the biopsy with tweezers, and with the help of curved scissors, gradually strip away the biopsy from the deeper tissue toward the other end of the parallel incisions. As the opposite end is approached, the biopsy comes off in the tweezers completely separated from the deeper tissue. Be careful not to touch the surface of the biopsy with the tweezers.

4) Gently hold the tissue with the tweezers, and clear away the superficial blood with a piece of gauze. Then place the tissue in the fixative solution of 10% buffered formalin.

5) Normally two sutures are required to close the biopsy wound.

6) Write on the bottle the name of the patient, chart number, lesion, and location from where the biopsy has been taken. Then send the biopsy to the pathologist for evaluation.

2. Punch Biopsy Procedure

The punch biopsy is often used in multiple screening when ideal clinical facilities are not always available. It is advocated when the lesion is uniform in appearance, the area to be biopsied is not very large, and the adjacent normal tissue is not required for comparison.

1) Anesthetize the lesion area with a 2% lidocaine hydrochloride anesthetic solution. Give the injection by local infiltration around the lesion and not directly into it.

2) Place the biopsy punch on the central area of the lesion and rotate it in a clockwise direction until some muscle tissue is included.

3) With the tweezers, lift up the tissue slightly and with curved scissors pointing initially downward and later upward, cut away the tissue from the deeper muscle tissue.

4) Gently hold the tissue with the tweezers, and clear away the superficial blood with a piece of gauze.

5) Drop the bipsy, thus cleaned, into the bottle containing a fixative solution of 10% buffered formalin.

6) Write on the bottle the name of the patient, chart number, lesion, and location from where the biopsy has been taken. Send the biopsy to the pathologist for evaluation.

The punch normally should not be turned in an anticlockwise direction, and the whole procedure should be completed without removing the punch from the tissue site. This continuous procedure is advocated to avoid overlapping of punch cuttings of the tissue, which would eventually be reflected in the microscopic examination. The rotating of the punch in a reverse direction also produces a distorted biopsy. During the entire procedure care must be taken to handle the biopsy gently, since rough handling even with an overfirm tweezer grip may produce compression of the epithelium, giving false histological findings. The biopsy should be deep enough to include a part of the connective tissue, since a superficial biopsy of only the epithelium may not reveal the desired information [5].

3. Excision Biopsy Procedure

Excision biopsy emcompasses total removal of the entire lesion specimen for histopathological examination. Lesions of 1 cm or less are ideal for an excisional biopsy.

1. Anesthetize the lesion area with a 2% lidocane hydrochloride anesthetic solution. Give the injection by local infiltration around the lesion and not directly into it.
2. Using a surgical scalpel, make an elliptical incision around the lesion with cuts converging to a "V" in the underlying normal tissue.
3. Now hold the tissue with tweezers and gently dissect it out.
4. Gently hold the tissue with tweezers, and clear away the superificial blood with a piece of gauze. Then place the tissue in the fixative solution of 10% buffered formalin.
5. Place sutures to close the biopsy wound.
6. Write on the bottle the name of the patient, chart number, lesion and location from where the biopsy has been taken. Then send the biopsy to the pathologist for evaluation.

During the entire procedure care must be taken to see that biopsy incisions are cleanly cut with sharp instruments to prevent tearing and distortion of tissues. The incision should be precise, deep, and narrow rather than broad and shallow [5].

References

1. Silverberg, E.: "Cancer Statistics – 1982", CA.: 32:15–29, 1982
2. Beahrs, O.H., et al.: Manual for Staging of Cancer – 1978, Ed. 2, (Whiting Press: Rochester, MN.), 1978
3. Miller, D., et al.: Cancer – A Manual for Practitioner, Ed. 5, (American Cancer Society: Boston, MA), 1978
4. Hamner, J.E., III: Management Guidelines for Head and Neck Cancer, Ed. 2, (N.I.H. Publication No. 80-2037: Bethesda, MD), 1979
5. Hamner, J.E., III: Chapter on "Oral Cancer". In: Oral Medicine (Lynch, M.A., ed.), Ed. 7, (J.B. Lippincott Co.: Philadelphia, PA), 1977
6. Cancer Facts and Figures – 1981, (American Cancer Society: New York, NY), 1981
7. Million, R.R., Cassisi, N.J., and Wittes, R.E.: Chapter on "Cancer in the Head and Neck". In: Cancer: Principles and Practice of Oncology (DeVita, V.T., Hellman, S., and Rosenberg, S., editors), Ed. 1, (J.B. Lippincott Co.: Philadelphia, PA), 1982
8. Silverman, S., Jr. and Galante, M.: Oral Cancer, Ed. 4, (University of California: San Francisco, CA), 1974
9. Silverman, S., Jr. and Griffith, M.: "Smoking Characteristics of Patients with Oral Cancer and the Risk for Second Oral Primary Cancers", J.A.D.A. 85:637–640, 1972
10. Shafer, W.G., Hine, M.K., and Levy, B.M.: Oral Pathology, Ed. 3, (W.B. Saunders Co.: Philadelphia, PA), 1974
11. Myers, M.H. and Hankey, B.F.: Cancer Patient Survival Experience, (N.I.H. Publication No. 80-2148: Bethesda, MD), 1980
12. Correa, J.N., et al.: "Carcinoma of the Floor of the Mouth", Amer. J. Roentgenol, 99:302–312, 1967
13. Lefall, L.D. and White, J.E.: "Cancer of the Oral Cavity in Negroes", Surg. Gynecol. Obstet. 120:70–72, 1965
14. Brown, R.L., et al.: "Snuff Dippers' Intraoral Cancer: Clinical Characteristics and Response to Therapy", Cancer 18:2–13, 1965
15. Mehta, F.S., Pindborg, J.J., and Hamner, J.E., III: Oral Cancer and Precancerous Conditions in India, Ed. 1, (Munksgaard: Copenhagen, Denmark), 1971
16. Mehta, F.S., Daftary, D.K., Gupta, P.C., et al.: "Tobacco Habits and Oral Cancer", Science Today 13:27–30, 1978

17. Pindborg, J.J., Mehta, F.S., Gupta, P.C., et al.: "Reverse Smoking in Andhra Pradesh, India: A Study of Palatal Lesions Among 10, 169 Villagers", Brit. J. Cancer 25:10–20, 1971
18. Gupta, P.C., Mehta, F.S., Daftary, D.K., et al.: "Incidence Rates of Oral Cancer and Natural History of Oral Precancerous Lesions in a 10-Year Follow-up Study of Indian Villagers", Comm. Dent. Oral Epidemiol. 8:287–333, 1980
19. Pindborg, J.J.: Atlas of Diseases of the Oral Mucosa, Ed. 3, (W.B. Saunders and Co.: Philadelphia, PA), 1980
20. O'Brien, P.H. and Catlin, D.: "Cancer of the Cheek (Mucosa)", Cancer 118:1392–1398, 1965
21. Jacobson, S. and Shear, M.: "Verrucous Carcinoma of the Mouth", J. Oral Pathol. 1:66–75, 1972
22. Totten, R.S.: Chapter on "Tumors of the Oral Cavity, Pharynx, and Larynx: Pathologic Aspects". In: Cancer of the Head and Neck (Rubin, P., ed.), Current Concepts in Cancer – Number 30, J.A.M.A. 215:5–6, 1971
23. Koss, L.G., et al.: "Some Histological Aspects of Behavior of Epidermoid Carcinoma-in-situ and Related Lesions of the Uterine Cervix: A Long-term Prospective Study", Cancer 16:1160–1211, 1963
24. Kripe, M.L. and Sass, E.R.: National Cancer Institute Monograph #50: International Conference on Ultraviolet Carcinogenesis. (N.I.H. Publishing: Bethesda, MD), 1977
25. Lane-Brown, M.M. and Melia, D.F.: "A Genetic Diathesis to Skin Cancer", J. Invest. Dermatol. 61:39–41, 1973
26. Gordon, D. and Silverstone, H.: "Deaths from Skin Cancer in Queensland, Australia". In: The Biologic Effects of Ultraviolet Radiation, (Urbach, F., ed.), Ed. 1, (Pergamon Press: New York, NY), 1969
27. Scott, E.L. and Straf, M.L.: Chapter on "Ultraviolet Radiation as a Cause of Cancer". In: Origins of Human Cancer. Book A – Incidence of Cancer in Humans, (Hiatt, H.H., Watson, J.D., and Winsten, J.A., editors), Ed. 1, (Cold Spring Harbor Laboratories: Cold Spring Harbor, NY), 1977
28. Robbins, S.L.: Pathology, Ed. 3, (W.B. Saunders Co.: Philadelphia, PA), 1967
29. Lever, W.F.: Histopathology of the Skin, Ed. 3, (J.B. Lippincott Co.: Philadelphia, PA), 1961
30. Sober, A.J.: "Melanoma Fact Sheet", CA. 29:276–279, 1979
31. Elwood, J.M. and Lee, J.A.H.: "Recent Data on Epidemiology of Malignant Melanoma", Semin. Oncol. 2:149–154, 1975
32. Sober, A.J., Fitzpatrick, T.B., and Mihm, M.C.: "Primary Melanoma of the Skin: Recognition and Management", J. Amer. Acad. Dermatol. 2:179–197, 1980
33. Gellin, G.A., Kopf, A.W., and Garfinkel, L.: "Malignant Melanoma: A Controlled Study of Possible Associated Factors", Arch. Dermatol. 99:43–48, 1969
34. Chaudhry, A.P., Hampel, A., and Gorlin, R.J.: "Primary Malignant Melanoma of the Oral Cavity", Cancer 11:923–928, 1958
35. Trodahl, J.N. and Sprague, W.G.: "Benign and Malignant Melanocytic Lesions of the Oral Mucosa: An Analysis of 135 Cases", Cancer 25:812–823, 1970
36. Clark, W.H.: Chapter on: "A Classification of Malignant Melanoma in Man Correlated with Histogenesis and Biological Behavior". In: The Pigmentary System. (Pergamon Press: London, England), 1967
37. Clark, W.H., From, L., Bernardino, E., and Mihm, M.C.: "The Histogenesis and Biologic Behavior of Primary Malignant Melanomas of Skin", Cancer Res. 29:705–726, 1969
38. Fitzpatrick, T.B.: Personal Communication
39. Sober, A.J., Fitzpatrick, T.B., Mihm, M.C., et al.: "Early Recognition of Cutaneous Melanoma", J.A.M.A. 242:2795–2799, 1979
40. Mihm, M.C., Fitzpatrick, T.B., Lane-Brown, M.M., et al.: "Early Detection of Primary Cutaneous Malignant Melanoma", N.E.J.M. 289:989–996, 1973
41. Craig, R.M., Glass, B.J., and Rhyne, R.R.: "Malignant Melanoma: Metastasis to the Tonsil", J.A.D.A. 104:893–894, 1982
42. Holland, J.F., and Frei, E.: Cancer Medicine, Ed. 1, (Lea & Febiger: Philadelphia, PA), 1973

43. Sober, A.J.: "Immuniology and Cutaneous Malignant Melanoma", Int. J. Dermatol. 15:1–18, 1976
44. Gorlin, R.J. and Goldman, H.M.: Thoma's Oral Pathology, Ed. 6, (C.V. Mosby Co.: St. Louis, MO), 1970
45. Small, I.A. and Waldron, C.A.: "Ameloblastoma of the Jaws", Oral Surg. 8:281–297, 1955
46. Stanley, H.R. and Diehl, D.L.: "Ameloblastic Potential of Follicular Cysts", Oral Surg. 20:260–268, 1965
47. Lucas, R.B.: Pathology of Tumors of the Oral Tissues, Ed. 1, (Little, Brown, & Co.: Boston, MA), 1964
48. Sprouge, J.D.: "Odontogenic Tumors", Oral Surg. 24:392–403, 1967
49. Kramer, I.R.H.: "Ameloblastoma: A Clinico-Pathological Appraisal", Brit. J. Oral Surg. 1:13–28, 1963
50. McMillan, M.D. and Smillie, A.C.: "Ameloblastomas Associated with Dentigerous Cysts", Oral Surg. 51:481–496, 1981
51. Hertz, J.: "Adamantinoma: Histopathologic and Prognostic Studies", Acta Chir. Scand. 102:405–432, 1952
52. Hertz, J.: "Adamantinoma: Studies in Histopathology and Prognosis", Acta Med. Scand. 142 (Suppl.):529–556, 1952
53. Stafne, E.C.: Oral Roentgenographic Diagnosis, Ed. 2, (W.B. Saunders Co.: Philadelphia, PA), 1963
54. Campbell, J.A.H.: "Adamantinoma Containing Tissue Resembling Granular Cell Myoblastoma", J. Pathol. Bact. 71:45–59, 1956
55. Gorlin, R.J., et al.: "Odontogenic Tumors", Cancer 14:73–101, 1961
56. Tsukada, Y., De la Paras, and Pickren, J.: "Granular Cell Ameloblastoma with Metastasis to the Lung", Cancer 18:916–925, 1965
57. Hodson, J.J.: "Observations on Origin and Nature of Adamantinomas with Special Reference to Certain Mucoepidermoid Variations", Brit. J. Plast. Surg. 10:38–59, 1957
58. Shafer, W.G. and Spring, A.W.: "Ameloblastoma: Report of a Case", Oral Surg. 7:32–37, 1964
59. Sonesson, A.: "Odontogenic Cysts and Cystic Tumors of the Jaws: Roentgendiagnostic and Patho-anatomic Study", Acta Radiolog. 81 (Suppl.):1–59, 1950
60. Bernier, J.L. and Tiecke, R.W.: "A Compliation of the Material Received by the Registry of Oral Pathology", J. Oral Surg. 9:341–348, 1951
61. Carr, R.F. and Halperin, V.: "Malignant Ameloblastomas from 1953 to 1966: Review of the Literature and Report of a Case", Oral Surg. 26:541–522, 1968
62. Lee, R.E., et al.: "Ameloblastoma with Distant Metastases", Acta Pathol. 68:23–29, 1959
63. Hoke, H.F. and Harrelson, A.B.: "Granular Cell Ameloblastoma with Metastasis to the Cervical Vertebrae", Cancer 20:991–999, 1967
64. Sugimura, M., et al.: "Malignant Ameloblastoma with Metastasis to the Lumbar Vertebrae", J. Oral Surg. 27:350–357, 1969
65. Vorzimer, J. and Perla, D.: "Instance of Adamantinoma of the Jaw with Metastases to the Right Lung", Amer. J. Pathol. 8:445–454, 1932
66. Becker, R. and Pertl, A.: "Zur Therapie des Ameloblastoms", Deutsch. Zahn, Mund., Kieferheilk. 49:423–436, 1967
67. Pizer, M.E. and Hamner, J.E., III: "Odontogenic Tumors: A Survey of Their Manifestations in Childhood", Clin. Pediat. 6:593–597, 1967
68. Giasanti, J.S., Someren, H., and Waldron, C.A.: "Odontogenic Adenomatoid Tumor (Adenoameloblastoma)", Oral Surg. 30:69–86, 1970
69. Courtney, R.M. and Kerr, D.A.: "The Odontogenic Adenomatoid Tumor: A Comprehensive Study of Twenty New Cases", Oral Surg. 39:424–435, 1975
70. Bedrick, A.E., Solomon, M.P., and Ferber, I.: "The Adenomatoid Odontogenic Tumor: An Unusual Clinical Presentation", Oral Surg. 48:143–145, 1979
71. Schosnagle, D.C. and Someren, A.: "The Ultrastructure of the Adenomatoid Odontogenic Tumor", Oral Surg. 52:154–161, 1981
72. Philipsen, H.P. and Birn, A.: "The Adenomatoid Odontogenic Tumor, Ameloblastic

Adenomatoid Tumor, or Adenoameloblastoma", Acta Pathol. Microbiol. Scand. 75:375–398, 1969
73. Sprouge, J.D.: "The Adenoameloblastoma", Oral Surg. 23:470–482, 1967
74. Lucas, R.B.: "Tumor of Enamel Organ Epithelium", Oral Surg. 25:143–149, 1957
75. Stafne, E.C.: "Epithelial Tumors Associated with Developmental Cysts of the Maxilla: Report of Three Cases", Oral Surg. 1:887–894, 1948
76. Miles, J.F.: "Adenoameloblastoma of the Maxilla", J. Oral Surg. 21:432–434, 1963
77. Gorlin, R.J. and Chaudhry, A.P.: "Adenoameloblastoma", Oral Surg. 11:762–768, 1958
78. Shear, M.: "Histogenesis of the Tumor of Enamel Organ Epithelium", Brit. Dent. J. 112:494–498, 1962
79. Takagi, M.: "Adenomatoid Ameloblastoma: An Analysis of Nine Cases by Histopathologic and Electron Microscopic Study", Bull. Tokyo Med. Dent. Univ. 14:487–506, 1967
80. Smith, R.R.L., Olson, J.L., Hutchins, G.M., et al.: "Adenomatoid Odontogenic Tumor: Ultrastructural Demonstration of Two Cell Types and Amyloid", Cancer 505–511, 1979
81. Hatakeyama, S. and Suzuki, A.: "Ultrastructural Study of Adenomatoid Odontogenic Tumor", J. Oral Pathol. 7:295–310, 1978
82. Lee, K.W.: "A Light and Electron Microscopic Study of the Adenomatoid Odontogenic Tumor", Int. J. Oral Surg. 3:183–193, 1974
83. Pindborg, J.J.: "Calcifying Epithelial Odontogenic Tumors", Acta Pathol. Microbiol. Scand. 111 (Suppl.):71, 1956
84. Pindborg, J.J.: "Calcifying Epithelial Odontogenic Tumor", Cancer 11:838–843, 1958
85. Pindborg, J.J.: "The Calcifying Epithelial Odontogenic Tumor: Review of the Literature and Report of an Extra-osseous Case", Acta Odont. Scand. 24:419–430, 1966
86. Vickers, R.A., et al.: "Amyloid-containing Odontogenic Tumors", Oral Surg. 20:476–480, 1965
87. Ranlov, P. and Pindborg, J.J.: "The Amyloid Nature of the Homogenous Substance in the Calcifying Epithelial Odontogenic Tumor", Acta Pathol. Microbiol. Scand. 68:169–174, 1966
88. Gardner, D.G., et al.: "Calcifying Epithelial Odontogenic Tumor: An Amyloid Producing Neoplasm", Oral Surg. 26:812–823, 1968
89. Gon, F.: "The Calcifying Epithelial Odontogenic Tumor: Report of a Case and a Study of Its Histogenesis", Brit. J. Cancer 19:39–50, 1965
90. Zimmerman, D.C. and Dahlin, D.C.: "Myxomatous Tumors of the Jaws", Oral Surg. 11:1069–1080, 1958
91. Hamner, J.E., III, Gamble, J.W., and Gallegos, G.J.: "Odontogenic Fibroma", Oral Surg. 21:113–119, 1966
92. Wesley, R.K., Wysocki, G.P., and Mintz, S.M.: "The Central Odontogenic Fibroma", Oral Surg. 40:235–245, 1975
93. Heimdal, A., Isacsson, G., and Nilsson, L.: "Recurrent Central Odontogenic Fibroma", Oral Surg. 50:140–145, 1980
94. Bhaskar, S.N.: Synopsis of Oral Pathology, Ed. 1, (C.V. Mosby Co.: St. Louis, MO), 1961
95. Gardner, D.G.: "The Central Odontogenic Fibroma: An Attempt at Classification", Oral Surg. 50:425–432, 1980
96. Bruce, K.W. and Royer, R.Q.: "Central Fibromyxoma of the Maxilla", Oral Surg. 5:1277–1281, 1952
97. Pincock, L.D. and Bruce, K.W.: "Odontogenic Fibroma", Oral Surg. 7:307–311, 1954
98. Thoma, K.H. and Goldman, H.M.: "Central Myxoma of the Jaw", Amer. J. Orthodont. Oral Surg. 33:532–540, 1947
99. Schultz, L.W. and Vazirani, S.L.: "Central Fibromyxoma of the Mandible", Oral Surg. 10:690–695, 1957
100. Gundlach, K.K.H. and Schulz, A.: "Odontogenic Myxoma: Clinical Concept and Morphological Studies", J. Oral Pathol. 6:343–358, 1977
101. Prout, R.E.S. and Hodson, J.J.: "Analysis of the Mucopolyscaccharide of a Myxoma of the Mandible", Nature 218:99–100, 1968
102. Hodson, J.J. and Prout, R.E.S.: "Clinical and Histochemical Characterization of Mucopolysaccarides in a Jaw Myxoma", J. Clin. Pathol. 21:582–589, 1968

103. Harrison, J.D.: Odontogenic Myxoma: Ultrastructural and Histochemical Studies", J. Clin. Pathol. 26:570–582, 1973
104. Westwood, R.M., Alexander, R.W., and Bennett, D.E.: "Giant Odontogenic Myxofibroma: Report of a Case with Histochemical and Ultrastructural Studies and a Review of the Literature", Oral Surg. 37:83–92, 1974
105. White, D.K., Chen, S., Mohnac, A.M., and Miller, A.S.: "Odontogenic Myxoma: A Clinical and Ultrastructural Study", Oral Surg. 39:901–917, 1975
106. Goldblatt, L.I.: "Ultrastructural Study of an Odontogenic Myxoma", Oral Surg. 42:206–220, 1976
107. Hendler, B.H., Abaza, N.A., and Quinn, P.: "Odontogenic Myxoma: Surgical Management and Ultrastructural Study", Oral Surg., 47:203–217, 1979
108. Gorlin, R.J., Chaudhry, A.P., and Pindborg, J.J.: "Odontogenic Tumors: Classification, Histopathology, and Clinical Behavior in Man and Domesticated Animals", Cancer 14:73–101, 1961
109. Barros, R.E., Dominquez, F.V., and Cabrini, R.L.: "Myxoma of the Jaws", Oral Surg. 27:225–236, 1969
110. Ghosh, B.C., Huvos, A.G., Gerold, F.P., and Miller, T.R.: "Myxoma of the Jaw Bones", Cancer 31:237–240, 1973
111. Cohen, P.B. and Gamble, J.W.: "Maxillary Resection for Odontogenic Myxoma: Report of a Case", J. Oral Surg. 35:573–577, 1977
112. Hamner, J.E., III: "Ameloblastic Fibroma", (Armed Forces Institute of Pathology C.P.C. #9–64: Washington, D.C.), 1965
113. Shafer, W.G.: "Ameloblastic Fibroma", J. Oral Surg., Anes., Hosp. Dent. Serv. 13:317–321, 1955
114. Couch, R.D., Morris, E.E., and Vellios, F.: "Granular Cell Ameloblastic Fibroma: Report of 2 Cases in Adults with Observations on Its Similarity to Congenital Epulis", Amer. J. Clin. Pathol. 37:398–404, 1962
115. Waldron, C.A., Thompson, C.W., and Conner, W.A.: "Granular Cell Ameloblastic Fibroma", Oral Surg. 16:1202–1213, 1963
116. White, D.K., Chen, S., Hartman, K.S., et al.: "Central Granular-cell Tumor of the Jaws (The So-called Granular-cell Ameloblastic Fibroma)", Oral Surg. 45:396–405, 1978
117. Carr, R.F., Halperin, V., Wood, C., et al.: "Recurrent Ameloblastic Fibroma", Oral Surg. 29:85–90, 1970
118. Trodahl, J.N.: "Ameloblastic Fibroma – A Survey of Cases from The Armed Forces Institue of Pathology", Oral Surg. 33:547–558, 1972
119. Huebsch, R.F. and Stephenson, T.D.: "Recurrent Ameloblastic Fibroma in a 3-year Old Boy", Oral Surg. 9:707–714, 1956
120. Tanaka, S., Mitsui, Y., Mizuno, Y., and Emori, S.: "Recurrent Ameloblastic Fibroma", Oral Surg. 33:944–950, 1972
121. Sawyer, D.R., Nwoku, A.L., and Mosadomi, A.: "Recurrent Ameloblastic Fibroma: Report of Two Cases", Oral Surg. 53:19–23, 1982
122. Bernier, J.L.: Tumors of the Odontongenic Apparatus and Jaws, (Armed Forces Institute of Pathology: Washington, D.C.), 1960
123. Thoma, K.H. and Goldman, H.M.: "Odontogenic Tumors: Classification Based on Observations of Epithelial, Mesenchymal, and Mixed Varieties", Amer. J. Pathol. 22:433–471, 1946
124. Hamner, J.E., III and Pizer, M.E.: "Ameloblastic Odontoma: Report of Two Cases", Amer. J. Dis. Child. 115:332–336, 1968
125. Gorlin, R.J., Meskin, L.H., and Brodey, R.: "Odontogenic Tumors in Man and Animals: Pathologyic Classification and Clinical Behavior – A Review", Ann. N.Y. Acad. Sci. 108:722–771, 1963
126. Hooker, S.P.: "Ameloblastic Odontoma: An Analysis of 26 Cases", Oral Surg. 24:375–376, 1976
127. Slootweg, P.J.: "An Analysis of the Interrelationship of the Mixed Odontogenic Tumors – Ameloblastic Fibroma, Ameloblastic Fibro-odontoma, and the Odontomas", Oral Surg. 51:266–276, 1981

128. Archard, H.O.: "Ameloblastic Odontoma", (Armed Forces Institute of Pathology C.P.C. #128), 1962
129. Gould, J.F.: "Complex Odontoma: Three-Year Follow-up of Tooth Movement", Oral Surg. 45:175–177, 1978
130. Howell, R.M. and Burkes, E.J.: "Malignant Transformation of Ameloblastic Fibro-odontoma to Ameloblastic Fibrosarcoma", Oral Surg. 43:391–401, 1977
131. Kegal, R.F.C.: "Adamantine Epithelioma", Arch. Surg. 25:498–528, 1932
132. Villa, V.G.: "Ameloblastic Sarcoma in the Mandible: Report of a Case", Oral Surg. 8:123–129, 1955
133. Pindborg, J.J.: "Ameloblastic Sarcoma in the Maxilla: Report of a Case", Cancer 13:1074–1080, 1960
134. Cina, M.T., Dahlin, D.C., and Gores, R.J.: "Ameloblastic Sarcoma: Report of Two Cases", Oral Surg. 15:696–700, 1962
135. Tashinoglu, M. and Ozerzifonlu, S.: "Ameloblastik Odontosarkom", Odonto-Stomatologi Dergisi 3:14–22, 1964
136. Dahlin, D.C. and Ivins, J.C.: "Fibrosarcoma of Bone: A Study of 114 Cases", Cancer 23:35–41, 1969
137. Hatfifotiadis, D., Govedaros, K., and Economou, T.: "Adamantinoblasko Sarcoma Ano Anathon", Stomatologia (Athenai) 28:189–195, 1971
138. Peychl, L. and Sazama, L.: "Adamantinosarcoma of the Maxilla: Report of a Case", Neoplasma 18:403–406, 1971
139. Forman, G. and Garrett, J.: "Ameloblastic Sarcoma: Report of a Case", J. Oral Surg. 30:50–54, 1972
140. Leider, A.S., Nelson, J.F., and Trodahl, J.N.: "Ameloblastic Fibrosarcoma of the Jaws", Oral Surg. 33:559–569, 1972
141. Adekeye, E.O., Edwards, M.B., and Goubran, G.F.: "Ameloblastic Fibrosarcoma: Report of a Case in a Nigerian", Oral Surg. 46:254–259, 1978
142. Fullmer, H.M.: "The Organization of the Dental Supporting Tissues". In: Chemical and Structural Organization of the Teeth, (Miles, A.E.W., ed.), (Academic Press: New York, NY), 1968
143. Hamner, J.E., III, Scofield, H.H., and Cornyn, J.: "Benign Fibro-osseous Jaw Lesions of Periodontal Membrane Origin: An Analysis of 249 Cases", Cancer 22:861–878, 1968
144. Fullmer, H.M. and Lillie, R.D.: "The Oxytalan Fiber: A Previously Undescribed Connective Tissue Fiber", J. Histochem. Cytochem. 6:425–430, 1958
145. Fullmer, H.M.: "Observations on the Development of Oxytalan Fibers in Dental Granulomas and Radicular Cysts", Arch. Pathol. 70:59–67, 1960
146. Fisher, A.K. and Fullmer, H.M.: "Oxytalan Fibers in Ameloblastomas", Oral Surg. 15:246–248, 1962
147. Hamner, J.E., III and Fullmer, H.M.: "Oxytalan Fibers in Benign Fibro-ossesous Jaw Lesions", Arch. Pathol. 82:35–39, 1966
148. Stafne, E.C.: "Cementoma: A study of 35 cases", Dent. Survey 9:27–31, 1933
149. Zegarelli, E.V. and Ziskin, D.E.: "Cementomas: A Report of 50 Cases", Amer. J. Ortho. and Oral Surg. 29:289–292, 1943
150. Bernier, J.L. and Thompson, H.C.: "The Histogenesis of the Cementoma", Amer. J. Orthodont. Oral Surg. 32:543–555, 1946
151. Scannell, J.M.: "Cementoma", Oral Surg. 2:169–180, 1949
152. Fòntaine, J.: "Periapical Fibro-osteoma or Cementoma", J. Canad. Dent. Assn. 21:10–20, 1955
153. Chaudhry, A.P., Spink, J.H., and Gorlin, R.J.: "Periapical Fibrous Dysplasia (Cementoma)", J. Oral Surg., Anes., Hosp. Dent. Serv. 16:483–488, 1958
154. Kline, S.N., Spatz, S.S., et al.: "Large Cementoma of the Mandible", Oral Surg. 14:1421–1426, 1961
155. Wertheimer, F.W., Driscoll, E.J., and Stanley, H.R.: "True Attached Cementoma with Root Canal Involvement", Oral Surg. 14:630–634, 1961
156. Jaffe, H.L.: Tumors and Tumorous Conditions of the Bones and Joints, (Lea & Febiger: Philadelphia, PA.), 1958

157. Whiteside, T.E. and Ackerman, L.V.: "Desmoplastic Fibroma", J. Bone Joint Surg. 42-A:1143–1155, 1960
158. Scheer, G.E. and Kuhlman, R.E.: "Vertebral Involvement by Desmoplastic Fibroma", J.A.M.A. 185:669–670, 1963
159. Griffith, J.G. and Irby, W.B.: "Desmoplastic Fibroma", Oral Surg. 20:269–275, 1965
160. Dahlin, D.C. and Hoover, N.W.: "Desmoplastic Fibroma of Bone: Report of Two Cases", J.A.M.A. 188:685–687, 1964
161. Rabhan, W.N. and Rosai, J.: "Desmoplastic Fibroma: Report of Ten Cases and Review of the Literature", J. Bone and Joint Surg. 50-A:487–502, 1968
162. Hinds, E.C., Kent, J.N., and Fechner, R.E.: "Desmoplastic Fibroma of the Mandible: Report of a Case", J. Oral Surg. 27:271–274, 1969
163. Hovinga, J. and Ingenhoes, R.: "A Desmoplastic Fibroma of the Mandible", Int. J. Oral Surg. 3:41–44, 1974
164. Wagner, J.E., Lorandi, C.S., and Ebling, H.: "Desmoplastic Fibroma of Bone", Oral Surg. 43:108–111, 1977
165. Main, D.M.G.: "Fibroma of the Mandible", Brit. J. Oral Surg., 3:172–175, 1966
166. Phemister, D.B. and Grimson, K.S.: "Fibrous Osteoma of the Jaws", Ann. Surg. 105:564–583, 1937
167. Spjut, H.J., Dorfman, H.D., Fechner, R.E., and Ackerman, L.V.: Tumors of Bone and Cartilage, Fasicle 5, (Armed Forces Institute of Pathology: Washington, D.C.), 1970
168. Lichtenstein, L.: "Benign Osteoblastoma", Cancer 9:1044–1052, 1956
169. Jaffe, H.L.: "Benign Osteoblastoma", Bull. Hosp. Joint Surg. 17:141–151, 1964
170. Dahlin, D.C. and Johnson, E.W., Jr.: "Giant Osteoid Osteoma", J. Bone Joint Surg. 36-A:559–572, 1954
171. Johnson, L.C.: Personal Communication
172. Lichtenstein, L. and Sawyer, W.: "Benign Osteoblastoma: Further Observations and Report of Twenty Additional Cases", J. Bone Joint Surg. 46-A:755–765, 1964
173. Kramer, H.S.: "Benign Osteoblastoma of the Mandible", Oral Surg. 24:842–851, 1967
174. Hamner, J.E., III: Unpublished Data
175. Jones, W.A.: "Familial Multilocular Cystic Disease of the Jaws", Amer. J. Cancer 17:946–951
176. Caffey, J. and Williams, J.L.: "Familial Fibrous Swelling of the Jaws", Radiology 56:1–13, 1951
177. Jones, W.A.: "Further Observations Regarding Familial Multilocular Cystic Disease of the Jaws", Brit. J. Radiol. 56:1–13, 1951
178. Jones, W.A., Gerrie, J., and Pritchard, J.: "Cherubism – A Familial Fibrous Dysplasia of the Jaws", J. Bone Joint Surg. 32-B:334–347, 1950
179. Waldron, C.A.: "Familial Incidence of Bilateral Giant Cell Tumors of the Jaw", Oral Surg. 4:198–207, 1951
180. Bruce, K.W., Bruwer, A., and Kennedy, R.L.J.: "Familial Intraosseous Fibrous Swellings of the Jaws (Cherubism)", Oral Surg. 6:995–1014, 1953
181. Talley, D.B.: "Familial Fibrous Dysplasia of the Jaws", Oral Surg. 5:1012–1019, 1952
182. McDonald, R.E. and Shafer, W.G.: "Disseminated Juvenile Fibrous Dysplasia of the Jaws", Amer. J. Dis. Child. 89:354–358, 1955
183. Small, I.A.: Familial Osseous Dysplasia of the Jaws", J. Oral Surg. 16:35–45, 1958
184. Anderson, D.E., McClendon, J.L., and Cornelius, E.A.: "Cherubism – Hereditary Fibrous Dysplasia of the Jaws. I. Genetic Consideration; II. Pathologic Considerations", Oral Surg. 15, Suppl. 2:5–42, 1962
185. Burland, J.G.: "Cherubism: Familial Bilateral Osseous Dysplasia of the Jaws" Oral Surg. 15, (Suppl. 2):43–48, 1962
186. Peters, W.J.N.: "Cherubism: A Study of Twenty Cases from One Family", Oral Surg. 47:307–311, 1979
187. Hamner, J.E., III and Ketcham, A.S.: "Cherubism: An Analysis of Treatment", Cancer 23:1133–1143, 1969
188. Thompson, N.: "Cherubism: Familial Fibrous Dysplasia of the Jaws", Brit. J. Plast. Surg. 12:89–103, 1959

189. Topazian, R.C. and Costich, E.R.: "Familial Fibrous Dysplasia of the Jaws (Cherubism): Report of a Case", J. Oral Surg. 23:559–566, 1965
190. Jones, W.A.: "Cherubism: A Thumbnail Sketch of Its Diagnosis and A Conservative Method of Treatment", Oral Surg. 20:648–653, 1965
191. Seward, G.R. and Hankey, G.T.: "Cherubism", Oral Surg. 10:952–974, 1957
192. Hamner, J.E., III: "The Demonstration of Perivascular Collagen Deposition in Cherubism", Oral Surg. 27:129–141, 1969
193. Aiken, H.E.: "Cherubism", Amer. J. Dis. Child. 103:697–701, 1962
194. Brannin, D.E.: "Bilateral Giant Cell Tumors of the Mandible in Siblings", J. Oral Surg. 12:247–251, 1954
195. Waldron, C.A.: "Comments", J. Oral Surg. 23:566–568, 1965
196. Fleuchaus, P.T.: "Cherubism Treated by Curettage and Autogenous Bone Chips: Report of a Case", J. Oral Surg. 25:347–355, 1967
197. Albright, F., et al.: "Syndrome Characterized by Osteitis Fibrosa Disseminata, Areas of Pigmentation, and Endocrine Dysfunction with Precocious Puberty in Females", N.E.J.M. 216:727–746, 1937
198. Lichtenstein, L.: "Polyostotic Fibrous Dysplasia", Arch. Surg. 36:874–893, 1938
199. Lichtenstein, L. and Jaffe, H.L.: "Fibrous Dysplasia of Bone", Arch. Pathol. 33:777–816, 1942
200. Reed, R.J.: "Observations on Bone Maturation and Fibrous Dysplasia of Bone", Bull. Tulane Med. Fac. 19:45–53, 1965
201. Reed, R.J. and Hapy, D.M.: "Benign Nonodontogenic Fibro-osseous Lesions of the Skull", Oral Surg. 10:214–227, 1965
202. Tillman, H.H., Silverman, L., and Shklar, G.: "Fibrous Dysplasia of Bone with Other Developmental Abnormalies", J. Oral Surg. 23:149–155, 1965
203. Gutman, D., Gellei, B., and Laufer, D.: "Fibrous Dysplasia of the Maxilla and Zygoma Treated by Intraoral Approach: Report of a Case", J. Oral Surg. 25:367–370, 1967
204. Pritchard, J.J.: Chapter in: The Biochemistry and Physiology of Bone, (Bourne, G.H., ed.), Academic Press: New York, NY), 1956
205. Frost, H.M.: "Observations on Fibrous Dysplasia and Lamellar Bone", Henry Ford Hosp. Med. Bull. 8:199–207, 1960
206. Ramsey, H.E., Strong, E.W., and Frazell, E.L.: "Progressive Fibrous Dysplasia of the Maxilla", J.A.D.A. 81:1388–1391, 1970
207. Jaffe, H.J.: "Giant Cell Reparative Granuloma, Traumatic Bone Cyst, and Fibrous (fibro-osseous) Dysplasia of the Jaw-bones", Oral Surg. 6:159–175, 1953
208. Jacoby, J.K.: The Giant Cell of Reparative Granuloma, M.S. Thesis, Indiana University, 1965
209. Waldron, C.A. and Shafer, W.G.: "The Giant Cell Reparative Granuloma of the Jaws: An Analysis of 38 Cases", Aner. J. Clin. Pathol. 45:437–447, 1966
210. Austin, L.T., Jr., Dahlin, D.C., and Royer, R.Q.: "Giant-cell Reparative Granuloma and Related Conditions Affecting the Jaw-bones", Oral Surg. 12:1285–1295, 1959
211. Waldron, C.A.: "Giant Cell Tumors of the Mandible and Maxilla", Oral Surg. 14:809–827, 1961
212. Brightman, V.J.: "Benign Tumors of the Oral Cavity". In: Oral Medicine (Lynch, M.A., ed.), Ed. 7, (J.B. Lippincott Co.: Philadelphia, PA), 1977
213. Jaffe, H.L. and Lichtenstein, L.: "Solitary Unicameral Bone Cyst with Emphasis on the Roentgen Picture, the Pathology, and the Pathogenesis", Arch. Surg. 46:1004–1025, 1942
214. Biesecker, J.L., Marcove, R.C., et al.: "Aneurysmal Bone Cysts: A Clinico-pathologic Study of 66 Cases", Cancer 26:615–625, 1970
215. Bernier, J.L. and Bhaskar, S.N.: "Anurysmal Bone Cyst of the Mandible", Oral Surg. 11:1018–1028, 1958
216. Daugherty, J.W. and Eversole, L.R.: "Aeurysmal Bone Cyst of the Mandible: Report of a Case", J. Oral Surg. 29:737–741, 1971
217. Ellis, D.J. and Walters, P.J.: "Aneurysmal Bone Cyst of the Maxilla", Oral Surg. 34:26–32, 1972

218. Oliver, L.: "Aneurysmal Bone Cyst: Report of a Case", Oral Surg. 35:67–76, 1973
219. Reyneke, J.P.: "Aneurysmal Bone Cyst of the Maxilla", Oral Surg. 45:441–447, 1978
220. Rappaport, I., Shiffman, M.A., and Greaney, E.M.: "Parathyroid Disease", Oral Surg. 17:802–811, 1964
221. Rosenberg, E.H. and Guralnick, W.C.: "Hyperparathyroidism", Oral Surg. 15, (Suppl. 2):84–94, 1962
222. Paget, J.: "On a Form of Chronic Inflammation of Bones (Osteitis Deformans)", Transactions of the Medical Chirurgical Society 60:37–64, 1877
223. Harrison, T.R.: Principles of Internal Medicine, Ed. 3, (McGraw-Hill Book Co.: New York, NY), 1958
224. McKusick, V.A.: Heritable Disorders of Connective Tissue, Ed. 2 (The C.V. Mosby Co.: St. Louis, MO), 1960
225. Aschner, B.M., et al.: "A Genetic Study of Paget's Disease (Osteitis Deformans) in Monozygotic Twin Brothers", Acta Genet. Med. Gemell. 1:67–79, 1952
226. Woodward, H.Q.: "Long Term Studies of the Blood Chemistry in Paget's Disease of Bone", Cancer 12:1226–1237, 1959
227. Wilner, D. and Sherman, R.S.: "Roentgen Diagnosis of Paget's Disease (Osteitis Deformans)", Dent. Rad. Photo. 43:47–59, 1970
228. Smith, N.H.H.: "Monostotic Paget's Disease of the Mandible Presenting with Progressive Resorption of the Teeth", Oral Surg. 46:246–253, 1978
229. Richardson, J.F., Fine, M.A., and Goldman, H.M.: "Fibrosarcoma of the Mandible: A Clinico-pathologic Controversy", J. Oral Surg. 30:664–668, 1972
230. Hamilton, I.: "Fibrosarcoma of the Lower Jaw", Aust. New Zealand J. Surg. 15:54–59, 1945
231. Saw, D.: "Fibrosarcoma of the Maxilla: Report of a Case with Histochemical Studies", Oral Surg. 47:164–167, 1979
232. Clark, R.L. and Martin, R.G.: "Fibrosarcoma: Management and End Results", In: 6th National Cancer Conference Proceedings, (J.B. Lippincott Co.: Philadelphia, PA), 1970
233. Garrington, G.E., Scofield, H.H., Cornyn, J., and Hooker, S.P.: "Osteosarcoma of the Jaws: Analysis of 56 Cases", Cancer 20:377–391, 1967
234. Cahan, W.G., Woodard, H.Q., Higinbotham, N.L., et al.: "Sarcoma Arising in Irradiated Bone", Cancer 1:3–29, 1948
235. Sabanas, A.O., Dahlin, D.C., et al.: "Postradiation Sarcoma of Bone", Cancer 9:528–242, 1956
236. Phillips, T.L. and Sheline, G.E.: "Bone Sarcomas Following Radiation Therapy", Radiology 81:992–996, 1963
237. Kragh, L.V., Dahlin, D.C., and Erich, J.B.: "Osteogenic Sarcoma of the Jaws and Facial Bones", Amer. J. Surg. 96:496–505, 1958
238. Schofield, I.D.F. and Johnson, R.H.: "Osteosarcoma: An Example of the thickened Periodontal Ligament Space", J. Periodontol. 48:487–491, 1977
239. Dahlin, D.C.: Bone Tumors, Ed. 2, (Charles C. Thomas Publisher: Springfield, IL), 1977
240. Newland, J.R., and Ayala, A.G.: "Parosteal Osteosarcoma of the Maxilla", Oral Surg. 43:727–733, 1977
241. Jaffee, H.L. and Selin, G.: "Tumors of Bone and Joints", Bull. N.Y. Acad. Med. 27:165–174, 1951
242. Hoffman, S., Krolls, S.O., and Jacoway, J.R.: Intraosseous and Parosteal Cysts and Tumors of the Jaws, Second Series Fasicle, (Armed Forces Institute of Pathology: Washington, D.C.), (in press)
243. Slootweg, P.J.: "Clear-cell Chondrosarcoma of the Maxilla: Report of a Case", Oral Surg. 50:233–237, 1980
244. Caravolas, J.J., Piece, J.M., et al.: "Mesenchymal Chondrosarcoma of the Mandible", Oral Surg. 56:478–484, 1981
245. Joshi, K., Abrol, B.M., and Roy, S.: "Extraskeletal Mesenchymal Chondrosarcoma", Indian J. Pathol. Microbiol. 21:261–264, 1978
246. Batsakis, J.G.: "Salivary Gland Neoplasia: An Outcome of Modified Morphogenesis and Cytodifferentiation", Oral Surg. 49:229–232, 1980

247. Thackray, A.C.: Histological Typing of Salivary Gland Tumours, (World Health Organization Histological Classification of Tumours, No. 7: Geneva, Switzerland), 1972
248. Nicolatov, O., Harwick, R.D., et al.: "Ultrastructural Characterization of Intermediate Cells of Mucoepidermoid Carcinoma of the Parotid", Oral Surg. 489:324–336, 1979
249. Chen, S-Y: "Ultrastructure of Mucoepidermoid Carcinoma in Minor Salivary Glands", Oral Surg. 47:247–255, 1979
250. Nochomovitz, L.E. and Kahn L.B.: "Adenoid Cystic Carcinoma of the Salivary Gland and Its Histologic Variants", Oral Surg. 44:394–404, 1977
251. Abrams, A.M., Cornyn, J., et al.: "Acinic Cell Adenocarcinoma of the Major Salivary Glands: A Clinicopathologic Study of 77 Cases", Cancer 18:1145–1162, 1965
252. Abrams, A.M. and Melrose, R.J.: "Acinic Cell Tumors of Minor Salivary Gland Origin", Oral Surg. 46:220–233, 1978

Chapter 4. Pretreatment Evaluation

James E. Hamner, III, John M. Lore, Jr., and Donald P. Shedd

In order to treat cancer properly and adequately, it is essential that a thorough pretreatment evaluation of the patient be conducted. Specific points to be included will be discussed below. A summation of pretreatment evaluation is given in Fig. 4.1 and 4.2.

DETAILED HEAD AND NECK EXAMINATION

FINDINGS· (Illustrate detected lesion on the accompanying diagram sheets)

Normal	Abnor (check one)	Normal	Abnor. (check one)	Normal	Abnor. (check one)
___	___ Neck	___	___ Major Salivary Glands	___	___ Paranasal Sinus
___	___ Thyroid	___	___ Eyes (E.O.M., Pupils, Lids)	___	___ Ears
___	___ Scalp	___	___ Nose – External	___	___ Cranial Nerves
___	___ Face/maxilla	___	___ Nasal Cavity	___	___ Other (Trachea, Thyroid Cartilage)

ORAL PALPATION AND INSPECTION

Normal	Abnor (check one)	Normal	Abnor. (check one)	Normal	Abnor. (check one)
___	___ Lips	___	___ Gingiva	___	___ Base of Tongue
___	___ Buccal Walls	___	___ Mandible	___	___ Retromolar Trigone
___	___ Palate	___	___ Floor of Mouth	___	___ Tonsil
___	___ Dentition	___	___ Tongue	___	___ Oropharynx

MIRROR ENDOSCOPY

Normal	Abnor (check one)	Not seen/not done	Normal	Abnor (check one)	Not seen/not done
___	___ Base of Tongue	___	___	___ Arytenoids	___
___	___ Vallecula	___	___	___ Pyriform Sinuses	___
___	___ Epiglottis	___	___	___ Hypopharynx	___
___	___ Vocal Cords	___	___	___ Nasopharynx	___
___	___ Ventricles	___	___	___ Aryepiglottic Folds	___
___	___ Ventricular Bands	___	___	___	___

IMPRESSION

___ No Evidence of Disease　　___ Neoplastic lesion of head and neck　　___ Other (specify)

RECOMMENDATION

TUMOR EVALUATION

1 Site of Probable Origin (check one) (number after site is the recommended diagram to be completed)

___ Oral Cavity (2,3)	___ Larynx (1)	___ Maxillary Sinus (4,5)
___ Nasopharynx (5)	___ Nose (4,5)	___ Major Salivary Glands (4)
___ Oropharynx (3)	___ Cervical Esophagus (1)	___ Sinus except Maxillary (4,5)
___ Hypopharynx (1)	___ Cervical Trachea (1)	___ Unknown Primary (any that apply)

CLINICAL TUMOR STAGE

2. Primary Site (check one) (definitions on opposite page)

___T1S　___T1　___T2　___T2a　___T2b　___T3　___T4

3 Nodes (check one) (definitions on opposite page) Use diagram 6 for positive findings

___N0　___N1　___N2　___N2a　___N2b　___N2c　___N3　N3a　N3b　N3c

4 Distant Metastases (check one) (definitions on opposite page)

___M0　___M1

5 Tumor Grade/Histology (specify) ______

Hospital Name ______　Surgical Pathology Report No ______

FINAL TREATMENT DECISION

6 Check if any of the following factors were important in the final decision

___ Age	___ Respiratory	___ Metastases	___ Lesion Non-resectable
___ Occupation	___ Cardiac	___ Co-existing Malignancy	___ Other (specify)

7 Recommended treatment plan · Check all that apply (treatment given sequentially will be considered separate phases. If radio, chemo and/or immunotherapy are to be given simultaneously, they represent a common treatment phase.

Sequence of Treatment	Surgery			Radiation Therapy			Chemotherapy		Immunotherapy
	Primary	Nodes	Dist. Mets.	Primary	Nodes	Dist. Mets.	Systemic	Regional	
1st Phase									
2nd Phase									
3rd Phase									
4th Phase									

8 What is treatment objective? (check one)　___ Curative　___ Palliative

Completed By ______

Patient's Name ______　Date ______

Fig. 4.1. Detailed head and neck examination form

I. Medical History and Symptoms

In addition to the customary family history, past medical history (especially as it relates to cancer or other major medical problems), and present illness, a specific history of exposure to possible carcinogens is necessary. This history would include the use of alcohol and tobacco, exposure to radiation and chemicals, and other potential carcinogenic substances.

Particular emphasis should be placed on the patient's current symptomatology. A head and neck cancer patient can present with no symptoms, however, if dysphagia, loosened teeth, hoarseness, pain, or bleeding are present, they should be investigated throughly to determine the exact cause. Also the presence of a nonhealing ulceration, numbness, otalgia, changes in denture fit, unexplained facial pain, or the presence of a lump in the neck are all symptoms of significance.

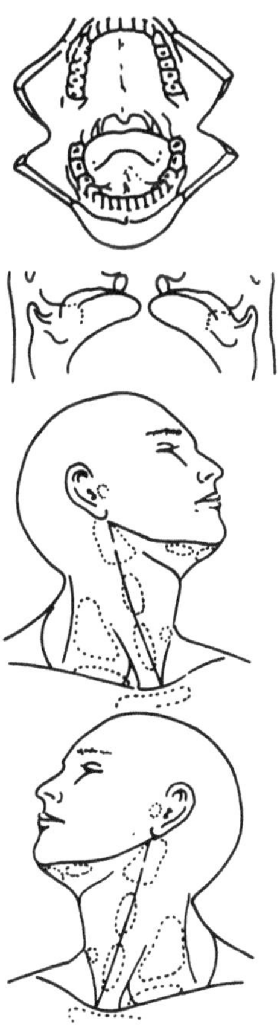

Patient's name.

Hospital no..

CLINICAL STATUS BEFORE TREATMENT ANYWHERE

Location of Tumor	Site of origin (check one)	Site(s) also involved
Lips:		
Upper	☐	☐
Lower	☐	☐
Buccal mucosa	☐	☐
Floor of mouth	☐	☐
Oral tongue	☐	☐
Hard palate	☐	☐
Gingivae.		
Upper	☐	☐
Lower	☐	☐
Retromolar trigone	☐	☐

Size of Tumor
<2 cm ☐ 2–4 cm ☐ >4 cm ☐

Characteristics of Tumor	Yes	No
Exophytic	☐	☐
Superficial	☐	☐
Moderately infiltrating	☐	☐
Deeply infiltrating	☐	☐
Ulcerated	☐	☐
Extends to or overlies bone	☐	☐
Gross erosion of bone	☐	☐
Radiographic destruction of bone	☐	☐
Involvement of Neighboring Regions		
Tonsillar pillar or soft palate	☐	☐
Nasal cavity or antrum	☐	☐
Nasopharynx	☐	☐
Pterygoid muscles	☐	☐
Soft tissues or skin of neck	☐	☐

Regional Lymph Nodes (check one only)

None	(N0)	☐			
Single homolateral <3 cm	(N1)	☐	Homolateral >6 cm	(N3a)	☐
Single homolateral 3–6 cm	(N2a)	☐	Bilateral*	(N3b)	☐
Multiple homolateral up to 6 cm	(N2b)	☐	Contralateral only	(N3c)	☐

*If bilateral nodes present, stage each side separately Right ______ Left ______

Distant Metastasis
None ☐ Lung ☐ Bone ☐ Liver ☐ Other (specify) ______

Histologic Cell Diagnosis
Squamous or epidermoid carcinoma ☐
Adenocarcinoma ☐
Other (specify) ______

Clinical Classification
T ______ N ______ M ______ Stage ______

Fig. 4.2. Site-specific data form for the oral cavity

II. Evaluation of Extent of Disease

A thorough general physical examination plus a detailed evaluation of the head and neck areas are required. This examination should include not only visual inspection, but palpation, both intraorally and externally. A bimanual examination is often of great value in assessing some of the upper neck and floor of mouth areas. A mirror evaluation of all areas of the pharynx and larynx is appropriate. Wherever pathology is identified, appropriate definition of areas of involvement, including measurements in centimeters is desirable.

Additional evaluation by radiologic and endoscopic means is necessary for many of the head and neck cancer sites. Radiologic evaluation may include xeroradiography of the soft tissues as well as x-ray evaluation of the bony structures, contrast evaluation, C.A.T. scans, and tomography of the pharynx and larynx. Diagnosis of all suspicious tumors requires microscopic confirmation. Biopsies should be carefully and precisely performed with a good record of the exact site from which each biopsy has been taken. Cell type and degree of maturity must be known when considering therapy.

Fine needle aspiration is a special method of biopsy, which is not to be used indiscriminately, and hence deserves some clarification of role at this point. Its success depends on both the surgeon and the pathologist knowing its restrictions and limitations. Only after a complete head and neck examination, should it be considered as an aid in determining the nature of a mass in the head and neck. Its main use is for tumors in the neck when metastatic disease is suspected, or when a primary lesion cannot be found. It is of distinct value when enlarged cervical nodes accompany a thyroid mass. When aspiration of such nodes reveals thyroid tissue, the diagnosis of metastatic cancer of the thyroid is virtually certain, realizing the extremely low incidence of normal thyroid tissue in cervical lymph nodes. In a lymphoma, needle aspiration may not provide a definitive diagnosis – and only a suggestion – an open biopsy may prove necessary. In tumors of the salivary glands, needle aspiration is used in selective situations, particularly when a positive diagnosis of a malignant tumor would significantly change the operative approach. If a chemodectoma is suspected, then the danger of hemorrhage must be weighed against the potential benefits to be gained by needle aspiration as opposed to other diagnostic measures, e.g., arteriography. At the very least, a 22 or 24-guage needle should be used first as a precautionary measure in such circumstances. Obviously, a pulsatile mass should not be aspirated.

III. Consultations

Total evaluation for diagnosis and pretreatment evaluation of head and neck cancer patients may require a multi-modality approach. Such consultation should be accomplished prior to the institution of definitive treatment. The number of consultants and their depth of involvement in individual patient management will vary. They may include any of the following specialities: dental, medical, surgical, radiotherapeutic, chemotherapeutic, diagnostic radiology, maxillofacial prosthodontic, anesthesiologic, psychiatric, rehabilitative medicine, and social work.

IV. Pretreatment Management

Customary pretreatment evaluation of the patient's general physical status should be performed, including liver profile and coagulation studies, when indicated. Depending on findings and the patient's status, additional studies may be necessary. Pulmonary status should be carefully evaluated and, if indicated, pulmonary function studies performed. If distant metastases are suspected, appropriate studies, such as liver scan, skeletal radiogram, and bone scan should be performed. It is particularly important to evaluate the nutritional status of head and neck cancer patients and provide any required special nutritional support. These patients are also frequently anemic and may require pretreatment transfusion. Arrangements for necessary dental care should be made. This action is especially important prior to initiation of radiation therapy and/or chemotherapy. If facial disfigurement or functional impairment is anticipated following surgery, then preoperative prosthodontic involvement should be arranged. Medical management of conditions such as coronary artery disease, chronic pulmonary insufficiency, or hepatic insufficiency, if they exist, should be undertaken prior to surgery in conjunction with a qualified internist. Psychological preparation of the patient and family is essential, and either the patient, his family, or both should be referred for psychological counseling, if deemed advisable prior to the initiation of therapy.

V. Informed Consent

Informed consent is absolutely essential. In order to obtain proper, legal informed consent from the patient, or if he/she is incompetent, from his/her guardian, it is necessary to communicate in understandable language and terms: the diagnosis, the alternative acceptable treatments that are available, the recommended treatment, its risks and likely sequelae, and the fact that no guarantee can be made by the doctor regarding either successful outcome or freedom from complications. Informed consent should be in writing and should be witnessed.

VI. Non-Standard Treatment

In any sizable group of cancer patients there will be a few individuals whose disease is advanced beyond a degree where standard treatment measures can be applied. For such patients, one of the options is no definitive treatment, and another is trial of new treatment approaches, primarily new chemotherapy or immunotherapy agents. Such treatment falls into the realm of clinical research and is managed in this context with appropriate safeguards and informed consent.

The following outline mechanism for head and neck cancer staging was presented and accepted by the American Joint Committee for Cancer Staging and End Results in 1976 and was revised in final form in 1978 [1].

VII. Rules for Classification

1. Clinical-Diagnostic Staging. The assessment of the primary tumor is based upon inspection and palpation of the oral cavity and neck. Additional studies may include plain, tomographic, and contrast roentgenograms, particularly evaluating bone invasion of the mandible or upper alveolus. Examinations for distant metastases include chest film, blood chemistries, blood count, and other routine studies as indicated.

2. Surgical-Evaluative Staging. Confirmation of the extent of disease is made by biopsy of suspected mucosal or submucosal spread, aspiration, or open biopsy of suspicious nodes. Biopsy of suspected distant metastases is desirable, but not required.

3. Postsurgical Treatment-Pathologic Staging. Complete resection of primary sites and radical nodal dissections allow for the use of this designation. Specimens that are resected after radiation and/or chemotherapy need to be especially noted.

4. Retreatment Staging. Utilization of available procedures noted above is required, particularly confirmation by biopsy since previous treatment by surgery or irradiation leads to scarring and induration. A reevaluation for distant metastases is important as well as T and N classifications [1].

VIII. TNM Classification [1]

1. Primary Tumor (T): (Oral)

TX No available information on primary tumor

T0 No evidence of primary tumor

TIS Carcinoma-in-situ

T1 Greatest diameter of primary tumor more than 2 cm, but not more than 4 cm

T3 Greatest diameter of primary tumor more than 4 cm

T4 Massive tumor more than 4 cmn diameter with deep invasion to involve antrum, pterygoid muscles, base of tongue, or skin of neck

2. Nodal Involvement (N)

Cervical Node Classification. – The following regional node classification is applicable to all malignant head and neck tumors. In clinical evaluation, the actual size of the nodal mass should be measured, and allowance should be made for intervening soft tissues. It is recognized that most masses over 3 cm in diameter are not single nodes, but are confluent nodes or tumor in soft tissues of the neck. There are three stages of clinically positive nodes: N1, N2, and N3. The use of subgroups a, b and c is not required, but is recommended. Midline nodes are considered as homolateral nodes.

NX Nodes cannot be assessed

N0 No clinically positive node

N1 Single clinically positive homolateral node 3 cm or less in diameter

N2 Single clinically positive homolateral node more than 3, but no more than 6 cm in diameter, or multiple clinically positive homolateral nodes, none more than 6 cm in diameter

- N2a Single clinically positive homolateral node more than 3 cm, but not more than 6 cm in diameter
- N2b Multiple clinically positive homolateral nodes, none more than 6 cm in diameter

N3 Massive homolateral node(s), bilateral nodes, or contralateral node(s)

- N3a Clinically positive homolateral node(s), one more than 6 cm in diameter
- N3b Bilateral clinically positive nodes (in this situation, each side of the neck should be staged separately; that is N3b: right, N2a; left, N1)
- N3c Contralateral clinically positive node(s) only

3. Distant Metastasis (M)

MX Not assessed

M0 No (known) distant metastasis

M1 Distant Metastasis present
Specify ______________________

Specify sites according to the following notations:

Pulmonary – PUL
Osseous – OSS
Hepatic – HEP
Brain – BRA
Lymph Nodes – LYM
Bone Marrow – MAR
Plura – PLE
Skin – SKI
Eye – EYE
Other – OTH

IX. Postsurgical Treatment Residual Tumor (R)

R0	No residual tumor
R1	Microscopic residual tumor
R2	Macroscopic residual tumor Specify ____________

X. Summary of Stage Groupings

Stage 1	T1 N0 M0
Stage II	T2 N0 M0
Stage III	T3 N0 M0 T1 or T2 or T3 N1 M0
Stage IV	T4 N0 or N1 M0 Any T N2 or N3 M0 Any T any N M1

XI. Common Departures from Sound Management [2]

Sound clinical management, as collectively developed over years of accumulated experience, is sometimes better expressed in negative rather than positive terms – either what should not be done, or pitfalls to avoid. It would, of course, be impractical to attempt any kind of exhaustive listing of departures from sound practive. However, a few that stand out as perhaps too often seen are itemized below for easy reference.

The following are cast in terms of *unsound* practices:

1. Open Biopsy of a Lump in the Neck Before Performing a Complete Head and Neck General Examination

(A) Discussion

An open biopsy will yield the histologic diagnosis, but in carcinoma it will usually:

2) encourage spread of tumor in the neck
3) make necessary the resection of a large area of overlying skin
4) interfere with the usual anatomic surgical planes relative to definitive therapy

(B) Prevention

Complete an adequate head and neck examination, including as indicated: direct endoscopy, plus x-ray evaluation of the mandible, sinuses, nasopharynx, larynx, and chest plus a general physical examination, including rectal and pelvic examination. When all of these fail to reveal the source of the primary tumor, then a needle aspiration is recommended, except in those patients in whom the clinical impression is that of a carotid body tumor, or other chemodectoma. If the needle aspiration fails, then open biopsy is justifiable and then, depending on circumstances, may preferably be performed in the operating room with frozen section.

2. Inadequate Incisional Biopsy of an Oral Cavity Lesion

(A) Discussion

Punch biopsy of localized areas of leukoplakia or erythroplakia may well miss the site of carcinoma and lead the physician and dentist to a false sense of security.

(B) Prevention

The localized area of leukoplakia or erythroplakia, not responding to conservative management within two to three weeks, usually is best totally excised. The specimen, properly marked as to orientation, is then submitted for serial histological sectioning.

3. Inadequate Excisional Biopsy of a Suspicious Oral Cavity Lesion

(A) Discussion

By and large, highly suspicious lesions are best evaluated prior to excisional biopsy by the physician who will eventually make the decision as to the best course of management, whether it be surgery, radiotherapy chemotherapy, or some combination of these modalities.

This evaluation is best achieved prior to any surgical intervention, so as to ascertain the size of the lesion, as well as its local extension and the presence or absence of metastatic disease. For example, inadequate excisional biopsy of a lesion of the floor of the mouth, may mask the actual extent of the tumor, as well as cause obstruction of Wharton's Duct, inducing enlargement of both submandibular salivary glands. This latter effect could be confused with possible metastatic spread to submandibular lymph nodes.

(B) Prevention

Initial evaluation prior to any type of surgical excision is best performed by the physician who will ultimately be responsible for the total management.

4. Failure to Review Previous Histopathologic Slides

(A) Discussion

At times, the physician responsible for the management of the patient with a head and neck neoplasm, which has been biopsied elsewhere, will in the face of expediency, rely solely of a written histopathologic report from an outside source. This occurs when a biopsy and histologic diagnosis have been performed at the time of original patient contact. Errors can occur when the personnel at the primary care facility simply have not had the exposure to some of the types of head and neck neoplasms. Evaluation of the degree of "malignancy" is most important. For example, in a muco-epidermoid carcinoma of a salivary gland, it is crucial to know whether the tumor is low grade or high grade. This "grading" not only influences prognosis, but it also is most important in the type of surgical management.

(B) Prevention

Request submission of all histologic slides and if necessary, blocks for further evaluation. The results may even indicate that an additional biopsy be performed.

5. Permitting a Single Histopathologic Benign Diagnosis to Override a Clinical Diagnosis of Carcinoma

(A) Discussion

At times, the clinical diagnosis of a malignant neoplasm is not substantiated by biopsy and histologic evaluation. The problem may lie with the choice of the location of the biopsy site. For example, if the biopsy is taken in an inflammatory area surrounding a neoplasm, or in the center of a necrotic area, or in the far periphery where only epithelial dysplasia is present – all will lead to histologic diagnosis of a non-malignant lesion. The other problem may rest with the paucity of histiologic sections taken through the block of tissue, thus missing the malignant cells.

(B) Prevention

It must be emphasized that a skilled clinician's impression on physical examination is more often right than wrong. The clinician, thus, must be wary of a benign diagnosis in the histologic evaluation for the above-mentioned reasons. Repeat biopsy, or total excision of the lesion, must be performed with explicit understanding by the pathologist that, if necessary, many serial sections be performed. It also may be necessary to have recourse to one or several repeat biopsies. Then, should all biopsies prove benign, such patients should be followed at close intervals until the diagnostic discrepancy is adequately resolved. Recourse to consultation may be advisable.

6. Biopsies of the Larynx, Hypopharynx, Nasopharynx, Esophagus, or Trachea Prior to Radiologic Studies

(A) Discussion

Biopsies of the above organ sites will often cause edema, and/or distortion of the neoplasm as far as its extent and size is concerned. Hence, radiologic studies, either in the form of plain soft tissue x-rays, tomograms, or contrast studies, can be erroneously interpreted, if performed following such biopsies.

(B) Prevention

If at all anticipated and practical, radiologic studies are best performed *prior* to biopsy of the areas in question to avoid this distortion.

7. Lack of Multidisciplinary Approach Where Indicated

(A) Discussion

A primary-care physician has the tremendous responsibility of the initial referral for definitive care of the patient with a head and neck neoplasm. At times these referrals are to other physicians who, although quite capable in their own discipline, are not well versed in the multi-discipline aspects of the management of head and neck malignant neoplasms.

(B) Prevention

Obviously, lesions frequently present with a choice of management which is clear cut, but even the slightest reservation, should be subjected to a broader scrutiny in the patient's best interest. Use of multi-disciplinary consultations or conferences should be stressed. The primary-care physician must be cognizant of this multi-discipline aspect and be sure that the physician he chooses to manage the patient is also cognizant of this multi-discipline approach. This latter physician in his basic training may have sufficient knowledge of the multi-disciplines involved or he may in fact, wish an additional consultation from the many varied disciplines in medicine and dentistry that relate to the proper management of head and neck cancer.

8. Tailoring the Scope of Surgical Resection to the Ability of the Surgeon Rather than to the Objective Requirements Imposed by the Lesion

(A) Discussion

It is a serious error when making a decision regarding the feasibility of surgical management of an extensive neoplasm, to render a verdict of non-resectability when, in fact, the problem rests with the physician or surgeon making the decision, who does not have the expertise or background regarding the necessary operation. Furthermore, in surgery tailoring the scope of excision to the ability of the surgeon, rather than to the objective requirements imposed by the character, location, and extent of the lesion is inexcusable.

(B) Prevention

It is realized that there often is a wide devergence of opinion regarding resectability. Nevertheless, the physician making the decision, must be well-versed in the various options and fully aware of what can and cannot be resected with reasonably satisfactory results. Clear-cut knowledge of the natural history of the disease is as important as knowledge of the surgical technique in making this decision.

9. A Compromise of the Ablative Phase of Surgery in Order to Accommodate Limited Reconstructive Skills

(A) Discussion

When the ablative surgery is modified to such an extent that adequate resection with reasonable free margins is jeopardized to accommodate wound closure, a surgical error is committed. The surgeon must be well versed both in the ablative phase and the reconstructive phase of surgical management. Otherwise, the likelihood of cure is compromised, or the patient is disabled. The reconstructive phase must at times take a somewhat back seat to the ablative phase, but never vise versa.

(B) Prevention

Complete training of the head and neck surgeon in all phases of ablative and reconstructive surgery is necessary.

10. Compromise of Surgical Margins Because Radiation Therapy or Chemotherapy Was or Is To Be Given

(A) Discussion

It is a sore temptation to limit the area of surgical resection because of a false sense of security, deriving from a favorable radiation therapy and/or chemotherapy result that has either already occured preoperatively or is anticipated post-operatively.

(B) Prevention

If radiotherapy and/or chemotherapy are utilized in combination with surgery, then it is important that the surgery encompass the same area that would have been resected had it been the sole treatment modality. It goes without saying that careful record keeping of the size and extent of the primary neoplasm, (at times with the use of tattoo) as well as the metastatic disease, is most important to prevent this error.

11. Performing the Right Operation on the Wrong Patient

(A) Discussion

This pitfall is closely allied with earlier items mentioned in certain respects, but primarily concerns itself with the definition of resectability versus operability. A neoplasm may be technically resectable, utilizing a specific surgical technique, yet the operation is not suited to the patient, or the patient may not be in such physical condition that he can tolerate the operation or the consequences of the operation. Actually, in head and neck surgery, there are very few general medical or general surgical problems which totally interdict surgical management; yet, there are contingencies, which influence the selection of a surgical procedure, e.g., a supraglottic laryngectomy may well be suited to the carcinoma of the larynx, but not suited to the patient who is elderly with chronic pulmonary insufficiency. The same principle may well apply also the use of a non-delayed deltopectoral flap in a severe arteriosclerotic and diabetic patient.

(B) Prevention

Careful evaluation of the total patient in regard to all vital functions, being certain that the patient can not only tolerate the operation, but also the anesthesia, as well as the sequelae of both is essential.

12. Assessing the Degree of Success or Failure of Radiation Therapy on the Basis of the Response of the Lesion During or Immediately on the Completion of Treatment

(A) Discussion

There is a tendency among some physicians to decide prematurely that radiotherapy has failed when upon completion of this modality, disease is still present. Along the same line of thought is the error of deciding that the neoplasm under treatment will not eventually have a successful outcome when early or midway through the treatment, the response has been slow. Conversely, a rapid response during radiotherapy is sometimes improperly used as a justification to reduce total dosage. A high rate of response of a neoplasm does not have implications for the dose necessary to sterilize the tumors.

(B) Prevention

Realize that radiotherapy response is varied during the course of treatment, and that this may not necessarily indicate the final outcome. Upon completion of the planned full course of treatment, a four-to-six-week interval should lapse before re-biopsy is performed.

13. Failure to Realize the Implication of the "Condemned Mucosa" or Multiple Primary Syndrome

(A) Discussion

Especially in patients with multiple areas of leukoplakia and/or erythroplakia, multiple primaries are not only a possibility, but actually a probability. Even in the absence of these possible precancerous lesions, multiple primaries are a distinct possibility in a patient who already has one squamous cell carcinoma of the head and neck. This clinical entity is somewhat more common in the heavy tobacco and/or alcohol user. These are the patients who demonstrate the condemned mucosa. Tendency to "zero in" on the site of the first or original primary in follow-up examination is only natural, and often a follow-up and repeat complete head and neck examination is bypassed, and thus, other lesions are all too frequently overlooked.

(B) Prevention

A complete head and neck examination must be performed at frequent intervals in all patients who have demonstrated a primary squamous cell carcinoma of the head and neck.

14. Failure to Perform a Complete General Physical Examination As Well As a Complete Head and Neck Examination

(A) Discussion

Unfortunately, the division of human anatomy into various regions, for example, head and neck, chest, abdomen, and pelvis, is not respected by neoplastic disease, nor for that matter, by infectious disease or trauma. A mass in the neck may not necessarily represent primary disease above the clavicle. The primary disease may be in the chest, breast, abdomen, pelvis, ovaries, or urinary bladder, or elsewhere.

(B) Prevention

In addition to a complete head and neck examination, a complete physical examination is a sine qua non for diagnosis and must be performed prior to commencement of definitive management of a head and neck neoplasm. This includes digital rectal and pelvic examination.

15. Prolonged Watch-and-Wait Attitude in the Face of an Asymptomatic Mass

(A) Discussion

All too often either the patient, or primary-care physician may delay the evaluation of a mass in the head and neck, which is causing no pain or interference with the patient's normal function. This delay could be a disaster.

(B) Prevention

Any abnormal mass must be promptly and completely evaluated, and it is then usually removed, depending on the findings and diagnosis.

16. Inadequate Search for an Occult Primary

(A) Discussion

There are patients seen who have histologically proven involvement of cervical lymph nodes by squamous cell carcinoma without an apparent primary lesion. Such a patient should not be placed in this unknown primary category until he has had a completely adequate diagnostic workup.

(B) Prevention

The only admonition in this problem is to repeat complete head and neck examination and general physical examination with diagnostic studies including x-rays of the paranasal sinuses, nasopharynx, esophagus, and chest. Depending on the histologic findings on aspiration of the metastasis, other radiologic studies may be indicated. Areas to scrutinize extremely carefully if the metastasis is squamous cell carcinoma are the following: nasopharynx, (vault, lateral walls, and posterior choanae, including posterior edge of septum), tonsils, base of the tongue, pyriform sinuses, and inferior portion of the laryngeal surface of the epiglottis. If open biopsy is necessary after all else has failed, it may well be best performed in the operating room with frozen sections, so that depending on the circumstances and histologic diagnosis, a radical neck dissection can then be performed without delay.

At times, the location of the cervical metastasis may give an indication of the location of the primary tumor, e.g. posterior triangle node: Nasopharynx – (vault) and subdigastric node: floor of the mouth, tongue, oropharynx, hypopharynx, larynx, maxillary sinus, sphenoid sinus, and posterior portion of nasal septum.

17. Abandonment of the Patient with Neck Metastasis from an Undetectable Primary

Such a patient should not be abandoned, but should be given the benefit of definitive treatment. If the cancer in the neck node is well differentiated, and if the node is situated in the mid-neck, it may possibly represent a so-called branchiogenic carcinoma, although there has been uncertainty about the existence of this entity. In such an instance, radical neck dissection is indicated, with careful subsequent follow-up in a continued search for hidden primary. In some patients, the long-term repeat examinations will eventually disclose the primary tumor, one hopes, at a treatable stage. If the node shows undifferentiated squamous carcinoma, and if the node is at the periphery of the usual neck dissection, the management is more controversial. Some clinicians would advise neck dissections, and others would advocate radiation therapy. When the neck is irradiated in such circumstances, a judgement is necessary as to whether the ports should encompass the sites of a possible undisclosed primary; for example, nasopharynx or base of the tongue (refer to discussion under 14 for additional suggestions). Despite the ominous situation of the undiscovered primary, a significant number of such patients do achieve cure by both surgical and radiotherapeutic approaches.

18. Enucleation of Tumors of the Major Salivary Glands and Thyroid Gland

(A) Discussion

There has been in the past and continues at present the practice of enucleation of circumscribed tumors of the major salivary glands (usually the parotid) and of the thyroid gland. This procedure is inadequate, can spread disease, and makes subsequent surgery difficult.

Following enucleation of a benign mixed tumor from a salivary gland, the tumor will probably recur, and as it recurs, metaplasia to a malignant form can take place. Mixed tumors tend to recur because tumor cells usually infiltrate the fibrous tissue capsule. Enculeation of thyroid nodule can lead to several problems:

(i) Although frozen section may appear benign, final sections could be malignant. The secondary operation thereby necessitated is quite hazardous because of the possibilities of injury to the recurrent laryngeal nerve, and/or external branch of the superior laryngeal nerve, and/or loss of the parathyroid glands.
(ii) A second nodule, which was not perceptible, may be left behind. This latter nodule has on occasion proven to be the carcinoma.

(B) Prevention

With all tumors of the salivary gland and thyroid gland, the operation of choice is *total* lobectomy. With the parotid salivary gland, exposure of the 7th nerve is important. With the thyroid gland, exposure and preservation of the recurrent laryngeal nerve and preservation of the parathyroid glands and external branch of the superior laryngeal nerve are important.
In relation to thyroid lobectomy, the word "total" is stressed since it is suspected that all too often the surgeon calls an operation a total lobectomy when in fact a subtotal lobectomy has been performed. A portion of the thyroid lobe is apt to be left behind Berry's (posterior suspensory) ligament of the thyroid, if meticulous care is not exercised.

19. Treating a Patient with Antibiotics for an Extended Period of Time Without a Biopsy

(A) Discussion

It is not at all uncommon to see patients with tumors of the head and neck in whom the initial physician assumed an inflammatory lesion and prescribed antibiotics for extended periods of time.

(B) Prevention

Often, in such circumstances, following a reasonable period of no response, more careful examination of the lesion would mandate a biopsy and thereby avoid an unwarranted delay in beginning definitive treatment for cancer.

References

1. Beahrs, O.H., et al.: Manual for Staging of Cancer – 1978, Ed. 2, (Whiting Press: Rochester, MN), 1978
2. Lore, J.M. and Shedd, D.P.: "Common Departures from Sound Management". In: Management Guidelines for Head and Neck Cancer, Ed. 1, (Hamner J.E., III, ed.), (N.I.H. Publication No. 80-2037: Bethesda, MD), 1979

Chapter 5. Treatment

Donald P. Shedd, Luther W. Brady, Lawrence W. Davis, and
James E. Hamner, III

I. Surgical Treatment of Head and Neck Cancer

Donald P. Shedd

When feasible, the best management of cancer is to separate all the malignant tumor from the patient by surgical excision. The advantages of surgery are that the treatment is administered promptly and completed in a short interval of time. It permits pathologic definition of the extent of the cancer and accurate evalution of the margins of the excision. Pathologic evaluation is facilitated and enhanced if the surgeon provides a diagrammatic description of the surgical specimen. The disadvantages of surgery are the tissue loss required by emcompassing all of the tumor during excision, the consequent functional and cosmetic deformities that may ensue, and the usual physiological risks of any surgical procedure.

Cancers of the upper aerodigestive tract are characterized by local extention and invasion, with subsequent cervical lymph node metastasis. Regional lymph node involvement generally follows regular patterns according to the location of the primary tumor, although exceptions with bizarre spread do occur. A simple scheme for classification of neck nodes is indicated in Fig. 5.1, wherein

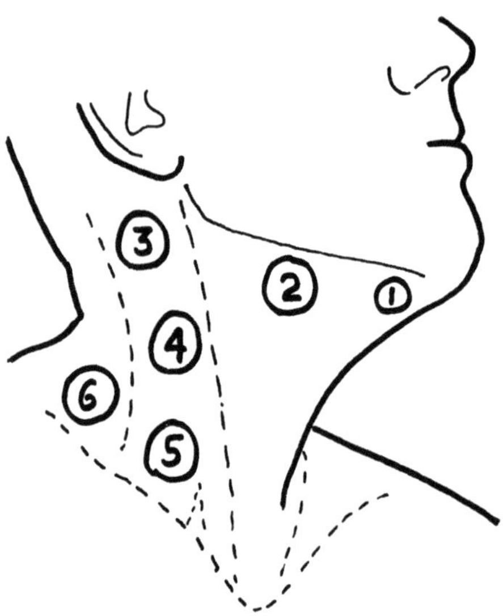

Fig. 5.1. Diagram showing major node zones in the neck: (*1*) submental, (*2*) submandibular, (*3*), (*4*), and (*5*) upper, middle and lower deep jugular respectively, and (*6*) posterior triangle

the major groups are submental, submandibular, deep jugular (upper, middle, and lower), and posterior triangle. Other zones in which involvement can occur from particular tumors are posterior auticular, juxta-parotid, retropharyngeal, pretracheal, and juxta-thyroid. Death results from the local disease more than from distant metastasis.

Squamous carcinoma of the upper aerodisgestive tract is relatively amendable to treatment, if accomplished early, with good survival figures in such patients. Despite educational efforts, however, a number of patients present with relatively advanced disease, and in these cases, cures are not often accomplished.

1. Oral Cavity Cancer

In recent years, significant improvement has been noted in results of treatment of oral cancer by both radiation therapy and surgery. For some oral sites, a variation of opinion on the respective role of the two methods exists, whereas for other sites some standardization of treatment concepts is emerging. Smaller cancers can be cured by either method. Far advanced lesions are seen which are incurable by any method. In between are moderately advanced cancers wherein the primary oral lesions may be curable by either skillful irradiation or extirpation, but wherein the tumor involvement of cervical nodes is best managed by radical neck dissection [1]. Many patients are candidates for composite operations, procedures in which the oral primary cancer is resected in continuity with the involved draining lymphatics, frequently including the mandible, depending on the location of the primary tumor. By modern reconstructive methods, the deformity and disability from such efforts can be minimized. Moderate disability is far more acceptable than the ravages of the uncontrolled cancer.

Studies are under way in various centers to determine whether the survival figures from operation can be increased by preoperative or postoperative radiation therapy; initial results are variable. One well-controlled study showed no significant reduction in post-operative local recurrence after radiation, and no increase in survival [2]. A second similar study did indicate some reduction in local recurrence, but this finding was accompanied by no gain in survival [3].

Cancer of the lip, when small, can be cured by radiation therapy or excision, but in the case of larger lesions, extirpation with immediate reconstruction provides good functional and cosmetic results.

Buccal mucosa is a site where circumscribed lesions are seen, curable by radiation therapy or adequate excision. Larger cancers require composite resection with reconstruction of the defect by pedicle grafts.

Cancers of the gingiva are seen which are exophytic and amendable to adequate local excision, including portions of bone according to clinical and radiologic evidence of involvement. More advanced lesions require segmental bone resection, hemimandibulectomy, or partial maxillectomy, depending on the extent of the lesion and its location.

Cancer of the floor of the mouth is a frequent lesion. It presents a special problem when the lesion involves the anterior portion of the mandible, since resection of this structure produces considerable deformity, a problem that is being solved by modern reconstructive techniques. Tumors of the lateral floor of the mouth are treated by adequate extirpation, usually with incontinuity neck dissection. A portion of the mandible is resected along with the tumor, if required by the position and extent of tumor.

Tongue cancer, occuring frequently on the lateral borders, can be managed by radiation therapy or by surgery. Moderate excisions of tongue, even hemiglossectomy, yield surprisingly little speech diability, provided the wound closure is such that the tongue is not bound down. Occasional patients with advanced lingual tumors require almost total glossectomy. Compensatory mechanisms can result in satisfactory recovery of speech.

Cancer of the hard palate usually requires excision of underlying bone, producing an opening into the antrum. This defect can be covered with a dental prosthesis, a maneuver that restores satisfactory swallowing and speech.

In reconstruction, some defects can be closed primarily. Small to medium sized oral mucosal defects, depending upon location, will heal satisfactorily with no effort at closure. For example, a defect of mucosa and periosteum over the hard palate will heal with a good result. Many defects, however, require closure with imported tissue, either free grafts or pedicle grafts. Tongue flaps are useful for closure of defects of moderate size. These reconstructive procedures must be viewed as major surgery in their own right and should not be undertaken by surgeons who are inexperienced with these techniques.

2. Pharyngeal Cancer

The conventional terms used in the United States for the three subdivisions of the pharynx are nasopharynx, oropharynx, and hypopharynx (Fig. 5.2). Alternate terms occasionally employed are epipharynx, mesopharynx, and laryngopharynx. Cancer in each of these states has distinctive features. From a historical viewpoint, evidence available on nasopharyngeal cancer from a study of skulls indicates that this disease existed in Egypt as far back as 3,000 B.C. and also in ancient Peru [4].

(A) Nasopharyngeal Cancer

Because of the anatomical location of the nasopharynx and the areas involved by tumor, radiotherapy plays the primary role in treatment. While the histologic types of tumors in the nasopharynx vary somewhat from other head and neck areas, including a higher frequency of lymphoepitheliomas and lymphomas, the predominant tumor is still an epidermoid carcinoma. Treatment must include all of the nasopharynx and its immediate contiguous areas of frequent spread and all of the lymph nodes in both sides of the neck with particular reference to the retropharyngeal nodes, which represent the first echelon of drainage

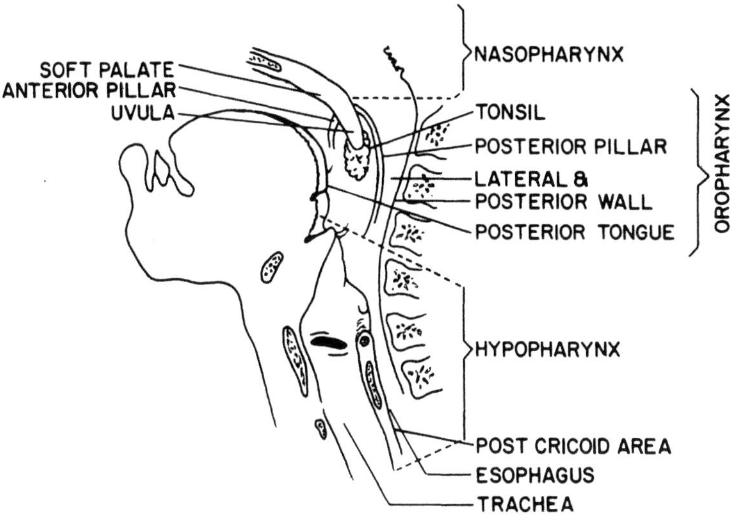

Fig. 5.2. Diagram of sagittal section of the head showing the pharynx and its divisions, as well as the larynx

from this site. The five-year survival rate is approximately 35%. Surgical salvage operations for persistent adenopathy in the neck, following control of the primary lesion, is appropriate in this selected situation [5, 6].

(B) Oropharyngeal Cancer

Carefully defined programs of integrated radiation therapy and surgical procedures for the treatment of cancer of the oropharynx have afforded substantial success [7]. Radiation therapy is frequently used for the primary lesions. Surgical extirpation of the primary tumor is done in selected circumstances, such as radiation failure or as a planned post-radiation operation in advanced leions. The approach to cervical nodes depends on the site and size of the primary and its histologic type. For example, in tonsillar cancer with small node involvement, an attempt would be made to achieve control by radiation therapy alone; whereas a patient with pharyngeal wall cancer with nodes would have radical neck dissection, if the primary cancer is controlled. Patients with soft palate and uvular lesions with small node involvement achieve 50% five-year survival by integrated radiation and surgery [8].

In some cancer centers one finds greater dependence on either radiation therapy or surgical treatment. Careful analysis of results, particularly of prospective studies, may in time provide a clear picture of the best approach to treatment of cancer in the oropharynx.

(C) Hypopharyngeal Cancer

Patients whose nutrition has suffered as a result of cancer in the laryngopharynx may require aggressive feeding measures as an adjunct to whatever method of treatment is used. Small cancers in this area can be cured by radiation therapy, particularly if they are exophytic. It is also possible to extirpate some of the small lesions in a manner that perserves laryngeal function, as demonstrated by Ogura [9]. It is important to know that a frequent characteristic of pharyngeal cancer is multicentricity and field cancerization, phenomena that can be recognized by in vivo staining pre-operatively or during operation with toluidine blue [10].

In the moderate sized hypopharyngeal cancers, and in those with node involvement which is not extensive, fair survival can be achieved by adequate composite operations in which the primary tumor is resected, usually with laryngectomy plus a radical neck dissection. Removal of sufficient pharyngeal wall may necessitate some method of reconstruction in which pedicle flaps of pectoral skin are used [11]. Patients who undergo such procedures have a temporary salivary fistula for a few weeks, during which time their nutrition is maintained by nasogastric tube feeding. At a second-stage operation, the fistula is closed, and swallowing is resumed. The pectoralis major myocutaneous flap is an alternative which eliminates the secondary operation.

For the more extensive lesions, results of surgical treatment alone are less satisfactory, and radiation therapy and surgery are used in various combinations [12]. Further studies of such approaches will determine the degree of improvement to be achieved by combinations over results obtainable by either method alone.

3. Laryngeal Cancer

The larynx is a complex structure, with intricate valves that not only produce speech sounds, but also control air flow, prevent aspiration, and permit straining, an act for which the closure of the glottis is a necessity (Fig. 5.3 and 5.4).

(a) Clinical Manifestations and Diagnosis

Very small tumors of the edge of the vocal cord can produce impressive alterations in voice and will lead to early recognition in an alert patient (Fig. 5.5).

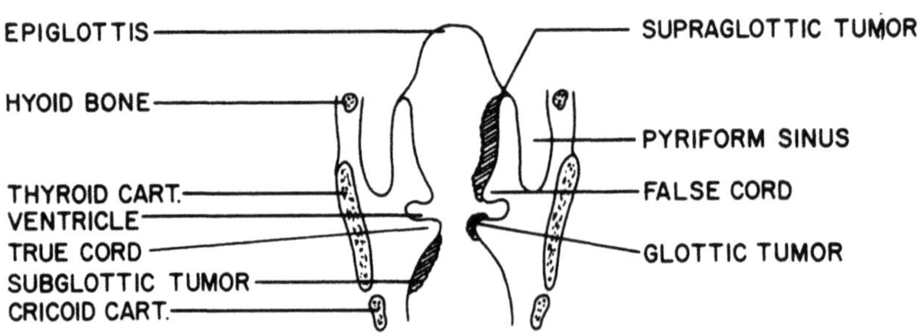

Fig. 5.3. Diagram of coronal section of the larynx showing anatomic landmarks and location of supraglottic, glottic, and subglottic tumors

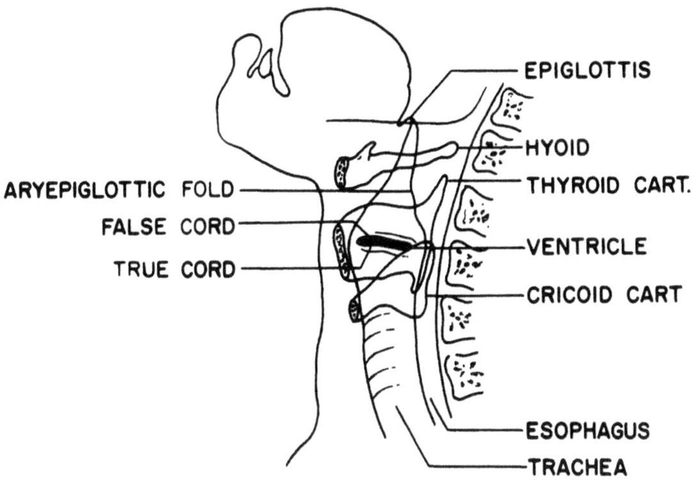

Fig. 5.4. Phantom sagittal view of the hypopharynx and larynx to demonstrate the cartilaginous framework and the anatomic structures

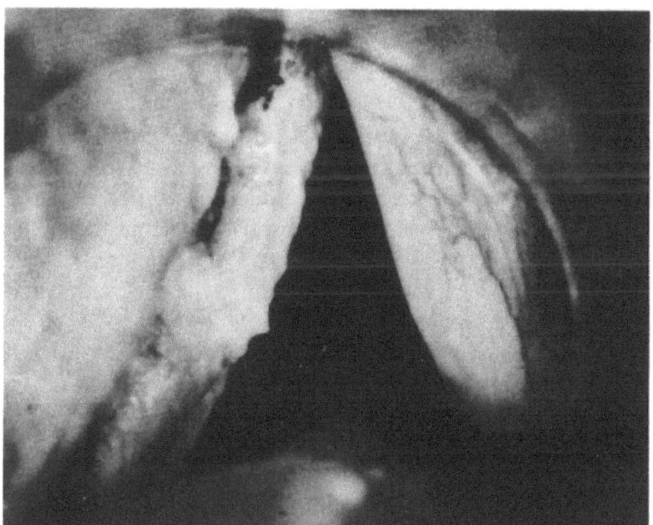

Fig. 5.5. Microlaryngoscopic view showing a normal right vocal cord and a verucous carcinoma of the left vocal cord

Supraglottic and subglottic tumors, however, can reach considerable size before the patient becomes concerned. Once suspected, the majority of laryngeal tumors can be seen by simple indirect laryngoscopy. Modern radiographic techniques, particularly laminography and computerized tomography, provide sufficient detail to permit definition of lesions within the larynx. Contrast studies, laryngography, provide additional information about the air passages. Histologic diagnosis is usually accomplished by biopsy at the time of direct laryngoscopy, which is done under topical or general anesthesia. Utilizing present day methods of suspension laryngoscopy, it is possible to study the fine details of mucosal change under magnification (laryngomicroscopy) and to perform a biopsy with precision in any area of abnormality. Such procedures, done under general anesthesia, permit adequate time for careful examination of the entire laryngeal and pharyngeal mucosa, and they more than compensate for the additional risk of general anesthesia.

(b) Treatment

At this point in time it is clear that a patient with cancer in the middle third of a completely mobile vocal cord has good prospects for cure by radiation therapy. At the other end of the scale, the chances for radiation cure are poor in a patient whose carcinoma has fixed the cord and extended around the anterior commissure, or in patients with advanced supraglottic and subglottic lesions. Patients such as these have a better hope for cure by total laryngectomy.

In between these extremes are patients in whom the decision is more difficult. There is question whether patients with beginning impairment of motion or early extension to the anterior commissure should have radiation therapy. One view holds that such patients should be treated by some form of partial laryngectomy, perserving vocal function. Another view is that such patients should have a trial of radiation therapy, followed by partial or total laryngectomy, if the radiation fails. Partial resections of larynx for lesions such as these are difficult operations, requiring considerable judgement and skill. It is clear that certain carefully selected patients with epiglottic cancer can undergo partial supraglottic laryngectomy, with adequate cure rates and preservation of function. The history of cancer surgery in other sites has demonstrated that problems arise when one begins to compromise with established, adequate cancer surgery such as total laryngectomy, but further evidence is defining the place for such endeavors in laryngeal cancer.

The work of Fletcher and associates indicates that there is a place in advanced supraglottic cancer for radiation therapy following surgery in an effort to increase the salvage [12].

(c) Management of Cervical Nodes

A patient with clinically involved nodes associated with laryngeal cancer should have appropriate regional lymphadenectomy done as a composite operation at the time of laryngectomy. Truly glotic cancers usually do not have node involvement, so that neck dissection can be omitted in most such patients. In patients with advanced supraglottic and subglotic tumors, the incidence of node involvement, even when not palpable, justifies radical neck dissection in association with the surgical treatment of the primary tumor.

(d) Rehabilitation

Patients who undergo laryngectomy can regain voice by various methods, the most convenient of which is esophageal speech. Unfortunately, about 40% of patients do not achieve this means of communication, and for this group, electronic devices are available. One of the early surgical approaches to restoring voice was that proposed by the Japanese surgeon, Asai, wherein a fistula is created from the tracheostoma to the oropharynx, through which air flows to produce sound [13]. Articulation by oral structures makes this sound into quite adequate speech. In recent years the procedure for voice rehabilitation described by Finger and Blum [14] has gained prominence. This involves making a fistula from the tracheostoma into the pharynx. The patient wears a prosthesis in the fistula to prevent leakage of ingesta. Digital occlusion of the stoma causes expired air to flow through the prosthesis into the pharynx, where sound is produced for speech. Experience reported to date concerning this approach has been quite favorable.

The one reported instance of transplantation of the the human larynx was done in Belgium with initial success, but reportedly the patient soon developed considerable tumor recurrence, presumably related to the use of immunosuppressive agents.

(e) Results

Nationwide survey data indicated an overall five-year survival rate for laryngeal cancer of 57%, with a rate of 76% for localized lesions and 29% for those with regional involvement [15]. In reports from specific institutions concerning treatment of purely glottic cancer in the middle-third of a mobile cord, the cure rates approach the 90% range, following radiation therapy.

4. Paranasal Sinus Cancer

Cancer in the sinuses presents problems because of its inaccessibility for diagnosis and treatment. Fortunately, neoplasms of this area are relatively rare.

(a) Management

Once the diagnosis has been made, and the extent of the tumor assessed, treatment planning begins. Those patients in whom the extent of disease is beyond cure will be determined by x-ray study, and in this inoperable group, radiation therapy is generally employed. In advanced but operable patients, attempts have been made to combine two modalities, to utilize radiation therapy as either a pre-operative or post-operative measure. The patients in whom a sinus cancer is moderately advanced, with extension beyond the site of origin, should have both radiation therapy and surgery in whatever sequence is appropriate for the particular lesion.

The operation done for antral cancer is a superior maxillectomy in which the eye must frequently be included because of involvement of the superior wall of the sinus. In tumors of the anterior inferior antrum the eye can be spared. Resection must on occasions be extended to include such areas as the cribriform plate. Extended resections with a combined external and intracranial approach have been devised as methods to deal with extensions of tumor [16].

The large defect from antrectomy is lined with a free skin graft, which reduces the contractural deformity of the cheek, and early insertion of a dental prosthesis permits resumption of speech and swallowing [17].

(b) Results

In a representative series of patients with paranasal sinus cancer, the early lesions showed five-year cures in the 18% to 35% range, but in the overall series the salvage was 10%, largely because so many of the lesions were of advanced stage. In patients with early lesions, who are treated for cure, a four-year survival of 44% has been reported [7].

This figure is indicative of progress being achieved in cancer centers by carefully planned programs integrating radiation therapy and surgical measures.

5. Salivary Gland Cancer

Embryologically, the salivary glands arise as outpouchings of the oral cavity. Tumors of these structures constitute a sizable fraction of the overall experience with head and neck neoplasms. Most salivary tumors are benign, in a ratio to malignant tumors of approximately six to one. Primary consideration in this presentation is given to malignant tumors except to mention that benign mixed tumors of the parotid in the past had a high recurrence rate after removal, largely because surgeons attempted to enucleate the tumor, an inadequate operation which left behind pseudopods of tumor. Present-day methods of adequate excision and careful facial nerve dissection are followed by very low recurrence rates in benign tumors.

(A) Anatomic Regions

Major salivary glands are paired and consist of the parotid glands, submandibular glands, and the sublingual glands.

(a) Parotid Gland

The gland lies immediately anterior and beneath the external ear on the lateral side of the face. Its lateral surface is convex and smoothly lobulated. The superficial layer of deep cervical fascia divides to completely encase the parotid gland and is referred to as the parotid fascia. The lateral surface of the gland is roughly triangular in shape, being wider above and narrowing to the tail which overlies the sternomastoid muscle and mastoid tip. Inferiorly, the gland is grooved by the posterior belly of the digastric muscle. Anteriorly, the gland overlies the mandible and it associated muscle. Posteriorly, the gland is immediately adjacent to the cartilaginous and bony segments of the external ear canal and the anterior inferior portion of the temporal bone. Medially, the gland is narrowed as it passes between the mandible anteriorly and the temporal bone posteriorly, but then it enlarges to form the deep or retromandibular portion of the gland. The parotid gland is in medial relation below the styloid process, the styloid muscle, the internal carotid artery, and the internal jugular vein. The stylo-mandibular ligament separates the gland above from the parapharyngeal space. The parotid duct emerges from about 1 cm below the zygomatic arch on the masseter muscle. The duct turns medially at the anterior boundary of the masseter muscle and pierces the buccal fat pad and buccinator muscle to enter the mouth opposite the second maxillary molar tooth. The facial nerve enters the parotid gland posteriorly and deep, immediately after giving off motor branches to the auricular and posterior digastric muscles. The nerve divides about $1^1/_2$ cm from the stylomastoid foramen to form the temporal-facial division above and the cervical-facial division below. The nerve continues to branch within the parotid gland and exits the gland anteriorly to innervate the muscles of facial expression. The parotid gland is richly invested with lymph nodes, which are located immediately under the parotid facia and within the substance of the gland [6, 18].

(b) Submandibular Gland

The submandibular gland is the second largest of the major salivary glands. Its external surface is finely lobulated in appearance and rounded in shape. It occupies the bulk of the submandibular triangle. Superficially, the gland is covered by skin, subcutaneous tissue, and platysma muscle and superficially by the deep cervical fascia. Medially, the gland is adjacent to the hypoglossus muscle posteriorly and the genioglossus muscle anteriorly and to the lingual and hypoglossal nerves. Anteriorly, the gland is indented by the mylohyoid muscle and overlaps it superficially. Posteriorly, the gland approximates the posterior belly of the diagastric and the stylohyoid muscles and the parotid gland. The duct arises from the deep surface of the gland and passes forward immediately to open into the anterior floor of the mouth. Post-ganglionic parasympathetic fibers to the submandibular gland arise in the submandibular ganglion, which is attached to the lingual nerve. There are no lymph nodes in the substance of the gland. Lymphatic drainage from these nodes is to the deep cervical lymphatic system [6, 18].

(c) Sublingual Gland

The sublingual gland is the smallest of the three major salivary glands. It is located deep to the mucous membrane of the floor of the mouth and is covered inferiorly by the mylohyoid muscle and laterally by the mandible. It lies on the genioglossus muscle. Posteriorly, it approximates the deep anterior projection of the submandibular gland. The sublingual gland has 10 to 12 small ducts, some of which empty into the submandibular duct and the rest into the anterior floor of the mouth. The lymphatic drainage is into the submandibular lymph nodes [6, 18].

Most benign tumors and the majority of malignant tumors remain confined to the involved salivary gland proper, although in time they can become massive. The more aggressive malignant types within the parotid will invade the facial or pterygoid muscles and/or encircle the mandible; approximately one-third

Table 5.1. Distribution of salivary gland tumors and percentage of each that are malignant [19]

Site	Tumor distribution in major salivary glands (%)	Proportion malignant (%)
1. Parotid Gland	85–90	20–25
2. Submandibular Gland	10–15	40–60
3. Sublingual Gland	1	80

invade and progress considerable distances along neural pathways, causing facial paralysis and extending intracranially. Submandibular direct extension may involve the platysma, digastric, or mylohyoid muscles, skin, mandible, floor of mouth, and/or pharyngeal wall. The lingual and hypoglossal nerves are also frequantly invaded [6, 7].

Cervical lymph node metastasis exists in roughly 15 to 20% of patients who present with major salivary gland malignant tumors. Squamous cell, undifferentiated, and high-grade mucoepidermoid carcinomas have a propensity for such metastasis. Proportionally more submandibular gland carcinomas than parotid gland carcinomas are found to metastasize to regional lymph nodes. Distant metastasis to lungs, long bones, etc. through hematogenous spread will also occur, though much less frequently than lymphogenous spread [6, 10, 17].

Table 5.1 illustrates the distribution of salivary gland tumors and the percentage within each that are malignant, as reported by Batsakis [19].

(B) Management

(a) Basic Principles

Surgical resection is the treatment of choice for controlling most of these tumors, with a combination of radiation therapy and surgery to be used in the very malignant neoplasms. The surgery to be performed depends on assessment of extent of the tumor in the gland.

Failure to recognize the salivary gland origin of the tumor and attempts at excision under local anesthesia often lead to tumor recurrences or injuries to the facial nerve.

Inoperable or recurrent disease may be managed with radiotherapy. Recent evidence suggests that neutron irradiation in preferable to conventional photon sources in the treatment of these tumors [6].

(b) Benign Adenomas

(i) Benign Mixed Tumor (Pleomorphic Adenoma). Mixed tumors are slow-growing and may be well-demarcated. About 90% arise in the parotid gland. A thin and often incomplete fibrous capsule encompasses the main body of the tumor through which project pseudopods of the tumor into the surrounding salivary gland. When these tumors are removed by simple enucleation, small nests of tumor are often left behind, and there is a high incidence of recurrence.

Because of this problem, the minimal surgical procedure for a mixed tumor of the parotid gland should be lateral lobectomy with dissection of the facial nerve. When the tumor involves the medial lobe, a total parotidectomy with facial nerve preservation should be performed [6].

(ii) Other. The papillary cystadenoma lymphomatosum, oxyphilic adenoma, and the other types of benign tumors should all be treated by surgical resection with preservation of the facial nerve.

(c) Carcinomas

(i) Acinic Cell Adenocarcinoma. The acinic cell adenocarcinoma arises almost exclusively in the parotid gland. Metastasis can be by either hematogenous or lymphogenous spread with the lung and bone being metastatic sites of predilection. This tumor is resected with a wide margin of normal parotid tissue. The surgery would be either a lateral lobectomy or total parotidectomy with sacrifice of any branches of the facial nerve which are in close proximity to the tumor. A radial neck dissection should be done if there is evidence of regional cervical lymph node metastasis. Radiation therapy can be used both for local recurrences and distant metastases. Chemotherapeutic agents might be considered for palliation for distant metastases [6].

(ii) Adenoid Cystic Carcinoma. This tumor, representing only 5% of parotid gland tumors, is uncommon in the parotid gland. However, adenoid cystic carcinoma occurs with a greater relative frequency in the minor salivary glands and smaller major salivary glands. It is the most common malignant tumor of the submandibular gland. Regardless of its site of origin, this tumor has a great tendency to invade nerves. There is a high frequency of pain and facial nerve paralysis when the tumor develops in the parotid gland. The tumor should be treated by wide surgical excision followed by post-operative radiation therapy. If the tumor arises within the parotid gland, a total parotidectomy, often requiring sacrifice of the facial nerve, is the surgical procedure of choice. In the submandibular and sublingual glands, any nerves in close proximity to the tumor should also be sacrificed. The long-term prognosis for this tumor is poor, even though many patients live longer than five years with their disease. The lungs are frequent sites of distant metastases. Chemotherapeutic agents, as well as radiation therapy, can be used for management of distant metastases [6, 17].

(iii) Mucoepidermoid Carcinoma. The parotid gland is most commonly involved by the mucoepidermoid carcinoma, which represents approximately 20% of all malignant tumors in this gland. This tumor is classified as either a low grade or high grade malignant tumor. A low grade mucoepidermoid carcinoma is characterized by slow growth and fairly frequent recurrences, but it rarely metastasizes. The high grade malignancy is a much more aggressive tumor with a higher rate of recurrence and frequent local and distant metastases. These tumors should be treated by wide surgical excision. In the parotid gland, any

branches of the facial nerve that are in close proximity to the tumor should be sacrificed. A radical neck dissection is performed for regional lymph node metastases. Post-operative radiation therapy should be considered for the larger tumors and for the high grade mucoepidermoid carcinoma [6, 10, 17].

(iv) Squamous Cell Carcinoma and Undifferentiated Carcinoma. These two tumors are rare in the major salivary glands and carry a poor prognosis. They should be treated with radical surgery followed by post-operative radiation therapy. When these tumors develop in the parotid gland, the surgery should include a total parotidectomy usually with sacrifice of the facial nerve, resection of any adjacent structures as indicated, and an ipsilateral radical neck dissection. Chemotherapy agents and radiation therapy may be used for palliation with distant metastases [6].

(v) Malignant Mixed Tumor. The diagnosis of malignant mixed tumor is a microscopic rather that a clinical diagnosis. About 5% of mixed tumors are malignant. The usual history for a patient with a malignant mixed tumor is that the tumor has been present for a number of years with or without recurrences and suddenly begins to grow rapidly over a 3–6 month period of time. Microscopically, malignant mixed tumors demonstrate localized destructive infiltrative growth and solid or nearly solid sheets of epithelial cells. The treatment for this neoplasm is radical wide surgical resection. If the tumor presents in the parotid gland, a total parotidectomy usually with sacrifice of the facial nerve should be performed. If there is clinical evidence of cervical lymph node metastases, a radical neck dissection is performed. Post-operative radiation therapy should be considered when the surgeon questions the adequacy of the operative procedure [6, 10, 17].

(C) Results

Survival in general is the range of 50% at five years for malignant salivary tumors, with a higher figure in the acinic cell adenocarcinomas and in the low-grade mucoepidermoid carcinomas. Five-year survival figures for cylindromas are not meaningful, because of the number of patients who live much longer than five years with either local recurrence or pulmonary metastasis. There is hope for improvement in these figures with earlier diagnosis and careful planning to be certain that the initial operation is of adequate scope.

6. Radical Neck Dissection

The operation known as a radical neck dissection is a unilateral cervical lymphadenectomy in which a block of tissue is removed from the level of the clavicle below up to the mandible above, from the trapezius muscle posteriorly to near the midline anteriorly. The sternocleidomastoid and omohyoid muscles are included as well as the internal jugular vein. It is clearly indicated in a patient who has oral cancer that has been controlled by radiation or by surgery, and who subsequently develops a mass in the ipsilateral neck. If such a patient later appears with a mass in the contralateral neck, a second neck dissection can be done. Certain patients are candidates for simultaneous bilateral neck dissection. These are patients with quite advanced disease. The morbidity and mortality expectations rise in such a category [17].

There has been an increasing trend in recent years toward modified neck dissections with preservation of the internal jugular vein, the spinal accessory nerve, the sternocleidomastoid muscle, or all three of these structures. Clinical judgement dictates when the modifications of the standard neck dissection are indicated.

Occasionally patients are seen with squamous cell carcinoma in cervical lymph nodes in whom a primary tumor cannot be found despite a thorough search. In this category, if carefully selected, a radical neck dissection may be justified, provided the subsequent surveillance is careful in a continued search for the primary source. If eventually found, the primary cancer usually is the upper aerodigestive tract.

The major danger in extensive head and neck surgery is rupture of the common or internal carotid artery. This misfortune can occur if the vessel becomes exposed following ischemic necrosis of the neck skin flap, a complication that is not completely avoidable. When the vessel ruptures, exsanguination occurs unless prompt tamponade is carried out. It is then necessary to ligate the artery, accepting the fact that neurologic sequelae and/or death will occur in a significant fraction of such patients. Carotid rupture is becoming less frequent as surgeons learn how the vessel can be protected by appropriate measures taken at the time of operation [17].

References

1. Staley, C.J.: "The Neck". In: Operative Surgery Principles and Technique: (Nora, P.F., ed.), (Lea & Febiger: Philadelphia, PA), 1972
2. Ketcham, A.S., Hoye, R., Chretien, P., and Kirkland, C.: "Irradiation 24 hours Preoperatively", Amer. J. Surg. 118:691–697, 1969
3. Strong, E.W.: "Preoperative Radiation and Radical Neck Disection", Surg. Clin. N. Amer. 49:271–276, 1969
4. Muir, C.S. and Shanmugaratnom, K.: Cancer of the Nasopharynx, (Med. Exam. Publ. Co.: Flushing, NY), 1967
5. Fletcher, G.H. and Million, R.R.: "Malignant Tumors of the Nasopharynx", Amer. J. Roentgenol, 93:44–55, 1965
6. Hamner, J.E., III, et al.: Management Guidelines For Head & Neck Cancer, Ed. 2, (N.I.H. Publication No. 80-2037: Bethesda, MD) 1979
7. Fletcher, G.H. and MacComb, W.S.: Cancer of the Head Neck, (Williams & Williams, C.: Baltimore, MD), 1967
8. Fletcher, G.H. and Lindberg, R.: "Squamous Cell Carcinoma of the Tonsillar Area", Amer. J. Roentgenol, 96:574–587, 1966
9. Ogura, J., Saltzstein, S.L. and Spjut, H.J.: "Conservation Surgery in Laryngeal and Pharyngeal Cancer", Laryngoscope, 71:258–276, 1961
10. Shedd, D.P. and Gaeta, J.F.: "In Vivo Staining of Pharyngeal and Laryngeal Cancer", Arch. Surg. 102:442–446, 1971

11. Bakamjiam, V.Y.: "Two-state Pharyngoesophageal Reconstruction with Pectoral Flap", Plast. Reconstru. Surg., 36:173–184, 1965
12. Fletcher, Jesse, R.H., et al.: "Radiation Therapy in Management of Carcinoma of the Supraglottic Larynx", Amer. J. Roentgenol, 108:19–26, 1970
13. Miller, A.H.: "First Experiences With Asai Technique for Vocal Rehabilitation After Total Laryngectomy", Ann. Otol., 76:829–833, 1967
14. Singer, M. and Blom, E.: "An Endoscopic Technique for Restoration of Voice After Laryngectomy", Ann. Orl., 89:529–533, 1980
15. Smith, R., Frazell, E., et al.: "American Joint Committee Stage Classification of Pharynx Cancer", Cancer, 16:1505–1520, 1963
16. Ketcham, A.S., Wilkins, R.H., et al.: "Combined Intracranial Facial Approach to Parnasal Sinuses", Amer. J. Surg., 106:698–703, 1963
17. Shedd, D.P.: Cancer of the Head and Neck", In: Cancer Medicine, (Holland, J.F.l and Frei, E., editors), (Lea & Febiger: Philadelphia, PA), 1973
18. Brash, J.C.: Cunningham's Textbook of Anatomy, E. 9, (Oxford University Press: Oxford, England): 1951
19. Batsakis, J.G.: Tumors of the Head & Neck: Clinical and Pathologic Considerations, (Williams & Williams, Co.: Baltimore, MD), 1974

II. Radiation Therapy in the Management of Head and Neck Tumors

LUTHER W. BRADY and LAWRENCE W. DAVIS

Shortly after the discovery of x-rays in 1895, radiation was used to treat head and neck tumors. It was not, however, until the development of megavoltage radiation therapy that this modality became a major part of the armamentarium in the management of these malignancies.

For small lesions of the head and neck region (T1 and 2) radiation therapy can be used effectively with generally excellent results and with preservation of the organ being irradiated. In these early lesions, radiation therapy is an alternative to surgery, and a number of factors such as the patient's general condition and preference must be considered in selecting the appropriate alternative. In addition, radiation therapy failures can often be effectively managed with surgical salvage.

Since advanced lesions of the head and neck offer a therapeutic challenge with moderately poor results with either radiation therapy or surgery, these lesions are frequently treated with a combined modality approach.

1. General Considerations

(A) Preoperative Radiation Therapy

Many radiation therapists have favored the use of preoperative radiation therapy when radiation therapy is combined with surgery. The rationale for this combination is that hypoxic tumors cells, which are contained in the central portion of most solid tumors, are less sensitive to the effects of radiation therapy than are the well-oxygenated cells of the surrounding normal structures. The peripheral extensions of the tumor are usually well oxygenated and, therefore, respond well to radiation therapy. These cells are the ones that could be left behind following a surgical resection. However, the bulky central mass of the tumor, the portion that is least sensitive to radiation therapy, is the portion most effectively managed surgically. Since the vascular supply is less disturbed prior to surgery, it is likely that the undisturbed tumor will be more responsive to the effects of radiation therapy than following surgery. In addition, cells that may be implanted into the surgical bed are the ones most likely to be made nonviable by radiation.

Preoperative radiation therapy fields should encompass the primary tumor and all the draining lymph node regions at risk. This will typically include both sides of the neck as well as the supraclavicular nodes. Radiation therapy doses have varied from 20 Grey in one week followed by immediate surgery to 50 Grey in five weeks with surgery delayed for three to six weeks [12, 14].

(B) Postoperative Radiation Therapy

Postoperative radiation therapy has generally been favored by the surgical community rather than the radiation therapy one. The rationale for using radiation therapy postoperatively is that the tumor can be adequately staged surgically and the status of the regional lymph nodes determined. The effect of radiation therapy on wound healing is avoided; therefore, the surgical procedure may be simplified.

The radiation therapy dose used is determined by the pathologic findings at the time of surgery. If all the tumor has been grossly and microscopically removed and all margins are free of disease, then 50 Grey in 5–6 weeks should be adequate. However, if there is any microscopic residual disease or if the capsule of any of the lymph nodes has been transgressed, then an additional 10 Grey boost should be added (total dose 60 Grey in 7–8 weeks.) If gross residual disease remains following resection, then the area of gross disease should be boosted to a total dose of 70 Grey in 7–8 weeks.

A multinstitution randomized study compared the relative merits of preoperative versus postoperative radiation therapy. Greater than 300 patients were randomized in the study. A preliminary report showed no significant differences in local control, complications or survival between the patients receiving postoperative versus preoperative radiation therapy. Local/regional success rates overall were 62%. The majority of patients died of their tumor with approximately 15% developing distant metastases without locally recurrent tumor [18].

(C) Interstitial Techniques

In accessible tumors, such as those in the anterior tongue, floor of mouth, and tonsillar region, radioactive sources may be placed directly into the tumor. Types of radioactive isotopes used include radium, iridium seeds and wires, gold and iodine seeds. Techniques which use radium and iridium require the removal of the radioactive sources after the calculated dose has been delivered (usually in 3–7 days). Techniques which use radioactive seeds result in a permanent implant, and the calculated dose of radiation is delivered over the effective life of the radioactive material. Small, well-differentiated tumors may be treated with only the use of an interstitial implant, while larger tumors or those less well-differentiated are treated with a combination of external irradiation and a supplemental boost to the tumor site using interstitial techniques.

(D) Treatment Volume

The volume irradiated should include the site of the primary tumor as well as areas of potential lymph node involvement. The extensiveness of the volume irradiated will depend upon the site of the primary tumor and its propensity to spread to regional nodes.

Factors to consider are the size and histologic differentiation of the primary and whether clinically palpable regional nodes are present. Treatment of tumors of the anterior tongue and floor of mouth would ordinarily include treatment of the submandibular and anterior cervical lymph nodes as a minimum.

With more posterior tumors such as those of the tonsillar pillars, in addition to the anterior cervical nodes, the posterior cervical lymph nodes should be irradiated if the primary tumor is a T_3 or greater. When ipsilateral lymph nodes are palpable, then the contralateral nodes should be irradiated.

When tumors arise in the pyriform sinus or lateral hypopharyngeal wall, then the retropharyngeal nodes should be irradiated, also.

Ordinarily the lower cervical and supracavicular lymph nodes are irradiated using a single anterior field. In patients with N_3 stage disease or with stage T_3 or 4 pyriform sinus tumors the upper mediastinum should be irradiated.

(E) Other Considerations

In all circumstances, the radiation therapy fields should be shaped to exclude the unnecessary irradiation of normal structures. In all circumstances, the dose to the spinal cord should probably be limited to 50 Grey given over five weeks. Since the primary morbidity of head and neck irradiation results from treatment of the salivary glands, primarily the parotid, this organ should be excluded from the field when feasible. The most disturbing late radiation effect to patients is dryness of the mouth. The chemical change in the composition of the saliva promotes dental caries; therefore, meticulous dental care is indicated for patients who are dentulous.

(F) Dental Care

According to Daly, patients may be placed into one of four groups according to the dental problems they present prior to irradiation.

Group 1 includes edentulous patients. They may require surgical removal of symptomatic problems such as cysts or retained root tips. These patients require instruction concerning trauma to the gingivae and the premature use of dentures.

Group 2 patients include those with poor dental hygiene and those whose teeth are beyond repair by ordinary dental procedures. Patients in this group usually require removal of all remaining teeth. Prior to irradiation, primary closures and surgical preparation of the alveolar ridges to support dentures should be done. Antibiotics are ordinarily used during the healing stage prior to the initiation of radiation therapy.

Group 3 patients include those whose dental condition is fair with teeth restorable by ordinary dental procedures. These patients require removal of any non-salvageable teeth and restoration of the remaining ones. These patients should be instructed in dental prophylaxis and in the use of custom-made fluoride carriers.

Group 4 includes those patients with good dental hygiene. These patients require training in dental prophylaxis, restoration of any careous teeth, and fitting for custom-made fluoride carriers.

When teeth are extracted prior to radiation therapy, the bone must be contoured so that primary closure is possible. Lose spicules and sharp projections should be removed. At least 10 days are required for adequate healing prior to the initiation of radiation therapy.

Dentulous patients should be instructed in a program of long-term fluoride treatment. Such treatments make the tooth surfaces less susceptible to the decay process. Such a program should include thorough cleansing of the teeth and fabrication of a custom-made mouth guard to provide local application of the fluoride solution. Such solutions can be compounded in the local pharmacy, and some are available commercially. Patients should cleanse their teeth prior to the placement of the carrier which is worn 5 min each day. The fluoride is then thoroughly rinsed from the mouth following its use. Such a program should continue indefinitely.

2. The Role of Radiation Therapy in Head and Neck Sites

(A) Lip

Carcinoma of the lip can be adequately treated with radiation therapy. Treatment fields are usually limited to the primary tumor with an adequate margin. Since such lesions are reasonably superficial, they can be treated either with orthovoltage irradiation or with electrons. Small lesions can be adequately treated and usually yield a minimal deformity of the lip. However, large lesions are frequently destructive, and some deformity is likely post-treatment. Such lesions are frequently treated surgically, and if there is any question of the surgical margins, radiation therapy should be used postoperatively [10].

(B) Anterior Tongue and Floor of Mouth

Small lesions of the oral cavity and floor of the mouth can be effectively treated with either irradiation or with surgery. The primary consideration should be the morbidity of the treatment and the defect associated with the primary management. T_1, well differentiated lesions, can be treated with only interstitial implants. However, larger lesions are ususally treated with external irradiation to a volume which includes the primary lesions and regional lymph nodes to a dose of approximately 50 Grey. This is then followed with a boost, using either a smaller photon field, electrons, or more often an interstitial implant. T_3 and T_4 lesions are frequently treated with a combination of radiation therapy and surgery.

T_1 and T_2 lesions have extremely satisfactory control rates with radiation therapy alone with those reported in the range of 85–95%. Even T_3 and T_4 lesions treated with radiation therapy and surgical salvage have reported five-year survival rates in excess of 50% [4, 9, 10].

(C) Gingiva

Because of the close proximity of the gingiva to the underlying bone, most of these tumors, even when very small, involve the adjacent bone. Therefore, most of these tumors are managed surgically. However, if the patient's condition precludes surgery, radiation therapy should be considered. Treatment fields should encompass the primary tumor with a minimum 2 cm margin and the adjacent lymph node draining areas. If any lymph nodes are palpable, then all the cervical and supraclavicular nodes should be included in the treatment field.

Because of the high likelihood of such tumors to involve bone, the possibility of a late radiation necrosis of the soft tissue and bone is high from the use of radiation therapy in the management of these tumors [10].

(D) Buccal Mucosa

Most tumors of the buccal mucosa are managed surgically since excision of the lesion and surgical repair of the defect can be accomplished with modest morbidity. However, if the patient's condition precludes the use of surgery, then radiation therapy should be considered. Lesions of the buccal mucosa can frequently be treated with an interstitial implant either used alone or in combination with external beam radiation therapy. If the lesion can be adequately encompassed with an interstitial implant, this is the preferable radiation therapy technique to use.

Results with radiation therapy for buccal mucosa and gingiva lesions have been reported from 33 to 90% depending on the extensiveness of the lesion. A majority of the radiation therapy failures can be subsequently salvaged by the use of surgery, bringing overall control rates to the range 90–100% [10].

(E) Oropharynx

(a) Retromolar Trigone

In the absence of trismus or bone involvement, the use of radiation therapy alone results in satisfactory control rates. However, if either of these unfavorable factors is present, then a combination of radiation therapy and surgery should be considered.

Treatment fields should include the primary tumor along with the cervical and supraclavicular lymph nodes bilaterally. When radiation therapy is used alone, doses in the range of 70.00 Gy in 7–8 weeks are necessary. Selective lesions can sometimes be treated with external radiation therapy and a boost using interstitial implants of radioactive material such as gold or iodine.

T_1 and T_2 lesions treated with radiation therapy alone have control rates in the range of 80 to 90% while T_3 and T_4 lesions have been variously reported from 40 to 80% [9, 11, 14].

(b) Tonsillar Fossa

Results with radiation therapy alone are comparable to surgery alone in the treatment of most stages of tonsillar fossa carcinoma. These range from in excess of 90% for T_1 and T_2 lesions to 40 to 60% for stage III and IV. A small proportion of radiation therapy failures can be salvaged with surgery.

Extensive lesions can best be managed with a combination of radiation therapy and surgery [4, 9, 11, 14].

Treatment fields should encompass the primary lesion as well as the cervical and supraclavicular lymph nodes bilaterally.

(c) Base of Tongue

Since the surgical excision of lesions of the base of the tongue often result in significant deformity and morbidity, radiation therapy should be considered as the primary means of management of such tumors. Small lesions can frequently be treated with a combination of external beam radiation therapy and interstitial implant, while larger lesions are usually treated with external radiation therapy only. As in the case of other lesions of the oral cavity and oropharynx, the cervical and supraclavicular lymph nodes bilaterally should be included in the radiation therapy treatment fields.

Control rates range from nearly 100% for small T_2 and T_1 lesions to 20–45% for more extensive ones. A small proportion of radiation therapy failures can be salvaged by subsequent surgery [11].

(F) Hypopharynx

Lesions arising in the lateral or posterior wall of the hypopharynx or in the pryiform sinus are frequently extensive and deeply infiltrating when initially diagnosed. Therefore, many of these lesions are poorly responsive to radiation therapy alone. Radiation therapy could be considered for the initial management of small lesions with surgery reserved for salvage. However, the more extensive ones should be managed with a combination of radiation therapy and surgery. Most patients presenting with hypopharyngeal tumors usually have clinically positive lymph nodes at the time of diagnosis. Therefore, the treatment fields should include not only the primary, but the cervical and supraclavicular lymph nodes bilaterally. A majority of the patients who fail do so at the site of the primary tumor, and five-year survivals for T_3 and T_4 lesions treated with a combination of radiation therapy and surgery are less than 50% [4, 15].

(G) Nasopharynx

Carcinomas of the nasopharynx are most commonly squamous cell carcinomas or the lymphoepitheloma variant. The radiotherapy techniques are similar for the two types of histologies, although the doses may be slightly lower with the latter type.

Very few tumors arising in the nasopharynx are detected at an early stage; therefore, most patients present with palpable cervical lymph nodes. Cranial nerve deficits occur through involvement of the retropharyngeal lymph nodes or by invasion of the base of the skull. Cranial nerve deficit and bony involvement are grave signs, and such patients have an extremely poor prognosis. A thorough clinical and radiographic evaluation is indicated to determine whether or not such involvement is present.

The treatment of such malignancies is largely within the province of radiation therapy. Treatment fields must include the base of the skull as well as the entire nasopharynx and retropharyngeal lymph nodes. Because of the high incidence of cervical lymph node metastases, both sides of the neck and the supraclavicular areas should be treated. Doses in the range of 60–65 Gy in $6^1/_2$–7 weeks are commonly used. An additional boost may be delivered to large bulky lesions.

In the absence of grave signs, five-year cure rates are reported in the range of 35–40%. The presence of cervical lymph nodes does not appear to adversely affect prognosis. However, with erosion of the base of the skull or with cranial nerve deficits, five-year survivals are only a few percent [1, 13, 19, 21].

(H) Larynx

Carcinomas which are limited to the vocal cord are well treated with radiation therapy with preservation of the normal voice. Because of the absence of lymphatic drainage of the vocal cord, spread of these localized lesions to lymph nodes should not occur. Cure rates for T_1 lesions are comparable to those reported for surgery, and while the control for T_2 lesions are slightly less favorable, with careful follow-up, patients developing recurrences can be salvaged with surgery.

Because hoarseness occurs very early in tumors of the glottis, most patients present with small, very curable tumors.

However, more extensive lesions with fixation of the vocal cord or extension to adjacent structure are best treated with a combination of radiation therapy and surgery.

Early lesions of the supraglottic or subglottic structures can also be managed with radiation therapy alone. However, most lesions in these regions are not detected as early since symptoms from the tumor are less pronounced; therefore, these primary tumors are more extensive at initial diagnosis, and cervical lymph node metastases are more common.

With tumors limited to the glottis treatment fields can be small, that is on the order of 6×6 cm. Since spread to regional lymph nodes is not likely, these regions need not be treated. Doses in the range of 60.00–70.00 Gy delivered in 6–8 weeks are indicated.

Five-year cure rates of approximately 90% are achieved with T_1 carcinomas of the glottis, while T_2 lesions have reported results of 75% with greater than 90% of patients surviving five years when surgical salvage is considered. Cure rates for supraglottic lesions are comparable in early stages; however, with T_3 and T_4 lesions treated by a combination of radiation therapy and surgery, control is variously reported from 40 to 80% depending on the extensiveness of the lesion [22].

(I) Salivary Glands

The majority of salivary gland tumors arise in the parotid. Tumors arising in any of the major salivary glands can be considered in a similar fashion.

Those involving the minor salivary glands can be generally treated in a fashion consistent with squamous cell carcinomas arising in the same area.

In general, there has been a lack of agreement of the effectiveness of radiation therapy in controlling tumors arising in the major salivary glands. As a result, the general management has been excision of the tumor with wide margins frequently followed by a course of radiation therapy. Recurrence rates following surgery alone are significant and have been variously reported from 20 to 50%. In addition, when the tumor margins are close or microscopically positive or if the histology is of an unfavorable type (adenoid cystic, squamous cell, or undifferentiated carcinoma), then the surgical failure rate rises to 50%. Also, approximately $^{1}/_{4}$ of the patients will suffer a permanent facial nerve damage. In view of control rates approaching 50% using wide local excision and postoperative radiation therapy, this combination appears to be the treatment of choice [2].

Since the recurrence in regional lymph nodes is unusual (approximately 10%), routine irradiation of the cervical lymph nodes is not recommended unless the histology is of an unfavorable subtype or lymph nodes are initially palpable.

Adenoid cystic carcinomas characteristically extend along the perineural structure to the base of the skull, and this must be considered when planning radiation therapy fields. Commonly, the treatment volume should include the entire parotid gland, the preauricular lymph nodes, and the retromandibular area.

Radiation therapy doses are similar to those used for squamous cell treatment modality or when it is used in combination with surgery.

(J) Paranasal Sinues

Most tumors of the paranasal sinues arise in the antrum. These are frequenly advanced at the time of diagnosis and many times involve the bony structures of the orbit. A thorough evaluation oft the extensiveness of the tumor using radiographic techniques including skull films, tomograms, and CT scanning is essential to determine whether or not the bony structures are involved.

Tumors of the antrum are best treated with a combination of radiation therapy and surgery unless factors are present which preclude the use of surgery. Tumors of the other paranasal sinues are commonly treated using only radiation therapy.

Because of the low incidence of cervical lymph node metastases, these regions are not commonly included in the treatment volume unless clinically palpable lymph nodes are present. With tumors of the maxillary antrum, if the floor of the orbit is not involved, then the eye can be excluded from the treatment field. However, if there is any evidence of involvement of the orbit, then the globe cannot be excluded. Multiple field treatment techniques must be planned to adequately encompass the tumor and to spare as much of the normal tissue as possible. Special treatment devices such as wedge filters are commonly employed. If the tumor involves the nasal cavity, then appropriate alterations in treatment technique must be used to adequately include this volume.

In contrast to treatment in other head and neck sites, late effects of radiation therapy can occur in the eye when this structure must be treated. Since the development of cataracts result from relatively small doses of radiation, a cataract may result several years following radiation therapy. When the entire eye must be included in the treatment volume, more serious sequelae occasionally occur such as cornea ulceration, which may require enucleation.

(K) Thyroid

Carcinoma of the thyroid is primarily managed by means of surgical techniques. In most cases, these tumors can be completely excised, and radiation therapy is not added.

If the tumor is incompletely excised or if distant metastases are present, the residual thyroid function should be ablated using I-131. Subsequently, the activity of any residual tumor or metastatic disease to incorporate radioactive iodine can be determined. If residual disease remains in the neck and the tumor either does not uptake I-131 or is of an undifferentiated histology, then postoperative radiation therapy should be considered. The treatment volume should include the primary tumor and the draining cervical lymph nodes.

(L) Unknown Primaries

Approximately 20% of patients present with palpable cervical lymph node metastases with no obvious site of the primary tumor. A thorough attempt is necessary to establish the primary site since this will aid in the proper treatment of such patients. The location of the palpable lymph node along with the knowledge of the areas that drain into it will provide some assistance in determining proper areas to investigate. A thorough history and physical examination should be performed along with endcoscopic examinations and biopsies of potential sites of the primary lesion.

If the site for the primary tumor cannot be identified, the treatment selection and technique can be influenced by the histology of the metastatic lymph node. Squamous cell carcinomas in the past have frequently been treated by radical neck dissection. However, radiation therapy offers an alternative treatment, especially if the lymph nodes are small. The treatment fields should encompass both sides of the neck and both supraclavicular areas [3].

If the lymph node arises from a malignant lymphoma, and a thorough workup to exclude other areas of lymphoma is done, then the selection of treatment fields and doses will depend on the subtype of lymphoma.

3. Treatment of Neck Nodes

There are a number of reports that have indicated that subclinical metastases to cervical lymph nodes can be adequately treated with radiation therapy doses in the range of 50 Gy given in five weeks. As the lymph nodes become larger, they become more difficult to control with radiation therapy alone, and the ultimate management of the cervical lymph nodes will be related to the management of the primary tumor. If the primary is being managed with surgery or a combination of radiation therapy and surgery, patients with palapble neck nodes will most often have a neck dissection, and the radiation therapy doses are selected to control subclinical metastatic deposits.

If the primary is being managed only with radiation therapy, then smaller lymph nodes can often be controlled using only radiation therapy. An assessment of the response at 50 Gy should give some indication of whether or not radiation therapy alone will be adequate. Palpable lymph nodes should be boosted to a total dose of 65–70 Gy in 7–8 weeks. However, if there is little response to radiation therapy when a dose of 50 Gy is delivered, then a neck dissection should be considered as part of the management of the cervical lymph nodes.

In addition, an assessment of the primary and lymph nodes can be made one to two months following a course of radiation therapy. If there is any indication of residual disease either in the primary site or cervical lymph nodes, then surgical removal of these areas should be planned [4, 20].

4. Late Effects of Radiation Therapy

Significant complications occur in fewer than 10% of the patients treated with full courses of radiation therapy for head and neck primary tumors. The development of late effects is related to the normal structures treated, the extensiveness of the volume irradiated, as well as the total dose delivered. When the oral cavity is irradiated, most patients will develop some disturbance of their taste, but this should be temporary. When the major salivary glands are included in the radiation therapy fields, some amount of dryness of the mouth will result. The degree of dryness and the amount of symptoms that result vary greatly with individual patients.

Lesions of the gingiva and floor of mouth which require large radiation therapy doses may result in necrosis of the soft tissue, and an occasional patient will develop necrosis of the mandible. In patients with tumors of these sites great care should be taken to avoid any trauma to these tissues such as through the use of poorly fitting dentures. If necrosis results, conservative management is indicated with medication to control pain. Surgical intervention should be considered as a last resort.

When radiation therapy is combined with surgery, there is a slight increase in those complications typically associated with the surgical procedure. These include such factors as delayed wound healing, fistula formation, and hemorrhage due to exposure of the cartoid artery [14, 18].

5. Future Approaches

Since local-regional failure for advanced head and neck tumors continues to be a significant problem, new approaches must be investigated to improve local control. Current areas of investigation include hypoxic cell sensitizers, radioprotectors, high LET radiations (neutrons and heavy ions), concurrent and sequential chemotherapy, and altered radiation fractionation [5–8, 16, 17]. While some of these techniques hold future promise, their value must be adequately studied through randomized trials. When local-regional failures are minimized, the management of distant metastasis is likely to become more important.

References

1. Chen, K.Y. and Fletcher, G.H."Malignant tumors of the nasopharynx", Radiology, 99:167–171, 1971
2. Davis, L.W. and Fazekas J. "Management of parotid neoplasms. The role of radiotherapy in carcinoma of the parotid gland." In: Controversy in Otolaryngology, (James B. Snow, ed. pp 95–106), (W.B. Saunders Co., Philadelphia), 1980
3. Brady, L.W. "Metastatic carcinoma of the neck from an occult primary tumor. Treatment with radiation therapy." In: Controversy in Otolaryngology, (James B. Snow, ed. pp 189–196), (W.B. Saunders Co., Philadelphia), 1980
4. Fazekas, J.T., Sommer, C. and Kramer, S. "Adjuvant intravenous methotrexate or definitive radiotherapy alone for advanced squamous cancers of the oral cavity, oropharynx, supraglottic larynx or hypopharynx. Concluding report of an RTOG randomized trial on 638 patients", Int. J. Radiation Oncology Biol. Phys., 6:533–541, 1980
5. Fazekas, J.T., Goodman, R.L. and McLean, C.L. "The value of adjuvant misonidazole in the definitive irradiation of advanced head and neck squamous cancer: an RTOG pilot study (#78-02)", Int. J. Radiation Oncology Biol. Phys., 7:1703–1708, 1981
6. Fu, K.K., Silverberg, I.J., Phillips, T.L. and Friedman, M.A. "Combined radiotherapy and multidrug chemotherapy for advanced head and neck cancer: results of a Radiation Therapy Oncology Group pilot study", Cancer Treat Rep, 63:351–357, 1979
7. Glick, J.H., Marcial, V., Richter, M. and Velez-Garcia, E. "The adjuvant treatment of inoperable Stage III and IV epidermoid carcinoma of the head and neck with Platinum and Bleomycin infusions prior to definitive radiotherapy: an RTOG pilot study", Cancer, 46:1919–1924, 1980
8. Glick, J.H., Fazekas, J.T., Davis, L.W., Rominger, J.C., Breen, F.A., Brodovsky, H.S. "Combined chemotherapy – radiotherapy for advanced, inoperable head and neck cancer. An RTOG pilot study", Cancer Clinical Trials, 1:129–136, 1979
9. Hamberger, A.D., Fletcher, G.H., Guillamondegui, O.M. and Byers, F.M. "Advanced squamous cell carcinoma of the oral cavity and oropharynx treated with irradiation and surgery", Radiology, 119:433–438, 1976
10. Lindberg, R.D. and Fletcher, G.H. "The role of irradiation in the management of head and neck cancer: analysis of results and causes of failure", Tumori, 64:313–325, 1978
11. Marcial, V.A. "Radiotherapy in carcinoma of the oropharynx", Advances in Medical Oncology, Res., Educ., 11:149–158, 1979
12. Marcial, V.A., Gelber, R., Kramer, S., Snow, J.B., Davis, L.W. and Vallecillo, L.A. "Does preoperative irradiation increase the rate of surgical complications in carcinoma of the head and neck? A Radiation Therapy Oncology Group report", Cancer, 49:1297–1301, 1982
13. Marcial, V.A., Hanely, J.A., Chang, C., Davis, L.W. and Moscol. J.A. "Split course radiation therapy of carcinoma of the nasopharynx: results of a national collaborative clinical trial of the Radiation Therapy Oncology Group", Int. J. Radiation Oncology Biol. Phys., 6:409–414, 1980
14. Marcial, V.A., Hanley, J.A., Ydrach, A. and Vallecillo, L.A. "Tolerance of surgery after radical radiotherapy of carcinoma of the oropharynx", Cancer, 46:1910–1912, 1980
15. Marks, J.E., Kurnik, B., Powers, W.E. and Ogura, J.H. "Carcinoma of the pyriform sinus: an analysis of treatment results and patterns of failure" Cancer, 41:1008–1015, 1978

16. Percarpio, B. and Fischer, J.J. "Irradiation of advanced head and neck cancer with large daily fractions", Radiology, 121:489–490, 1976
17. Rubin, P., Hanley, J., Keys, H.M., Marical, V. and Brady, L. "Carbogen breathing during radiation therapy. The Radiation Therapy Oncology Group study", Int. J. Radiation Oncology Biol. Phys., 5:1963–1970, 1979
18. Snow, J.B., Gelber, R.D., Kramer, S., Davis, L.W., Marcial, V.A. and Lowry, L.D. "Randomized preoperative and postoperative radiation therapy for patients with carcinoma of the head and neck: preliminary report", The Laryngoscope, 90:930–945, 1980
19. Thompson, R.W., Doggett, R.L.S. and Bagshaw, M.A. "Ten-year experience with linear accelerator irradiation of cancer of the nasopharynx", Radiology, 97:149–155, 1970
20. Votava, C., Gletcher, G.H., Jesse, R.H. and Lindberg, R.D. "Management of cervical nodes, either fixed or bilateral, from squamous cell carcinoma of the oral cavity and faucial arch", Radiology, 105:417–420, 1972
21. Wang, C.C. and Meyer, J.E. "Radiotherapeutic management of carcinoma of the nasopharynx. An analysis of 170 patients", Cancer, 28:566–570, 1971
22. Wang, C.C. "Treatment of glottic carcinoma by megavoltage radiation therapy and results", Amer. J. Roentgenol., 120:157–163, 1974

III. Chemotherapy

James E. Hamner, III

1. General Remarks

Chemotherapy for squamous cell carcinoma of the head and neck area involves the use of antineoplastic compounds such as antimetabolites, antibiotics, bifunctional alkylating agents, plant alkaloids, and heavy metal coordination complexes. The chemotherapy may be systemic or geared to a regional type of treatment. Since certain anticancer drugs possess the ability to attack widespread metastatic disease and possibly to augment the local effects of surgery and radiation therapy, there appear to be several points in the treatment management of head and neck cancers at which the possible use of chemotherapy should be considered.

Early chemotherapy programs for managing head and neck cancer limited its role to that of a palliative measure. The addition of chemotherapy to locally curable neoplasms, such as certain forms of breast cancer, suggests its possible benefit as an adjunct treatment in head and neck cancer [1]. At this point in time, the value of adjuvant chemotherapy in the treatment of squamous cell carcinoma of the head and neck is still in the theoretical stage [2].

Certain general principles apply for head and neck cancer patients who are to undergo chemotherapy. Patients with advanced head and neck cancer often already suffer from pain, intermittent bleeding, local infection, obstruction difficulties in speech and swallowing, and unpleasant odor. Because many of these particular cancer patients fall into the older age group or have been habitues of alcohol and tobacco abuse, they may consequently suffer from various nutritional, liver, kidney, pulmonary, and cardiac disorders. Therefore, patients about to undergo courses of chemotherapy may be in a rather tenuous medical condition before even embarking on chemotherapy. Every effort, thus, should be directed toward reversing any remediable maladies before compounding them by the use of cytotoxic drugs. Dehydration, malnutrition, vitamin deficiences, etc., should be managed vigorously.

The potential side effects of chemotherapy, particularly the deleterious effects on the bone marrow, the oral mucosa, the gastrointestinal tract, and less frequent complications involving the skin, cardiac, and pulmonary tissue must be considered in planning chemotherapy in each individual patient and in determining the appropriate time for the institution of such a modality. The major consideration in planning the addition of chemotherapy to, or substitution for, other modalities of treatment are: the stage of the disease, the degree of differentiation, and the histology of the tumor involved. The anatomic site of the primary cancer does not affect the choice of chemotherapy, except for consideration for intra-arterial infusion treatment [2].

The first, the most widely used, and the most studied antitumor agent for the treatment of carcinoma of the head and neck has been Methotrexate. It has been given in a variety of doses and schedules [3–8]. Methotrexate given at the more standard dose of either 20 mg per square meter intravenously or intramuscularly twice weekly, or 40 to 60 mg per square meter intravenously once a week, results in survival comparable to high dose Methotrexate therapy in those patients who respond to Methotrexate as a single agent. Cumulative data from the literature indicates a response rate in the range of 40–50%. Bone marrow reserve, white blood count, palatelet count, and evidence of mucositis, as well as drug interactions, are of critical importance in treating patients with Methotrexate [2].

In his review of the results obtained with intra-arterial infusion of Methotexat, Carter concluded that the slight possible increase in response rate over systemic drug administration was nullified by the increased substantial rate of catheter-induced complications such as bleeding, infection, and vessel occlusion leading to stroke [9, 10]. Before commencing therapy, normal renal function must be verified, since Methotrexate is excreted almost entirely by the kidneys.

In a multi-institutional clinical trial, Levitt et al. were unable to demonstrate a significant increase in response rate with moderate doses of Methotrexate and Leucovorin over that of Methotrexate alone [7]. The use of "high dose Methotrexate" followed by rescue therapy with Leuovorin is potentially extremely toxic. Failure to-give the rescue therapy properly results in severe bone marrow depression, mucositis, and in some instances, fatalities. It is recommended strongly that this regimen be used only in institutions where there has been prior experience with this mode of therapy and where both white cell and platelet transfusions are readily available. In all instances the dose of Methotrexate must be governed by the level of creatinine clearance and the blood level of Methotrexate. Since there has been no increase in the length of remission following this expensive and somewhat hazardous therapy, it cannot be recommended as a standard routine course of chemotherapy [2, 7].

Three specific chemotherapeutic agents have been used in combination with radiation therapy because of their effects on irradiated tissue.

(A) Hydroxyurea has been used as an S-phase specific agent in an attempt to synchronize cells, since with large dose single increment radiation cycles, cells in G2 are several times more responsive than non-synchronized cells. In addition, Hydroxyurea inhibits the enzymes necessary to repair sublethal injury. Its use in head and neck cancers has been studied extensively, however, its specific role at this point is difficult to determine [2].

(B) Actinomycin-D and Adriamycin, both inhibitors of protein synthesis, reduce the Sutton-Elkind curve of radiation therapy, giving an enhanced local antitumor effect. However, this action is not specific for neoplastic tissue. Nevertheless, both of these agents are known to augment an anticipated radiation response [2].

(C) Bleomycin has been reported to be synergistic when administered to patients receiving radiation therapy, particularly in those patients with well-differentiated squamous cell neoplasms. This agent, however, should not be given to patients beyond the sixth decade and causes, as its major significant toxicity, pulmonary fibrosis. It is thus contraindicated in patients with chronic restrictive pulmonary disease. While it may be administered intravenously, subcutaneously, or intramuscularly, the total dose should not exceed 400 units per square meter. The optimum dose is 10–15 units per square meter [2].

For carcinomas of the tongue, buccal mucosa, and maxillary sinus, intraarterial infusions of 5-Fluorouracil in combination with radiation therapy have been useful in carefully selected patients. This route of administration of chemotherapy should be undertaken, however, only by those who are familiar with and capable of managing the complications associated with the maintenance of arterial catheters. Brain necrosis, bilateral blindness, and cerebrovascular thromboses have all been reported in patients treated with intra-arterial infusion therapy [2].

The National Cancer Institute has funded numerous clinical trials of chemotherapy protocols, using multiple chemical agents in various combinations to treat advanced head and neck carcinoma. Examples of such combination trials include: (1) Cyclophosphamide, Adriamycin and Cis-diamminedichloroplatinum; (2) Methotrexate versus Methotrexate, Methyl CCNU, and Bleomycin; and (3) Cis-platinum, Oncovin, and Bleomycin versus Methotrexate.

In each of these respective trial studies, it was concluded that the combination therapy was not superior to standard Methotrexate therapy [11–13]. Since many of the response rates in such clinical trials are based on small numbers of accrued patients, most of the response rates should be regarded as approximate. All of the combination drug clinical trials should be considered investigational at this time.

2. Combined Treatment Modalities

The rationale behind combined treatment of cancer rests on the site or sites of failure when a single mode of treatment is employed. Of the three major treatment disciplines, surgery and radiation therapy have a high probability of local tumor control, although the probability decreases with increasing tumor volume. Systemic chemotherapy has a lower probability of control, primarily because the therapeutic ratio is limited by exposure of the normal cell renewal systems of bone marrow and GI tract to the antitumor agents. In order to improve the relatively lower cell kill factor or therapeutic ratio, several agents may be combined which have different normal tissue toxicities, but combined effect on the neoplasm [14].

Where local and/or regional persistence of the neoplasm is the only or a significant clinical problem, combinations of surgery and radiation have been shown to be of value. When such combinations are used, one must take into consideration the combined effect of each treatment involving the following principles: the dose of radiation therapy necessary to sterilize a tumor site is directly related to the volume of the tumor, i.e., the number of reproductively viable tumors cells in the treatment volume. Therefore, a sub-clinical or microscopic residual disease can be eradicated with a high probability with doses in the 5,000 rad range. This dose is well-tolerated by all except the most sensitive normal tissues. Small clinical masses of tumor require somewhat higher doses, which in general can be delivered and well-tolerated to limited volumes of most normal tissues. Large masses require doses in the 7,000–8,000 rad range, which may well exceed the normal local tissue tolerances, since larger masses also require treatment of larger volumes. Interstitital implantation of radioactive isotopes has undergone a renaissance in recent years in a effort to increase the tumor dose perferentially over the dose to normal tissues [14].

The combined use of surgery and radiotherapy (pre or postoperative) is recommended where the probability of residual disease is of significance and the normal tissues in the tumor area will be tolerant of modest levels of radiation. Specific circumstances in which it is believed that planned postoperative radiotherapy is indicated include:

(A) Disease at line of resection.
(B) Microscopic or gross disease at the superior and/or inferior margins of neck dissection, or extension of disease beyond the usual fascial planes of the neck dissection, and/or significant involvement of the deep surface of the sternocleidomastoid muscle.
(C) Multiple lymph nodes, microscopically positive, or nodes showing tumor extending through the lymph node capsule.
(D) Inferior tracheoesophageal, paratracheal, mediastinal, and/or superior parapharyngeal lymph nodes positive for carcinoma. In the event of positive superior parapharyngeal nodes, the radiation port may include the base of the skull [14].

References

1. Hellman, S., Harris, J.R., et al: "Cancer of the Breast". In: Cancer: Principles and Practice of Oncology, (DeVita, V.T., Hellman, S., and Rosenberg, S.A., editors), (J.B. Lippincott Co.: Philadelphia, PA.), 1982
2. Cooper, R.G. and Ellison, R.R.: "Chemotherapy". In: Management Guidelines for Head & Neck Cancer, (Hamner, J.E., III, editor), (N.I.H. Publication # 80-2037: Bethesda, MD.), 1979
3. Papac, R., Lefkowitz, E. and Bertino, J.R.: "Methotrexate (NSC-740) in Squamous Cell Carcinoma of the Head and Neck. II. Intermittent Intravenous Therapy", Cancer Chemother. Rep. 51:69–72, 1967
4. Lane, M., Moore, J.E., Levin, H., et al: "Methotrexate Therapy for Squamous Cell Carcinoma of the Head and Neck. Intermittent Intravenous Dose Program", J.A.M.A. 204:561–564, 1968
5. Leone, L.A., Albala, M.M. and Rege, V.B.: "Treatment of Carcinoma of the Head and Neck with Intravenous Methotrexate", Cancer 21:828–837, 1968
6. DePalo, G.M., DeLena, M., Molinari, R., et al.: "Clinical Evaluation of High Weekly Intravenous Doses of Methotrexate in Advanced Oropharyngeal Carcinoma", Tumori 56:259–268, 1970
7. Levitt, M., Mosher, M.B., DeConti, R.C., et al: "Improved Therapeutic Index of Methotrexate with Leucovorin Rescue", Cancer Res. 33:1729–1734, 1973

8. DeConti, R.C.: "Phase III Comparison of Methotrexate with Leucovorin Versus Methotrexate Alone Versus a Combination of Methotrexate Plus Leucovorin, Cyclophosphamide, and Cytosine Arabinoside in Head and Neck Cancer", Proc. Amer. Assoc. Cancer Res. 17:248, 1976
9. Carter, S.K.: "The Chemotherapy of Head and Neck Cancer", Semin. Oncol. 4:413–424, 1977
10. Goldsmith, M.A. and Carter, S.K.: "The Integration of Chemotherapy into a Combined Modality Approach to Cancer Therapy. V. Squamous Cell Cancer of the Head and Neck", Cancer Treat. Rev. 2:137–158, 1975
11. Creagan, E.T., Fleming, T.R., Edmonson, J.H.: "Cyclophosphamide, Adriamycin, and Cis-Diamminedichloroplatinum (II) in the Treatment of Patients with Advanced Head and Neck Cancer: Preliminary Comparison of Two Treatment Regimens", International Head and Neck Oncology Research Conference, Rosslyn, Virginia, Sept. 8–10, 1980
12. Lehane, D.E., Montaque, L., Stucky, W.J., et al: "A Comparison of Methotrexate with Methotrexate, Methyl CCNU, and Bleomycin in Patients with Advanced Squamous Cell Carcinoma of the Head & Neck Region" International Head and Neck Oncology Research Conference, Rosslyn, Virginia, Sept. 8–10, 1980
13. Al-Sarraf, M.: "The Clinical Value of Cis-Platinum, Oncovin, and Bleomycin (COB) Combination Versus Standard Single Agent in Advanced Epidermoid Cancer of the Head and Neck", International Head and Neck Oncology Research Conference, Rosslyn, Virginia, Sept. 8–10, 1980
14. Hamner, J.E., III: Management Guidelines for Head and Neck Cancer, (N.I.H. Publication # 80-2037: Bethesda, MD.), 1979

Chapter 6. Follow-Up

James E. Hamner, III

General Considerations

Periodic follow-up examinations are an essential part of the total management of the head and neck cancer patient. The following general guidelines are recommended as one acceptable regimen. For the first year following treatment, the patient should be seen and examined every month. During the second year the patient should be seen every two months; the third year, every three or four months; and during the fourth and fifth years, the patient should be seen semi-annually. Because the head and neck cancer patient is in a high risk category for developing a second primary cancer, these patients should continue to have annual complete physical examinations for life, including chest x-rays, clinical pathology laboratory work-ups, and oral/dental examinations.

The outcome status and long-term complications should be recorded at three or four month intervals. The presence or absence of recurrence, degree of regression or progression, and any evidence of regional or distant metastases should be noted. Figure 6.1 illustrates one follow-up form that has proven highly successful [1]. The general physical health should be noted as well as any specific problems or disabilities. If death has occurred since the patient's last office visit, the cause and contributing factors should be recorded. At the time of death, an autopsy should be encouraged to provide complete information on the cause of death and the extent of any possible contributory malignant disease.

Page 1 of 2

FIGURE 6 – 1

FOLLOW-UP REPORT

Log ID No. ________

Patient's Name ____
Last First

Physician's Name ______________________________ This Form Due___/___/___

1. Date of this follow up examination___/___/___
2. Patient status:
   ____Living Go on to Question #4
   ____Dead Go to Death Report Form
   ____Lost to follow up Go on to Question #3
3. Reason for the patient being lost to follow up:
   ____Moved without forwarding address
   ____Refusal to return for follow up examination
   ____Physically unable to return to office
   ____Other (specify______________________________
4. Check if patient has: ____Tracheotomy ____Control Fistula ____Spontaneous Fistula
   ____Requires tube feedings
5. What is the patient's disease status?
   ____No evidence of disease – Go on to Question #9
   ____Disease present either residually or new primary – Go on to Question #6
6. What is the primary tumor status?
   ____No evidence of disease ____Recurrence detected this visit
   ____Residual disease – regressing ____Uncertain
   ____Residual disease – stable ____New primary detected this visit
   ____Residual disease – progressing Site: ______________
7. What is the cervical node status? (check for both areas)

TREATED AREA	UNTREATED AREA
____No evidence of disease	____No evidence of disease
____Clinically regressing	____Clinically regressing
____Clinically stable	____Clinically stable
____Clinically progressing	____Clinically progressing
____Uncertain	____Uncertain

8. What is the extent of metastatic disease?
   ____No evidence of disease ____Detected this visit
   ____Suspected this visit Site: ______________
   Site: ______________ ____Continued presence
9. General disability assessment (check one of the following as to the patient's general status)
   ____Fully active
   ____Engages in work and other activity with difficulty
   ____Disabled; requires special care; can live at home
   ____Severely disabled; hospital or other care facility indicated

a

Fig. 6.1 a, b. Follow-up form example

Page 2 of 2

Patient's Name__________________ (Last only) Log ID No.________

10. Complete appropriate categories if patient has complaints or specific disabilities due to cancer and/or treatment (with protheses, if these are generally worn) Date of this Examination___/___/___

_____ No specific disabilities and complaints at this time

(Check for each disability category)

							Uncertain
Physical Appearance		Normal □	Slightly disfigured □		Noticeably Disfigured □	Greatly Disfigured □	□
Speech		Normal □	Intelligible □		Not Intelligible □	No speech □	□
Deglutition		Normal □	With diffigulty □		With pain □	Unable to Swallow □	□
			Solids easier □		Liquids easier □		
Mastication		Normal □	With difficulty □	With Pain □	Extremely limited □	Unable to Masticate □	□
Salivation		Normal □	Adequate □		Inadequate □	None □	□
Drooling		None □	Minimal □		Moderate □	Excessive □	□
Hearing	Left	Normal □	Minimal defect □		Moderate defect □	Deaf □	□
	Right	Normal □	Minimal defect □		Moderate defect □	Deaf □	□
Vision	Left	Normal □	Minimal defect □		Moderate defect □	Blind □	□
	Right	Normal □	Minimal defect □		Moderate defect □	Blind □	□
Nerve Defect		None □	Minimal □	Moderate □	Severe □	Total □	□
Shoulder Defect		None □	Minimal □	Moderate □	Severe □	Total □	□
Pain		None □	Minimal □		Moderate □	Severe □	□
Social Activity		Normal □	Curtailed □		Isolates self □		□
Emotional Status of Patient		Composed/ Accepting □	Somewhat depressed/ Difficulty in Coping □		Very depressed/ Unable to Cope □		□

11. Delayed complications not covered in above: (check where exists)

_____ Endocrine
_____ Pneumonia
_____ Fistula (unplanned)
_____ Stroke
_____ Lymphedema
_____ Skin Flap Necrosis
_____ Other Flap Necrosis
_____ Perichondritis
_____ Wound Infection
_____ Osteo Necrosis other than oral cavity

Oral Cavity
___ Loss of Taste
___ Soft Tissue Necrosis
___ Osteo Necrosis
Other
____
____
____
____
____

12. Consultations and Recommendations (give name, title, type of consult, and consultant's recommended treatment)
____
____
____
____
____
____
____
____
____

Completed by ________________
Date ________________

Fig. 6.1b

References

1. Hamner, J.E., III: Management Guidelines for Head and Neck Cancer, Ed. 2, (N.I.H. Publication No. 80-2037: Bethesda, MD.), 1979

Chapter 7. Rehabilitation

JAMES E. HAMNER, III and JOE B. DRANE

I. General Principles of Rehabilitation

JAMES E. HAMNER, III

A high degree of concern, attention, and effort must be directed at reconstructive and rehabilitative measures in order to minimize to the greatest possible extent the functional and cosmetic impairments, which often accompany the effective control of head and neck cancer.

The most effective rehabilitation begins with pre-planning and consultation with all disciplines that will ultimately be involved. These specialists include: (1) the prosthodontist, where a pre-operative tissue impression will facilitate production and prompt use of a prosthesis; (2) the speech pathologist, where voice impairment may be a sequela of treatment of laryngeal or oral cancer; (3) the dentist, for improvement of oral hygiene and preservation of sound dentition, particularly relating to radiation therapy; (4) the appropriate surgical team member, where reconstruction may require preparation and movement of tissues; and (5) finally, many patients benefit by psychosocial evaluation and counseling concerning many facets of their problems in readjustment. Rehabilitation (prosthetic and surgery) requirements should be considered at the time of initial treatment planning.

Common psychological problems of head and neck cancer patients include: (1) a great deal of anxiety around the issues of recurrence of the cancer; (2) depression and anxiety related to the change in body functions and body image as a result of the treatment for the cancer; (3) a process of mourning the loss of their body part or body function which requires resolution; (4) anxiety over any disfigurement of the body which will cause the patient to begin to withdraw from social contacts with family members or significant others; and finally, (5) a loss of self-esteem and self-worth with a fear of rejection from other people as a result of their disfigurement.

Suggestions on how to respond to these patient problems include the following considerations:

1. It is important that the emotions of these patients are legitimized. If they are experiencing a depression or anxiety, it is essential that the people working with them acknowledge that depression and anxiety and indicate to them that these emotions are appropriate for the type of experience that they have been through.
2. It is also equally necessary for these patients to feel supported as they are making attempts to work through the emotionality of their particular situation. This support can be rendered by anyone involved in the treatment process.

3. It is essential to the patient that they experience an accepting relationship by the people involved in their treatment. If a patient has been disfigured or has lost a function of a body part, it is important that the people around him make every effort to make him feel accepted as a person of worth and value.
4. Efforts should be made to replace the loss that each patient has experienced. If there has been disfigurement, efforts should be made to minimize that disfigurement through either a prosthesis or some other cosmetic method. If there has been a loss of body function, other mechanical means should be found to assist the patient to replace the loss.

Because of the severity of the loss of function experienced and also the visability of the disfigurement, family members often have a difficult time accepting and responding to the head and neck cancer patient in an appropriate, understanding, and caring manner.

Efforts should be made and recources made available to family members to assist them in understanding the processes that the patient has been through to help them with their own emotions in dealing with the patient and to guard against the tendency to withdraw from the patient, and thus, isolate the patient from social contact. The busy attending physician should build around him a team of psychosocial professionals to help care for the head and neck cancer patient in this very critical area.

Reconstruction and rehabilitation considerations must not compromise therapeutic objectives.

Careful attention to, and the provision of, needed rehabilitative measures, for example, temporary and permanent prostheses, dental care, speech therapy, surgical reconstruction, vocational counseling, psychological, and social services can have a salutary effect on the patient's quality of survival.

Despite maximum use of all of these measures, a significant number of head and neck cancer patients will have persisting disability. Some will need to depend upon the feeding tube long-term, and some may need a permanent tracheotomy. Certain of these disabilities are in such cases a necessary price to pay for control of an extensive cancer.

II. Maxillofacial Prosthetics

Joe B. Drane

The functional and esthetic rehabilitation of patients who have been treated for cancer of the head and neck area can vary from comparatively simple surgical closure of a small defect to an extremely complicated surgical and/or prosthetic restoration of form and function of an area involved in a gross defect.

The availability of maxillofacial prosthetic services which have steadily increased and improved over the past thirty years (Fig. 7.1) has opened doors to new areas of rehabilitation that were formerly not thought to be possible. These areas are the gross surgical defects that are the necessary sequela to the total removal of the cancer such as: mid-third of the face resections (Fig. 7.2)

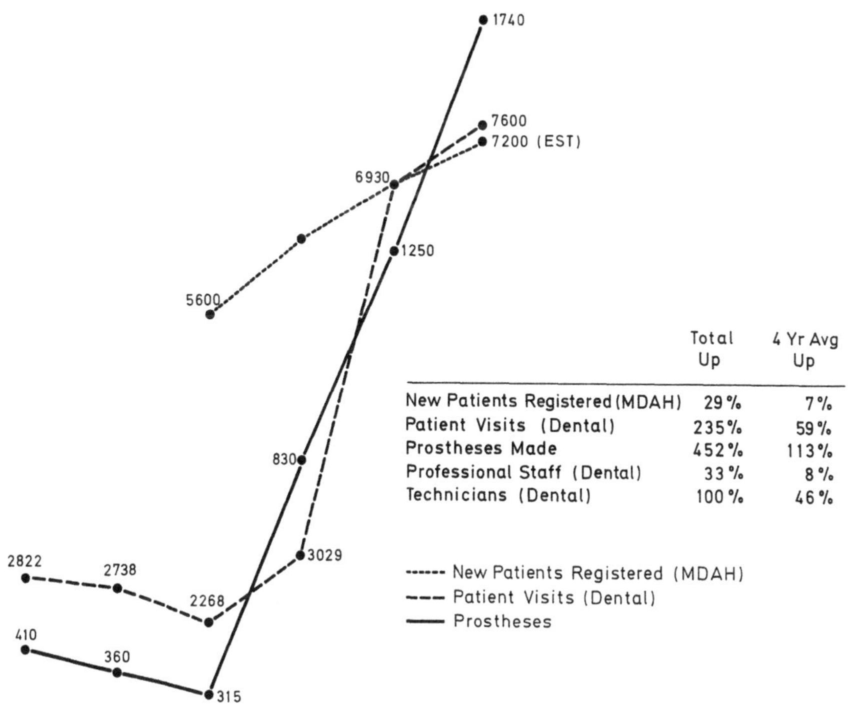

	Total Up	4 Yr Avg Up
New Patients Registered (MDAH)	29%	7%
Patient Visits (Dental)	235%	59%
Prostheses Made	452%	113%
Professional Staff (Dental)	33%	8%
Technicians (Dental)	100%	46%

1970	1971	1972	1973	1974	1975	
3	3	3	3	3.5	4	Professional Staff
3	3	3	4	4.5	6	Technicians
1	1	1	1	1	1	Hygienist

Fig. 7.1. Graph showing dental oncology activities

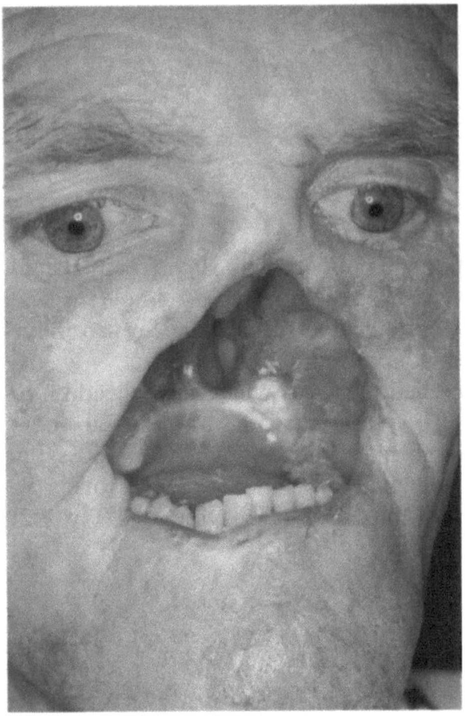

Fig. 7.2. Post surgical removal of cancer of mid third of face

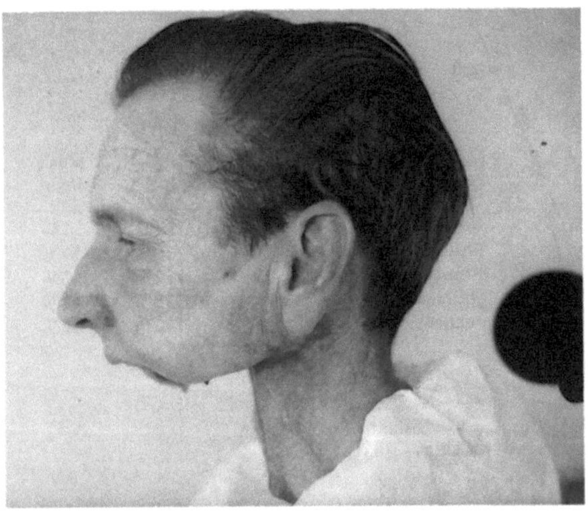

Fig. 7.3. "Andy Gump" resection

that include the upper lip, pre-maxilla and the nose; total removal of the mandible (Fig. 7.3), lower lip, skin and soft tissues of the lower face; resection of a portion or all of the maxilla (Fig. 7.4); orbital exenteration and skin graft covering the exposed bone (Fig. 7.5); resection of the external nose (Fig. 7.6); resection of the external ear (Fig. 7.7); resection of portions of the cranium (Fig. 7.8), and combinations of these defects (Fig. 7.9).

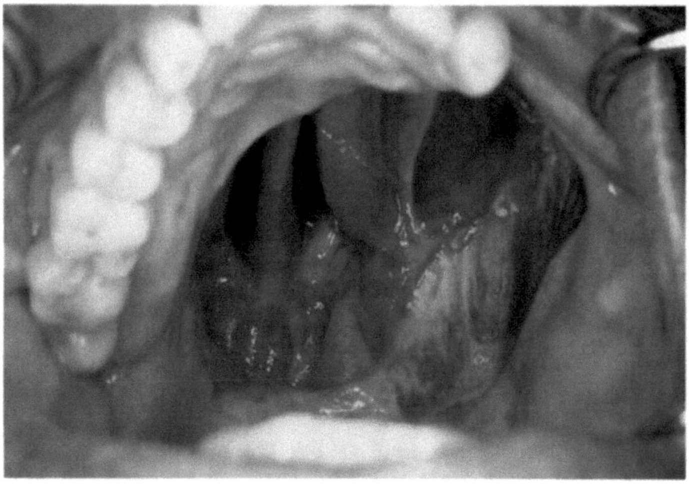

Fig. 7.4. Palatal defect following maxillary resection

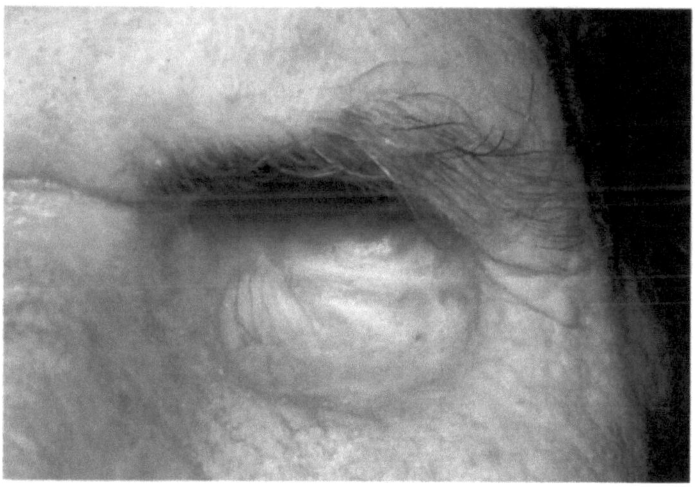

Fig. 7.5. Orbital defect and skin graft

Even though it might be possible to manage some of these defects such as nose reconstruction or ear reconstruction by plastic surgery procedures, patient factors often preclude that method of rehabilitation. Some of the patient factors to be considered are age, general health, prognosis of primary disease, financial situation, family situation, location of home related to location of medical facility, and availability of adequate speciality services by well trained competent surgeons.

For the above reasons, adequate maxillofacial prosthetic services should be available for patient care in all cancer treatment centers. At the M.D. Anderson Cancer Center where maxillofacial prosthetic services are readily available in the Department of Dental Oncology, one year's, activities from July 1, 1980

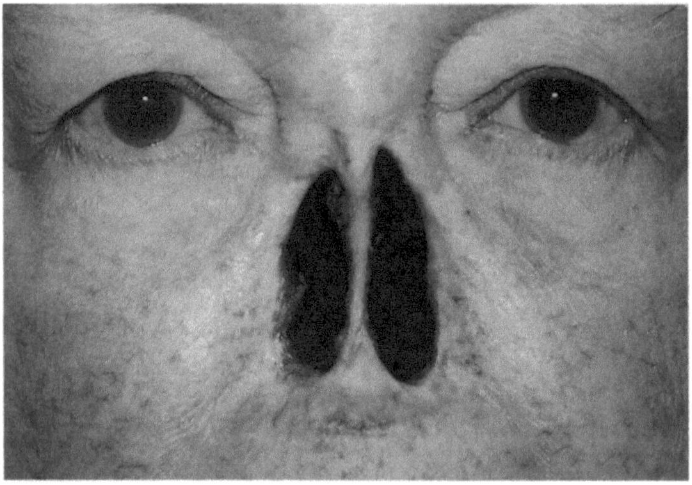

Fig. 7.6. Nasal defect following surgery

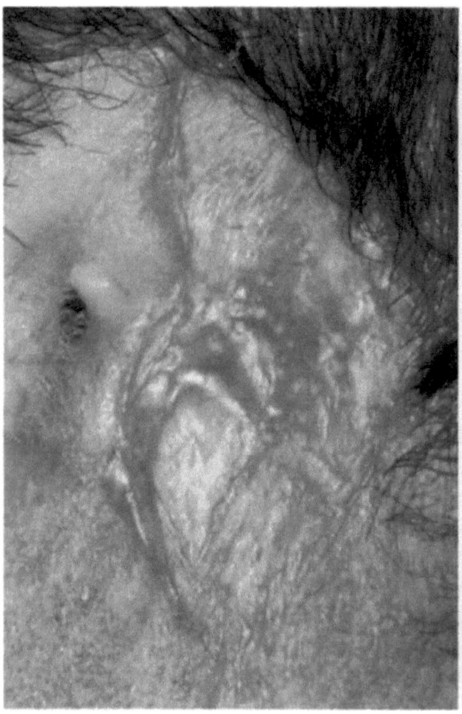

Fig. 7.7

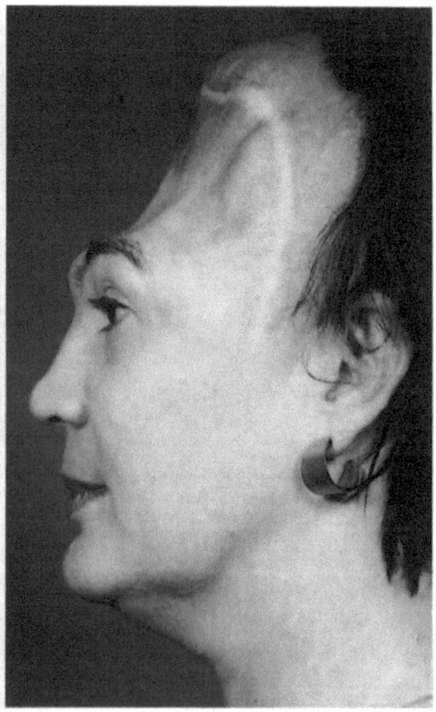

Fig. 7.8

Fig. 7.7. Ear defect with skin graft

Fig. 7.8. Frontal bone defect

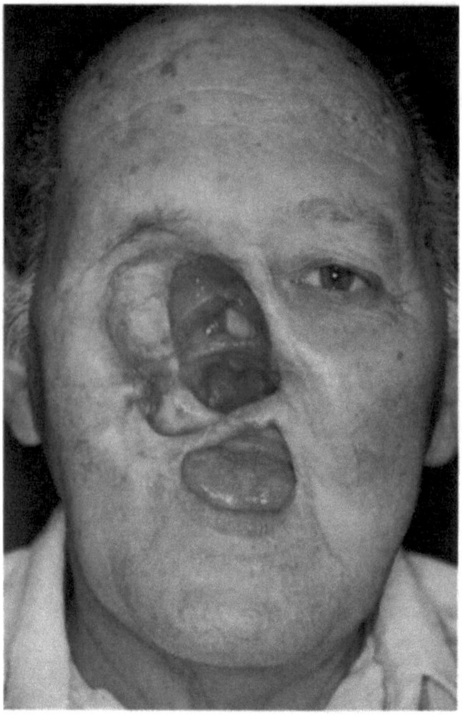

Fig. 7.9. Combination oral and facial defect

to June 30, 1981 resulted in over nine thousand patient visits involving twenty five hundred individual patients of which fourteen hundred were new patients. The services to these patients included the fabrication and insertion of over fourteen hundred prostheses and over nine thousand dental procedures that were necessary for the prevention of oral complications and the maintenance of oral health before, during, and following treatment of the patients' primary disease and their rehabilitation [1].

All head and neck patients should be seen by the maxillofacial prosthodontist with the surgeon and the radiotherapist on their initial and follow-up visits to the head and neck clinic. It is during these early visits that the appropriate treatment for the primary disease is decided on. Treatment may include surgery and/or radiotherapy and/or chemotherapy. At times, each of these modalities, or combined modalities, requires preparatory dental procedures and fabrication of treatment and protective prostheses before treatment of the primary disease is begun. This type of care is preventive rehabilitation, which is the best form of rehabilitation.

The preparatory procedures used in the care of patients to be treated surgically include oral prophylaxis (Figs. 7.10 and 7.11), elimination of foci of infection such as periapical abscesses of the teeth and periodontal lesions and the establishment of acceptable oral hygiene. This usually can be accomplished without causing any delay in the surgical procedures and has the benefit of

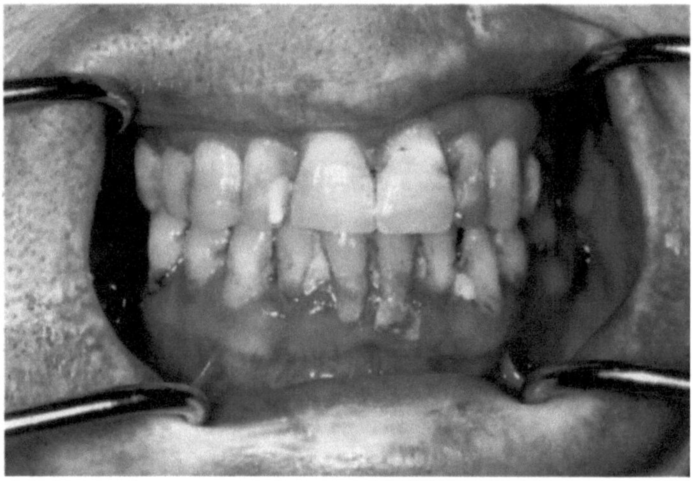

Fig. 7.10. Mouth before prophylaxis

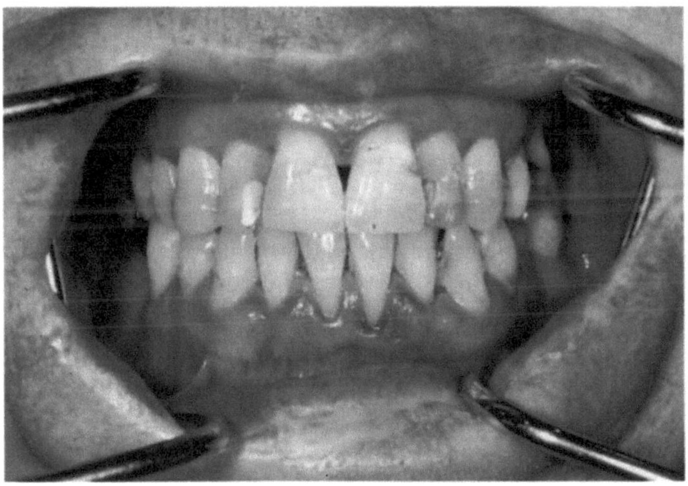

Fig. 7.11. Mouth following routine prophylaxis

reducing the possibility of infection and breakdown of the wound if the surgical procedure involves the lips or oral cavity.

Treatment prostheses such as surgical splints, stents (Fig. 7.12), surgical or immediate obturators (Fig. 7.13), and implant prostheses (Fig. 7.14) are also designed and fabricated for use during the primary surgical procedure. The use of these prosthetic aids can at times preclude the necessity of subsequent surgical procedures and can usually hasten healing and shorten necessary hospitilization. This is particularly true with the use of surgical obturators which was well documented by Nakamota [2] in a review of 120 maxillary resection patients at M.D. Anderson Hospital in 1971 (Table 7.1). His conclusions were:

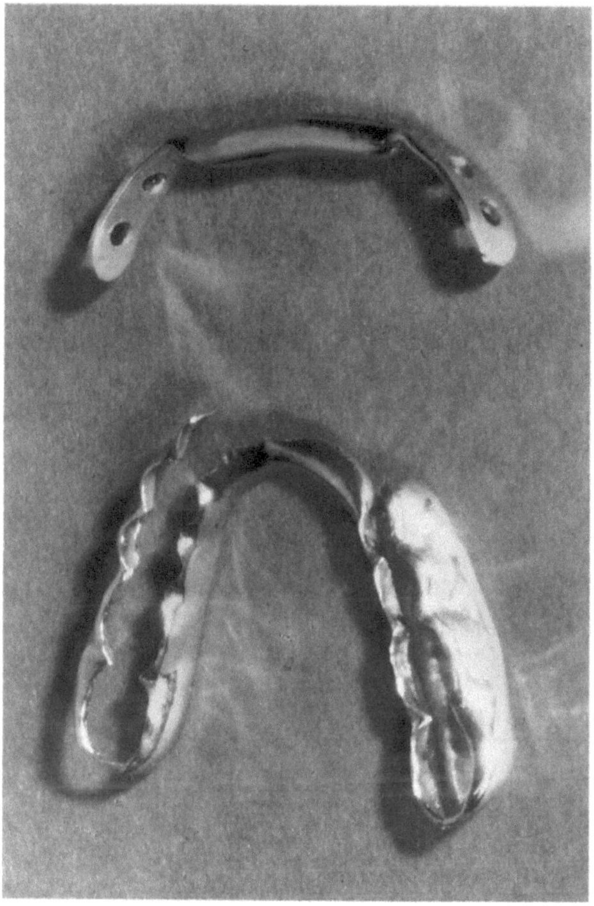

Fig. 7.12. Cast ticonium splint

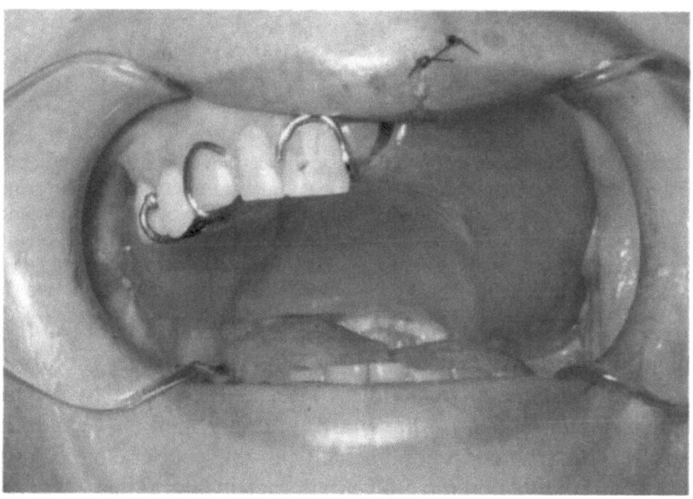

Fig. 7.13. Surgical obturator

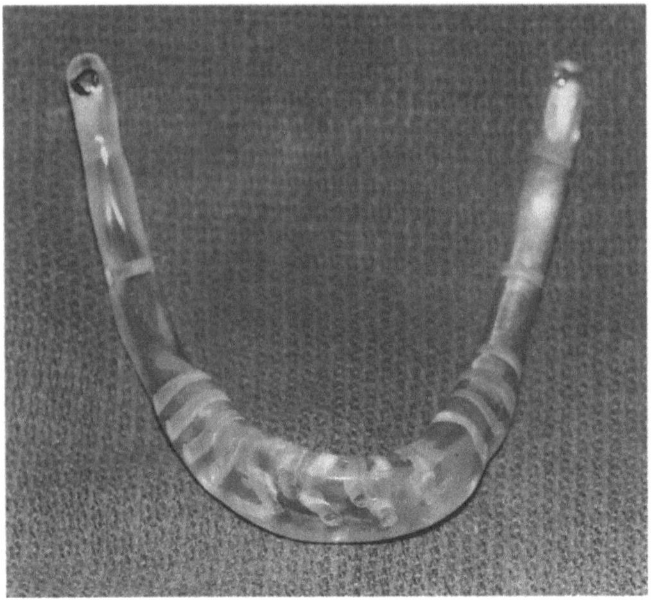

Fig. 7.14. Methyl methacrylate mandibular implant prosthesis

Table 7.1. 120 maxillary resection patients

	Entire group		
	Group A *no* imm. obt.	Group B imm. obt.	No. of days *shorter* stay by *group B*
Total average days from admission to discharge	22.7	14.2	*8.5*
Total average days from surgery to discharge	20.2	12.6	*7.6*

One of the prerequisites to be considered prior to maxillary resections in dentulous patients should be the construction of an immediate obturator. Close cooperation between the surgeon and maxillofacial prosthodontist can lead to extended benefits for all involved. The patient recovers faster and is discharged earlier. This reduces his financial obligations. The surgeon is able to use the bed space to treat other patients. If the patient's treatment is paid for by some sort of public aid, everyone benefits from the reduced total cost.

Implant prostheses are being used more frequently in recent years for the immediate replacement of portions of the mandible (Fig. 7.15). These are fabricated from chrome-cobalt cast metal or stainless steel as developed by Hahn [3], from methyl methacrylate, or from other inert materials such as Tantalum or Titanium. These are constructed preoperatively in the proper shape and size arrived at from measurements taken from cephalometric lateral head x-rays, occlusal intra-oral x-rays, and impressions of the face, cranium, and jaws. If

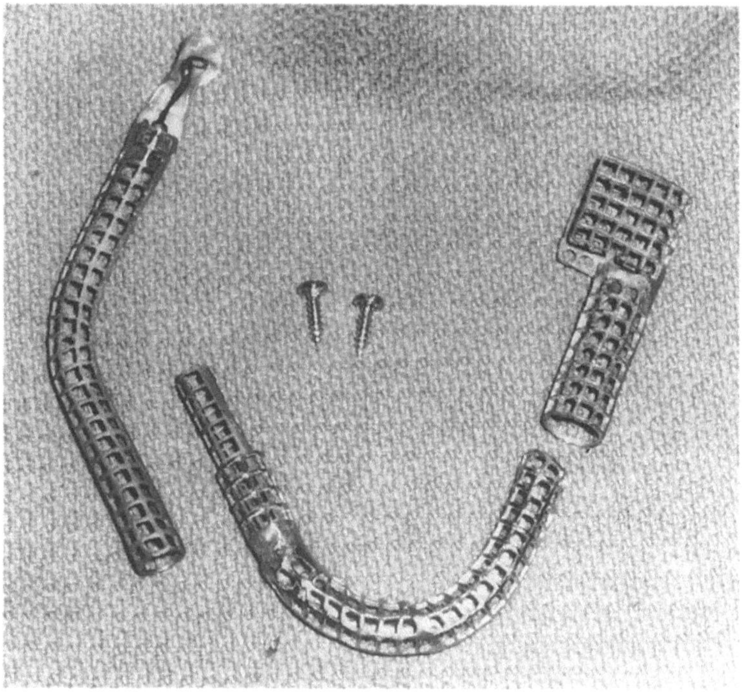

Fig. 7.15. Modified Hahn cast stainless steel mandibular implant with acrylic condyle

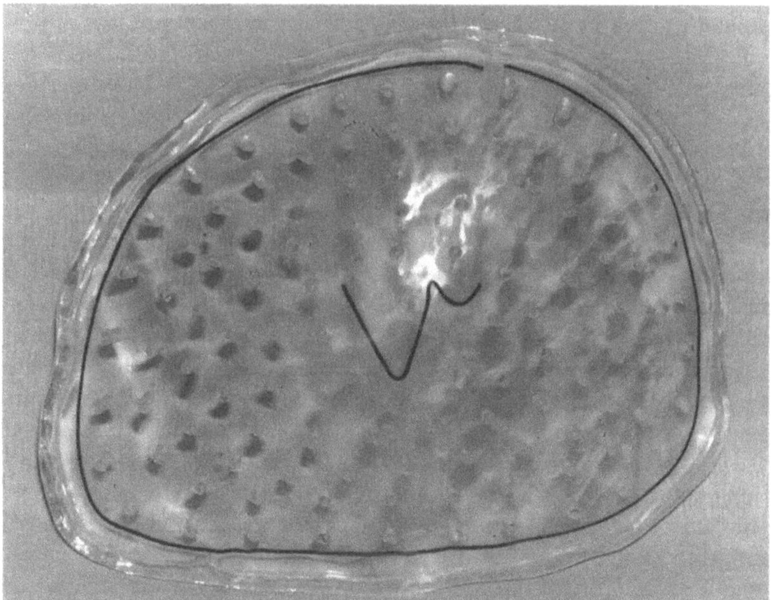

Fig. 7.16. Cranial implant made of methyl methacrylate with radiopaque markers

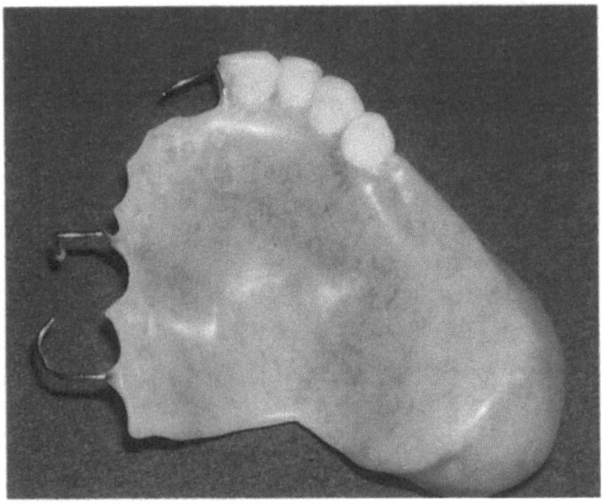

Fig. 7.17. Interim maxillary obturator

the implant is made of methyl methacrylate such as the cranial implants (Fig. 7.16), marker threads or other radio opaque material is embedded along the outer margins to make the implant visible on x-ray examination. Of prime importance for the successful use of implants in rehabilitation, in addition to the normal surgical requirements, is the ability for easy adjustment of the size and configuration of the prosthesis at the time of surgery, the ability to secure the prosthesis to the remaining portions of bone, and the immobilization of the jaw during the healing period. For cranial prosthetic replacement, tantalum or methyl methacrylate are the materials of choice. Metal implants however, should not be used in patients who will receive radiotherapy as part of their primary treatment. All implants larger than 5 cm in diameter should be perforated every centimeter with a No. 4 round dental bur to allow for an interchange of tissue fluids and to allow for an ingrowth of connective tissues into the implant. The perforated metal implants should be immersed in a 25% solution of hydrochloric acid to eliminate any ferrous contamination from the steel dental burs and metal dies used in the procedure.

Prostheses used during the treatment of patients by radiotherapy are classified as preventive prostheses and will not be discussed in this section even though as previously mentioned, by preventing disabling and disfiguring situations from occurring, they probably are one of the best forms of rehabilitation.

Many rehabilitative prostheses are made and used on a temporary basis during the period following initial healing of the wound but before the complete tissue changes have occurred (Fig. 7.17). Interim obturators are in this catagory and are made within 6 to 8 weeks following excision of the tumor. The actual time depends on patient factors, extent of resection, and whether the patient received pre or post operative radiation therapy. This type of obturator differs from the immediate or surgical obturator in that it extends into the surgical defect, thereby providing better obturation, improving the quality of the voice, enhancing retention and stability, and improving esthetics by the adding of artificial teeth to replace those lost due to the surgical resection. This also improves the patient's ability to masticate food and speak intelligibly.

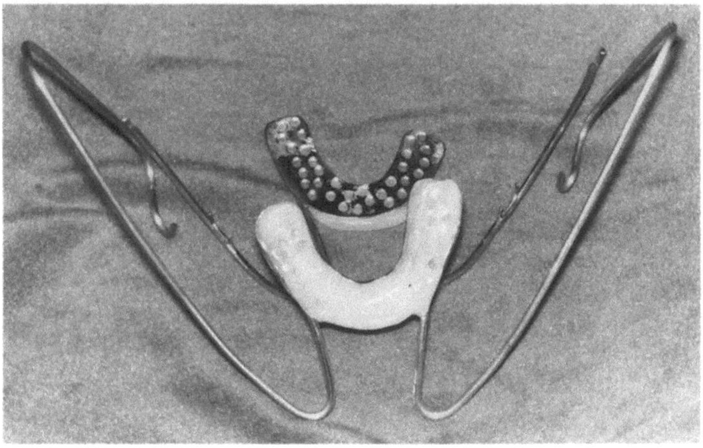

Fig. 7.18. Dynamic bite opener

One other type of intraoral interim prosthesis is the mandibular resection appliance. This prosthesis is needed to correct the centric relationship between the maxilla and mandible following resection of one side of the mandible. The remaining portion of the mandible usually deviates toward the resected side and rotates downward resulting in malocclusion of the teeth and inability to properly masticate food. This type of prosthesis is made in two parts, a removable maxillary and a removable mandibular segment. The upper portion includes a buccal guide plate or bar, and the lower segment has a guide arm which rides on the plate which holds the mandible in a centric relation during opening and closing movements. These prostheses need only to be used until the remaining muscles of mastication are retrained to accomplish their altered functions. Also, if the remaining portion of the lower jaw is immobilized by intermaxillary fixation at the time of resection and maintained in a centric relation during the following two to four weeks, there is generally no need for the resection prostheses.

Another temporary treatment prosthesis is the dynamic bite opener (Figs. 7.18 and 7.19). It is used quite successfully on patients who have undergone surgical and/or radiation treatments that involved the muscles of mastication and the temporomandibular joint and who subsequently develop trismus. The bite opener is made by adapting and indexing occlusal wafer plates to the maxillary and mandibular teeth and attaching metal rods shaped in such a way as to apply opening forces to the jaws by the use of elastic bands. The successful function of this prosthesis is based on the application of light, continuous pressure which fatigues the muscles, reduces the spasms, and allows the jaws to open. The use of the prosthesis is required usually for only a few weeks but may be needed periodically if the trismus persists or recurs.

The prostheses described above are some of the basic types. From these, many variations in technique, material, and function are made to meet the needs prior to and during treatment of the primary disease as well as the immedi-

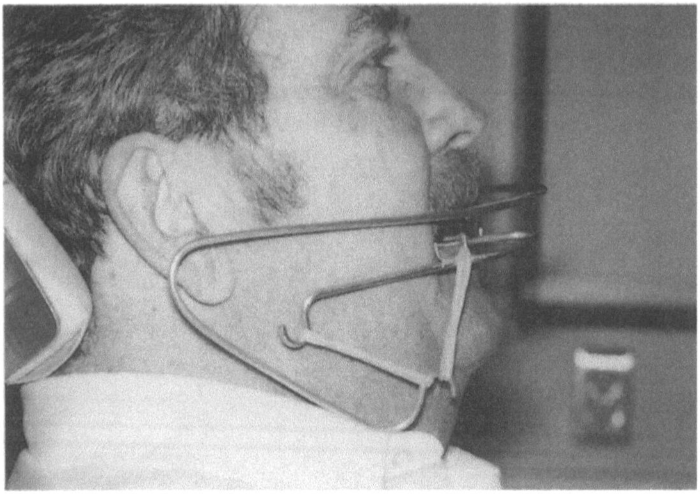

Fig. 7.19. Dynamic bite opener in place on patient

ate post treatment period. The next section is devoted to some of the various types of definitive, long term, maxillofacial prostheses used in rehabilitation.

For the head and neck cancer patient who has received good health care and management of his primary disease including preventive and interim rehabilitation, there often remains the problem of definitive or long term correction of necessary residual anatomical defects and functional disabilities. If, due to size, location, functional activity or specific patient factors, surgical rehabilitative procedures are not feasible, maxillofacial prosthetic rehabilitation can in many cases be quite satisfactory.

One such type of prosthesis is used in the post-irradiated patient (Fig. 7.20) whose salivary flow has been greatly reduced or eliminated entirely and who has not cooperated in the caries prevention program. Rampant caries progressively develops from the oral condition at time of radiation treatment (Fig. 7.21) to the condition two years post treatment (Fig. 7.22) and one year following that (Fig. 7.23) by which time the patient was malnourished due to his inability to masticate a regular balanced diet and was in generally poor health (Fig. 7.24). The remaining teeth were smoothed off, and overdentures were constructed (Figs. 7.25, 7.26). One per cent sodium fluoride gel was used each day inside of the denture base to prevent further decay. The patient has used these prostheses (Fig. 7.27) over the past five years, exfoliating a number of residual roots atraumatically, recovered his general health, and resumed a normal productive life (Fig. 7.28).

All dentures, whether complete or removable partial used for post-irradiated patients, should be constructed with as little trauma and irritation as possible. Impression materials that require heat or that have flavoring oils or other irritating components should not be used. Border extensions should be very carefully established so as not to impinge on the soft tissues in the muco-buccal folds. Flat plane teeth are desirable so as to minimize any cuspal interference and

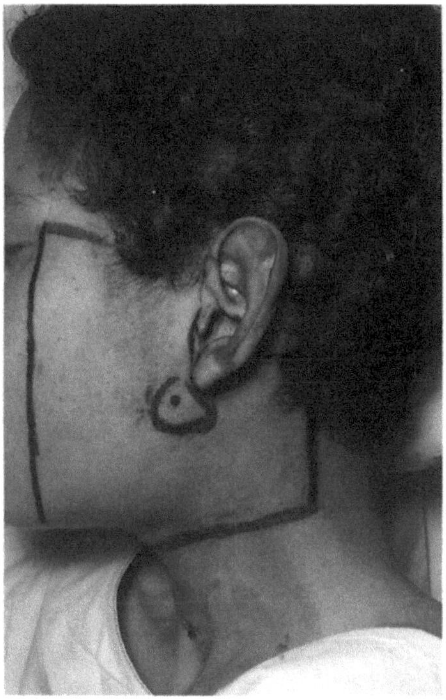

Fig. 7.20. Patient showing radiation fields

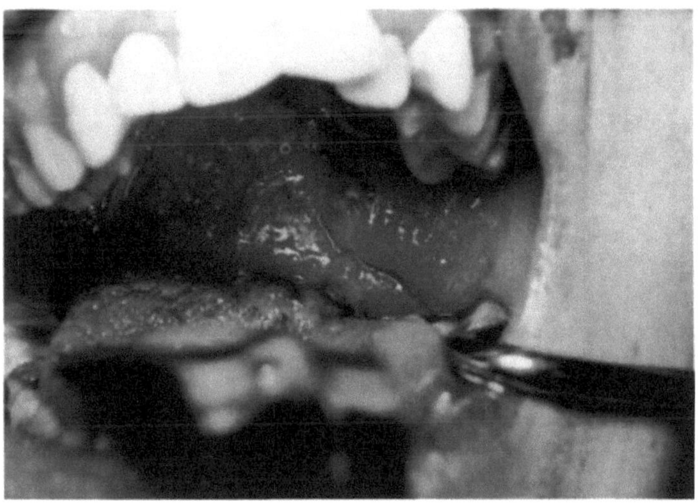

Fig. 7.21. Pretreatment view of lesion and condition of maxillary teeth

denture base movements on the supporting mucosa and on patients with extremely sensitive mucosa. The occlusal tables of the posterior teeth should be narrowed and the vertical dimension slightly reduced from normal in order to reduce the amount of vertical force on the supporting tissues.

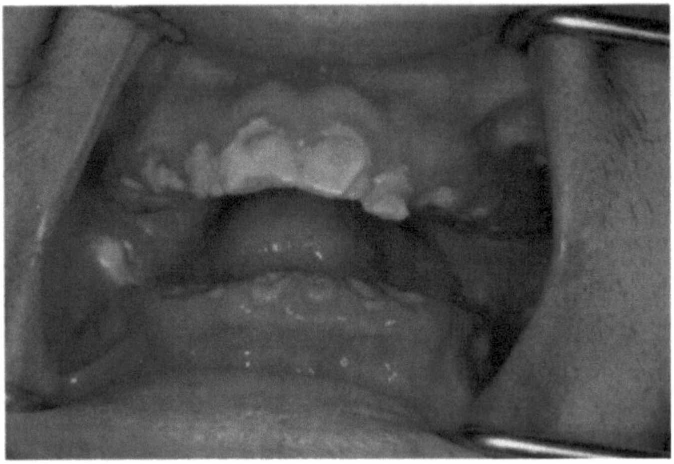

Fig. 7.22. Condition of maxillary teeth 2 years post-radiation therapy

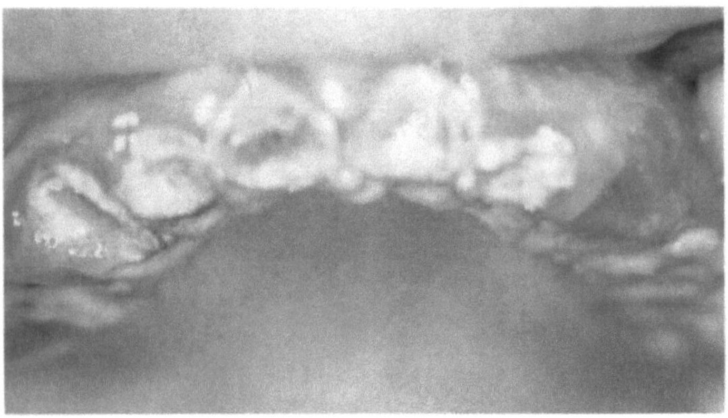

Fig. 7.23. Loss of crowns of maxillary teeth 3 years post-radiation therapy

Following insertion of the denture, follow up examinations should be done daily for the first week and close observation maintained for the next several weeks.

The advisability of this close post-insertion care was demonstrated by the retrospective study of 96 patients who had complete dentures constructed following radiation therapy for cancer of the head and neck region by Anderson [4]. In his discussion, he states that "the dentist should be willing to follow the patient for an adequate period of time following the insertion of complete dentures. One or two adjustment appointments is not sufficient."

Definitive, long term prosthetic rehabilitation of the surgically treated head and neck cancer patient can be quite varied as dictated by:

- the location of the defect – whether intra-oral, facial, or both.
- the size of the defect, and whether it involves esthetics, function, or both.

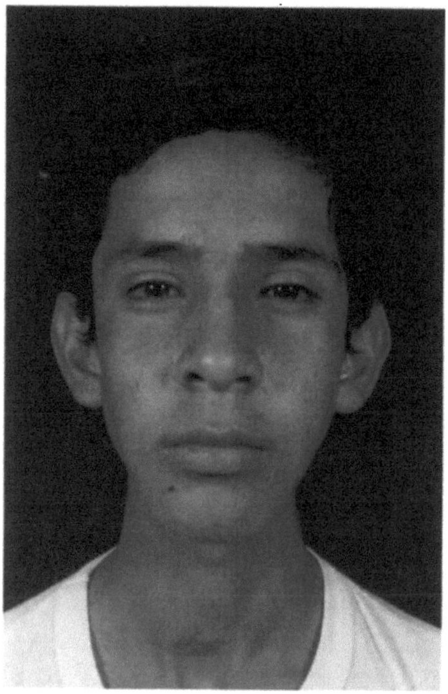

Fig. 7.24. Malnourished condition of patient 3 years post treatment

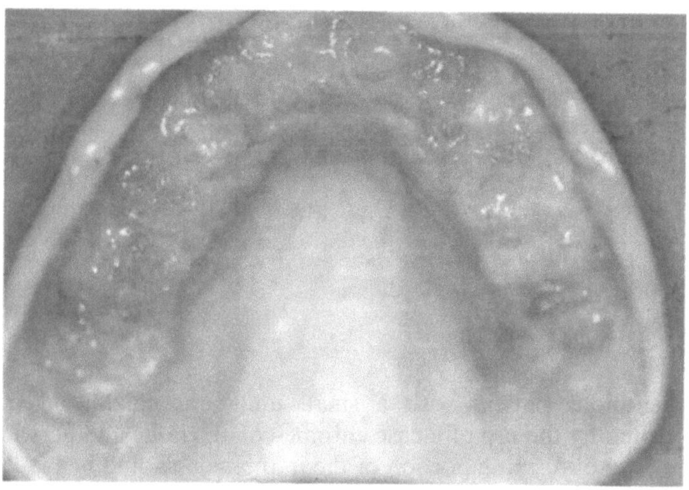

Fig. 7.25. Tissue surface of maxillary overdenture

Defects of the palate primarily involve loss of function – mastication of food – swallowing – and loss of ability to speak. These disabilities are permanent following resections of the maxilla, but can be corrected by the proper design and fabrication of maxillary, removable obturators. These obturators will vary in size and configuration according to the defect.

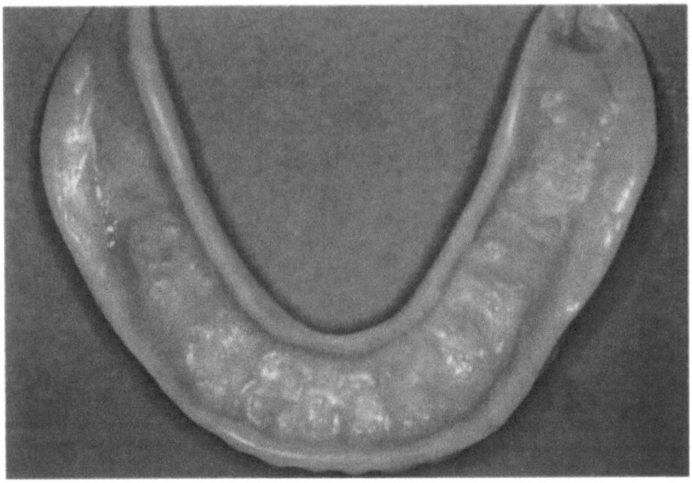

Fig. 7.26. Tissue surface of mandibular overdenture

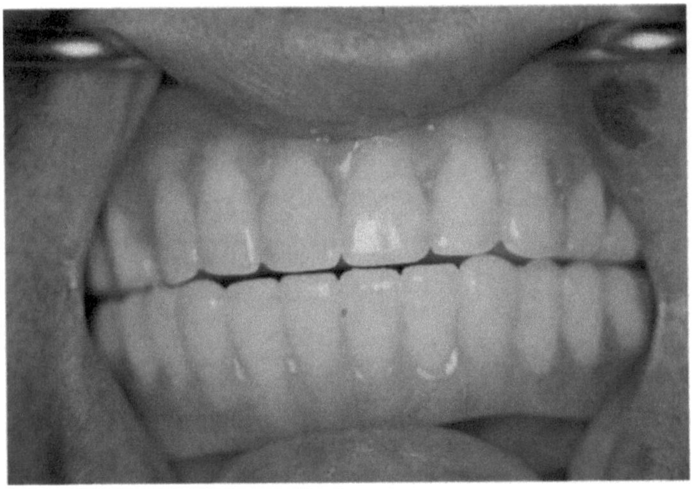

Fig. 7.27. Overdentures inserted

The partially edentulous patient with a small unilateral palatal defect (Fig. 7.29) may be treated by the use of a case chrome-cobalt frame and acrylic resin base (Fig. 7.30). The obturating portion of the impression should be made by border moulding with green stick compound (Fig. 7.31) and finishing the impression by using a heavy bodied rubber base material or Korecta wax (Kerr Manufacturing Co, Romulus, Mich.) (Fig. 7.32). The case is then processed as in a normal "altered cast" technique (Fig. 7.33), resulting in the completed obturator which reestablishes normal speech, deglutition, and esthetics (Fig. 7.34).

Large palatal defects (Fig. 7.35) may be corrected in the same manner as the small defects with the addition of "functional" final impression procedures.

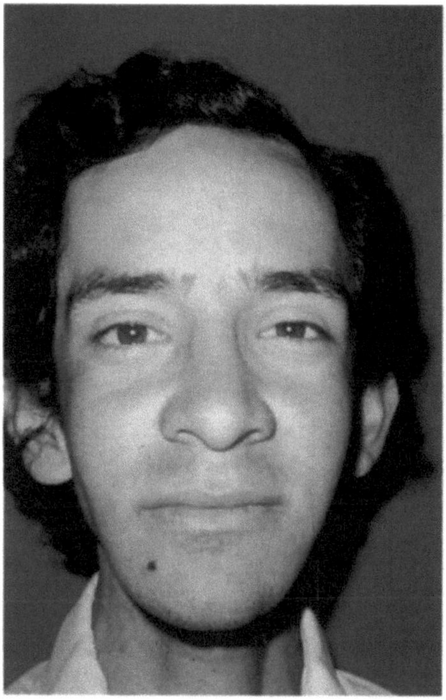

Fig. 7.28. Patient at present time

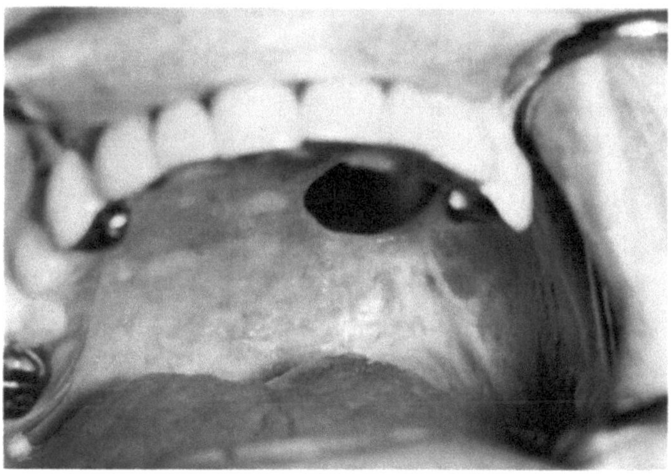

Fig. 7.29. Small palatal defect

These are accomplished by having the patient bend his head down on his chest, move it from side to side, and swallow while the rubber base or other wash material is setting. The frame and obturator are removed from the mouth and examined for accuracy. Any pressure areas should be relieved and repainted with Korecta wax and the procedure repeated until no more pressure areas

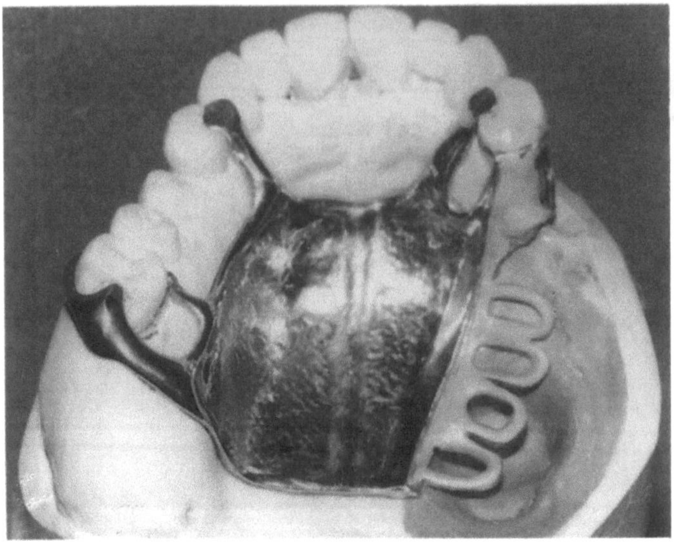

Fig. 7.30. Cast maxillary framework

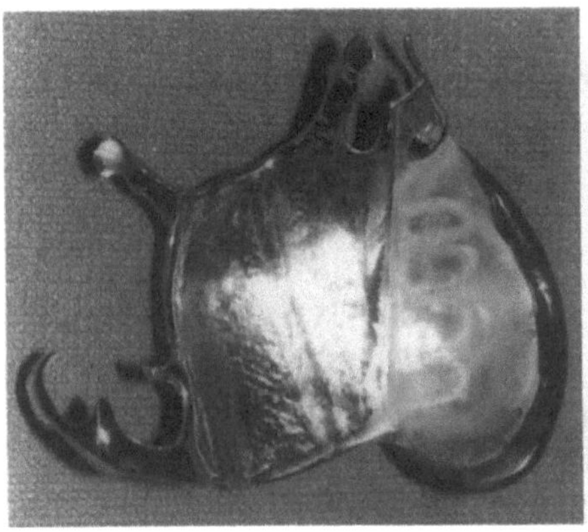

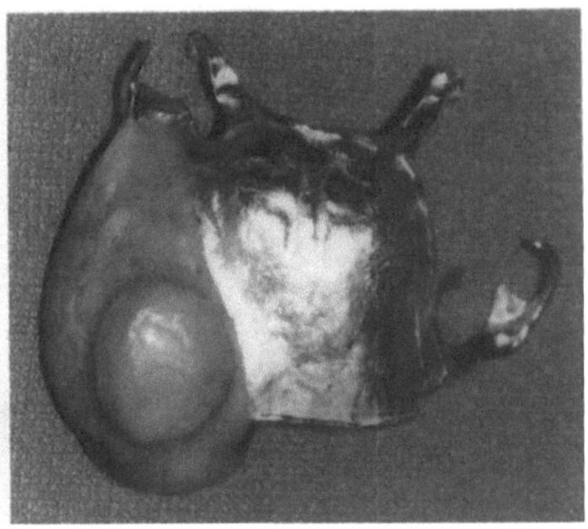

Fig. 7.31 **Fig. 7.32**

Fig. 7.31. Framework with acrylic base and border molding

Fig. 7.32. Framework with rubber base impression

are evident. The obturator is then invested and processed in the normal manner (Fig. 7.36). New records are made, the prosthesis is remounted on the articulator, and the occlusion refined. The completed prosthesis is then ready for delivery to the patient (Fig. 7.37).

Other palatal defects may involve only a portion of the soft palate (Fig. 7.38). These are often more difficult to correct than the larger defects due to fibrosing of the remaining soft tissues and change in muscle action.

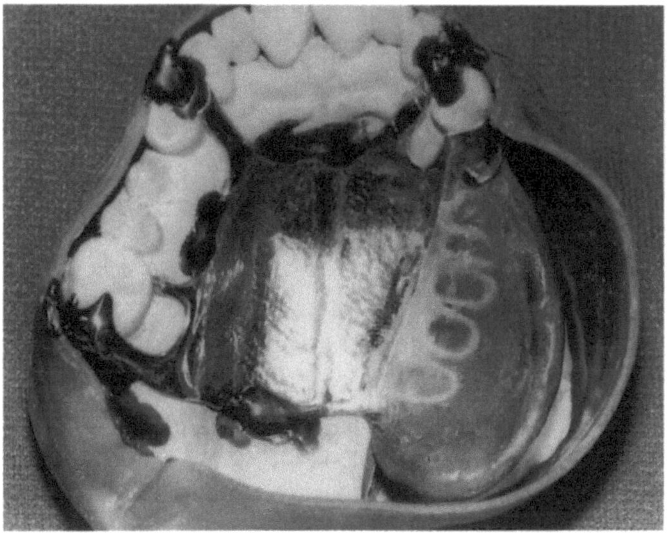

Fig. 7.33. Altered cast technique

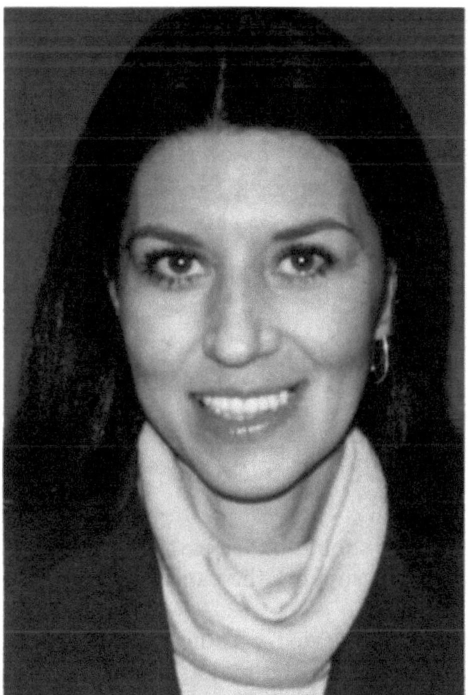

Fig. 7.34. Completed obturator inserted

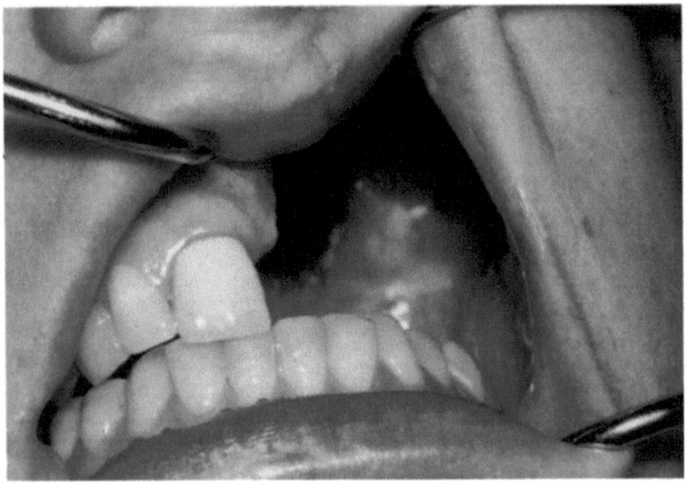

Fig. 7.35. Large palatal defect

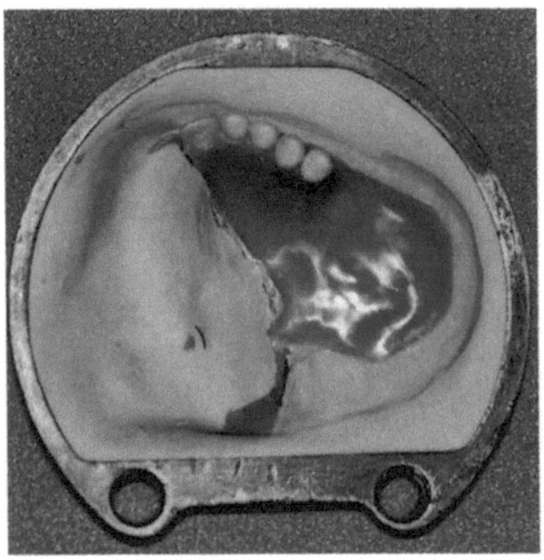

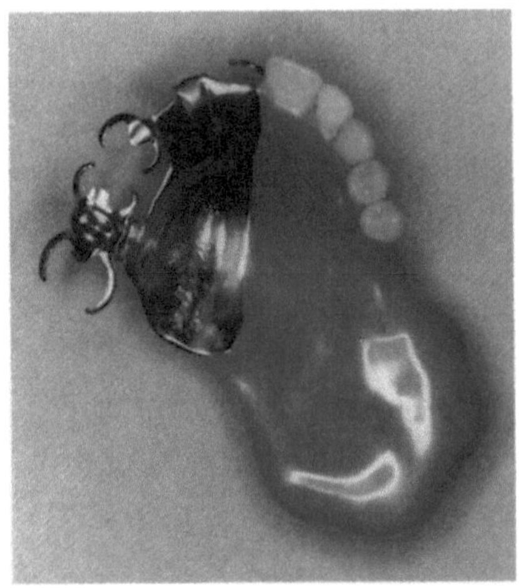

Fig. 7.36 **Fig. 7.37**

Fig. 7.36. Obturator flasked for final processing

Fig. 7.37. Processed obturator

The oral or carrier portion of the obturator should be very carefully designed (Fig. 7.39) with adequate clasping in order to support the cantilevered weight of the pharyngeal portion.

After the oral, cast framework is fitted and seated with no further adjustments needed, an acrylic resin core is attached to the major connector loop of the framework (Fig. 7.40). Compound tracing of the bulb is accomplished to determine the extent of the defect (Fig. 7.41). A functional impression is

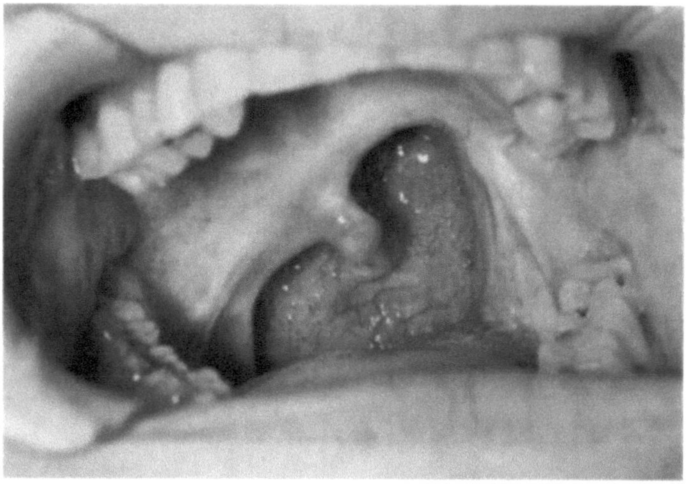

Fig. 7.38. Unilateral surgical defect of soft palate

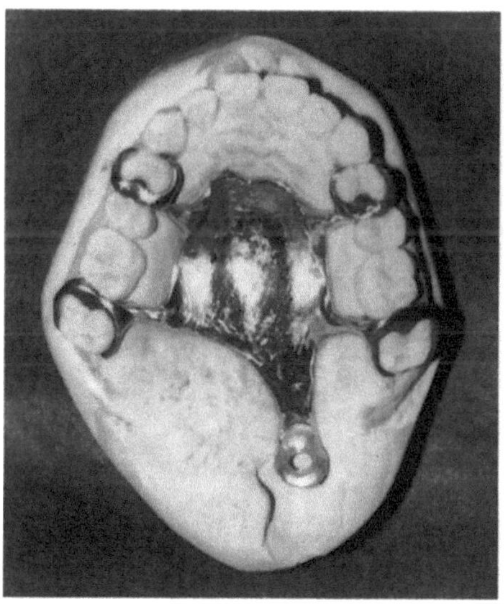

Fig. 7.39

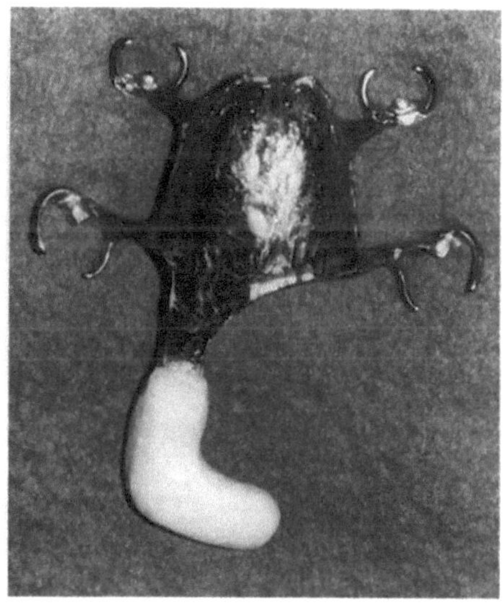

Fig. 7.40

Fig. 7.39. Cast framework showing adequate clasping for retention

Fig. 7.40. Acrylic resin core attached to framework

then made by using Korecta wax (Fig. 7.42), inserting in the mouth (Fig. 7.43), moving the head, and swallowing. The bulb is chilled, carefully removed from the mouth, and invested (Fig. 7.44). The processed obturator is polished (Fig. 7.45) and delivered to the patient (Fig. 7.46). This type of prosthesis corrects the functional disabilities of speech and swallowing, yet allows for normal nasal breathing while the palate is in rest position. This is accomplished by use of a functional impression technique.

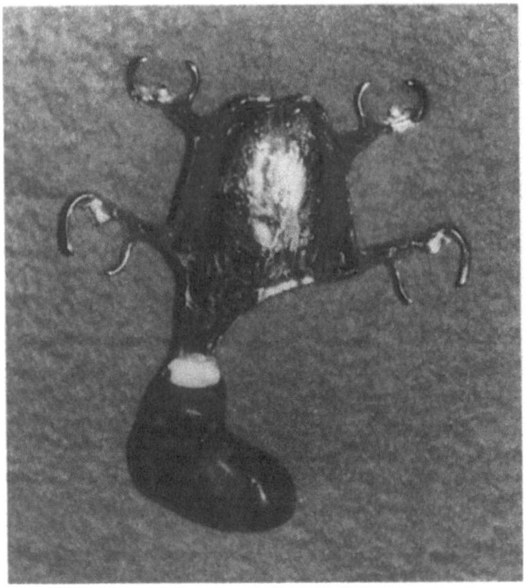

Fig. 7.41. Compound added to acrylic core

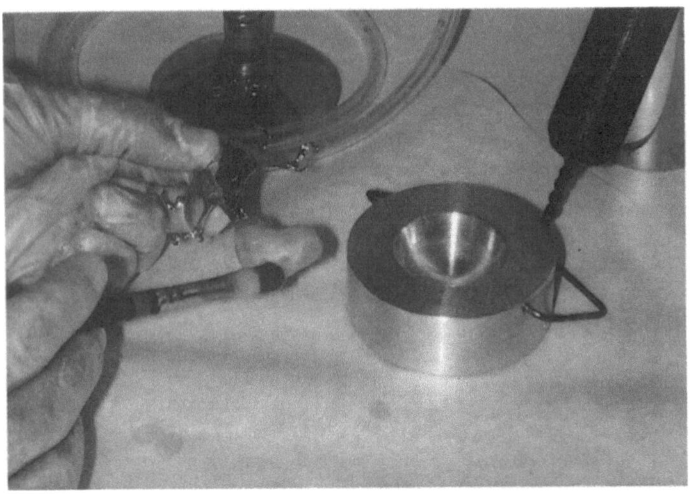

Fig. 7.42. Adding Korecta wax for functional tracing

Combination intra-oral and facial defects pose additional problems in rehabilitating the post-surgical cancer patient (Fig. 7.47). Usually the defects are much larger than single defects, involve more functional areas and more moving tissues. They also usually involve two or more separate prostheses which must be inter-related to each other. A mid-third of the face defect requires an intra-oral prosthesis which replaces the anterior palate, alveolar ridge, and teeth and which must be retained by clasping remaining posterior teeth. If the patient is edentulous, the problem of retention is further complicated and must be solved by the use of soft tissue undercuts or scar bands (Figs. 7.48 and 7.49),

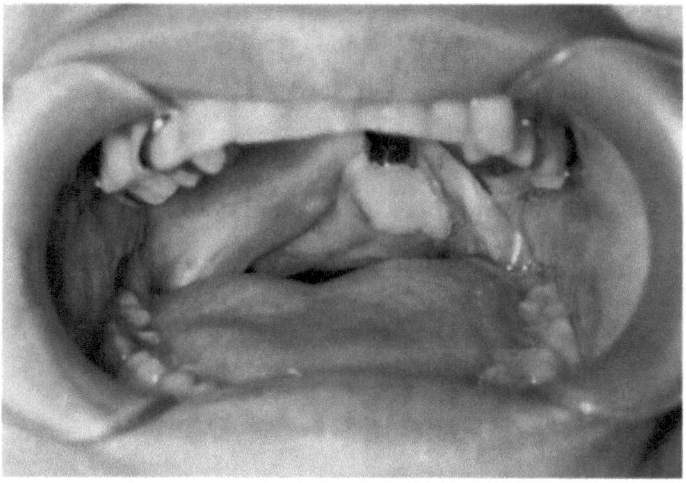

Fig. 7.43. Prosthesis inserted during functional tracing of bulb

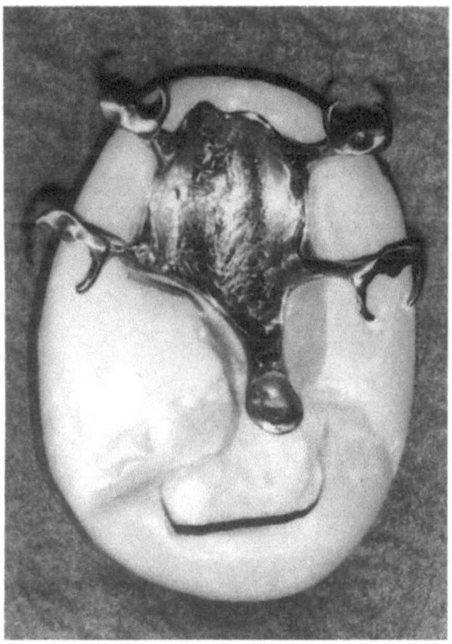

Fig. 7.44

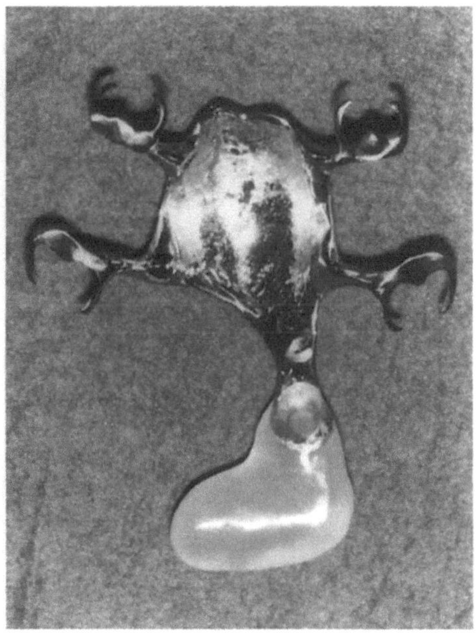

Fig. 7.45

Fig. 7.44. Bulb invested for processing

Fig. 7.45. Completed obturator with speech bulb

mechanical retention such as the use of springs attached to a mandibular prosthesis, attracting magnets embedded in the obturator bulb, and an orbital prosthesis or "button" retention of the lip portion of a facial prosthesis to the labial flange of the obturator (Figs. 7.50 and 7.51). The large facial and intra-

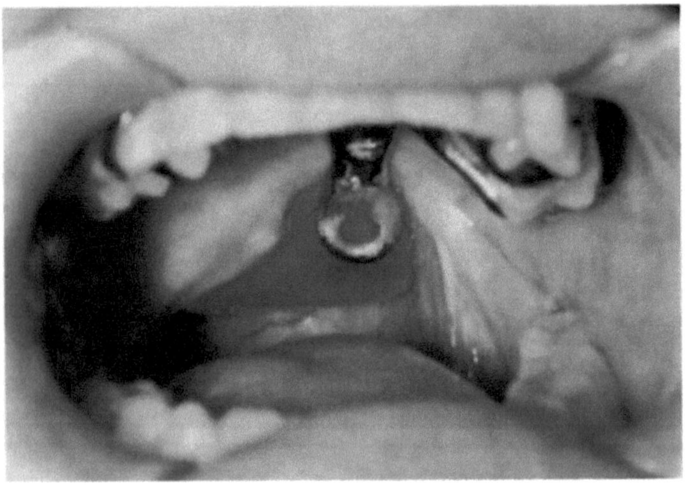

Fig. 7.46. Completed obturator inserted

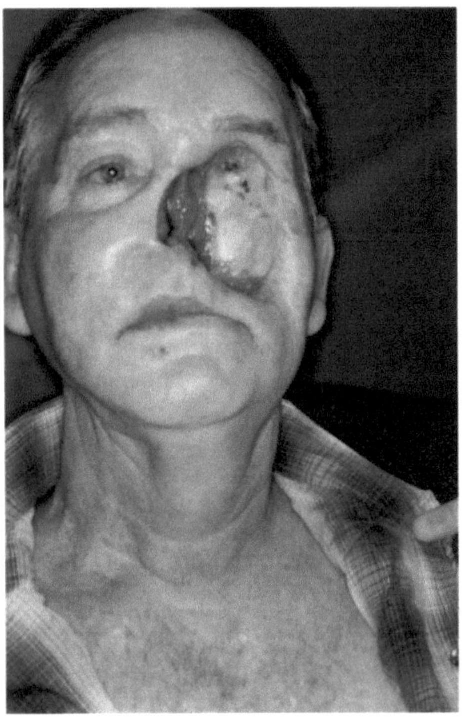

Fig. 7.47. Combination intraoral and facial defect

oral defects involving the mid-third and lower part of the face introduce additional problems of retention due to movements of the muscles of expression and mastication. If the prosthetic restoration of these facial defects and rehabilitation of the patient is to be satisfactorily accomplished, the technique must

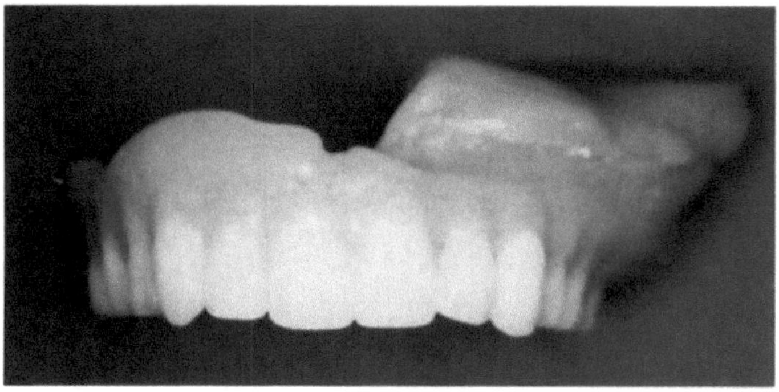

Fig. 7.48. Obturator with buccal and superior extension

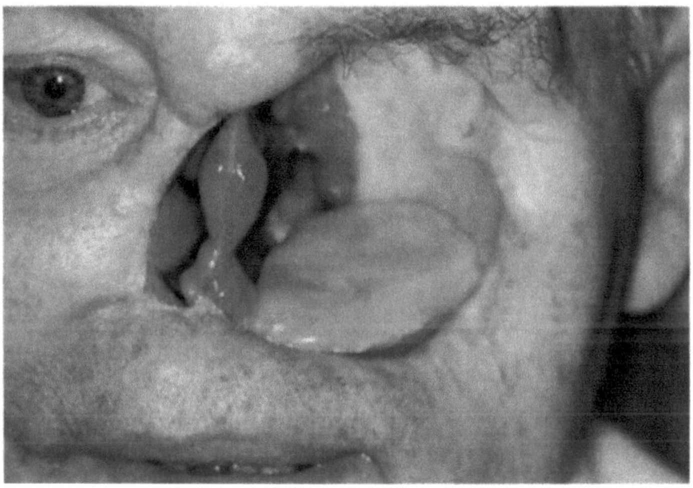

Fig. 7.49. Obturator inserted engaging defect undercuts

be comparatively simple, the materials must be biologically inert, and they must be fairly durable and easily cared for by the patient. Many materials are being used in different treatment centers which answer, to some extent, these requirements. An ideal material for all situations has not been found as yet, and due to different requirements of hardness, elasticity, and color stability in different parts of the same prosthesis, it may never be available. Polyvinylchloride (PVC), polyurethane, acrylic resin, and various types of silicones are the materials most widely used at the present time.

PVC is inexpensive and easy to fabricate. It is easy to match color to the various areas of the defect border. It has good "adheophilic" [5] properties. The material can be modified after curing by resoftening and surface tinting. The principle disadvantages are that it requires metal molds or glycerin bath for processing, and harmful gases are liberated during manufacture of the raw material.

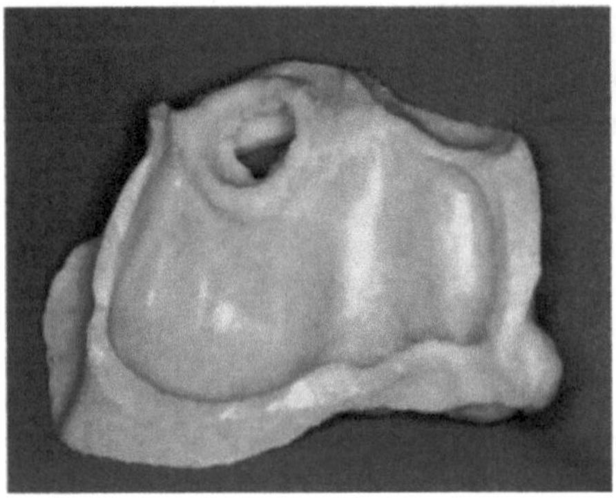

Fig. 7.50

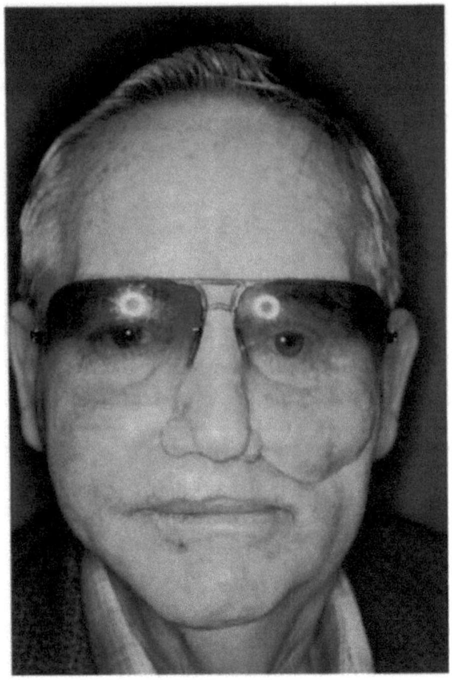

Fig. 7.51

Fig. 7.50. Tissue surface of facial prosthesis

Fig. 7.51. Prosthesis positioned over defect

Polyurethane has some excellent qualities, particularly its elasticity and skin like texture. It also has an undesirable aspect of undergoing spontaneous softening after processing which reduces the durability of the prosthesis significantly.

Acrylic resin is quite satisfactory for prostheses that do not require any elasticity or softness. It is light, has good color properties, and is very durable. It can also be readily altered or adjusted.

Several types of silicone have been used over a period of many years with varying degrees of success. The principle difficulties with using the heat cured silicone is that it must be freshly milled in order to be packed in metal molds, and the colors must be milled into the material "individually". The R.T.V. (Room Temperature Vulcanizing) silicones usually have poor edge tear resistance, and in some preparations, such as MDX-4210 (Dow Corning Corp.), the extreme sensitivity of the curing agents limits the practical use of the material.

Beginning with acrylic and PVC, all of these materials have been in use since the early 1950's. In 1976, Udagama [6] developed a technique using Silastic medical adhesive type A (Dow Corning Corp.) which is a preparation of methyl triacetoxy silane cross-linked silicone, for use as a margin seal material (Margi-Seal, M.D. Anderson Pharmacy, Houston, Tex.) (Figs. 7.52–7.57). This was a significant advancement in improving the esthetic quality of facial prostheses. With the addition of earth pigments in the proper base colors, the matrial can be packaged for dispensing to the patient for home use. The material is easily applied to the margins of the prosthesis when it is in place on the defect either by the patient or another person and acts both as an adhesive and to mask the obvious margins.

In 1977, Udagama developed and described the further use of Silastic medical adhesive silicone type A, as a material for fabricating the total prosthesis. This material is a translucent nonflowing paste. It contains no solvents or plasticizers and will cure at room temperature on contact with moisture in the air. The curing cycle can be shortened by processing at 185°F in a plaster or stone mold. Acetic Acid is liberated as the material cures, which makes a thorough rinsing of the prosthesis in warm water necessary after curing is complete before placing on the patient's face. Various improvements have been made in the use of this material by combining other materials such as kaolin and uncured MDX4-4210 (Dow Corning Corp.) silicone which lengthens the working time, allowing for easier incorporation of dry earth pigments or oil based pigments for proper base coloring and which makes the material more opaque. The addition of uncured MDX4-4210 to the type A adhesive in varying proportions also permits control of the hardness or softness of different parts of the prosthesis [7].

In fabricating a prosthesis of this type, stone molds are made of the finished sculpture, and the surfaces are painted with an alginate separating medium. This should be applied in a very thin even layer and thoroughly dryed. An even layer of type A adhesive (triacetoxy silane crosslinked silicone) is then applied to the mold surfaces with a camel's hair brush. This layer is translucent and gives depth and toughness to the outer skin of the prosthesis. Color flockings are sprayed onto various regions of this layer to match the color pattern of the patient's skin.

Approximately 10% by weight of dry kaolin is thoroughly mixed with uncured MDX4-4210 on a mixing pad. Various nontoxic earth pigments as well as flocking are mixed into the kaolinsilicone mixture in proper amounts to match the basic skin color of the patient. Different color mixtures can be placed in different regions of the mold to match the adjacent skin at that particular margin of the defect. Also varying amounts of type A silicone is added to the MDX mixture if a harder material is desired in a particular area of the prosthesis. The mold is then filled with a sufficient amount of the base color silicone mixture and closed. After the excess material is squeezed out, the mold is then placed in a clamp, and the prosthesis is cured at 185°F for approximately 10 h in a water bath.

After curing, the prosthesis is removed from the mold, the flash trimmed, and Hollister adhesive (Hollister Adhesive, Inc., Chicago, Ill.) placed on the tissue surface margins. The prosthesis is then placed over the defect. Any voids or errors can be corrected by adding correctly colored type A silicone mixed with kaolin, and the margins are then finished by the Margi-Seal technique.

The prosthesis should be worn in place for 24 h to allow for proper curing of the added Margi-Seal material after which it may be removed. At this time the surface may be further characterized by replacing on the patient's face, adding flocking if needed, adding long fibers to simulate arteriols, adding additional dry earth pigments, and individualizing the surface texture of an added thin layer of methyl triacetoxy silane crosslinked silicone.

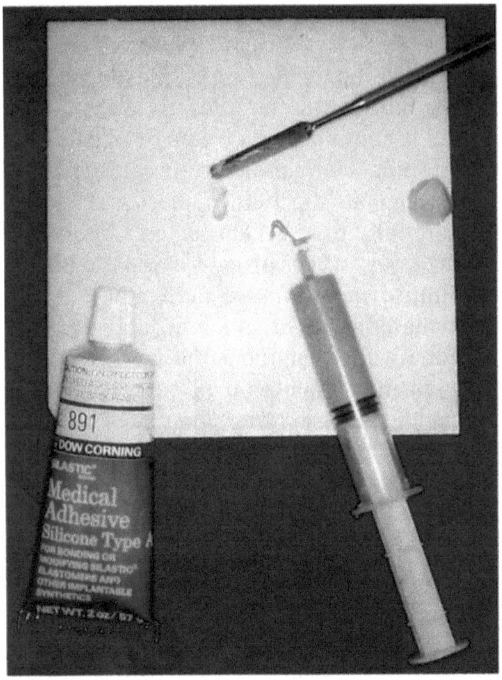

Fig. 7.52. "Margi-Seal" materials

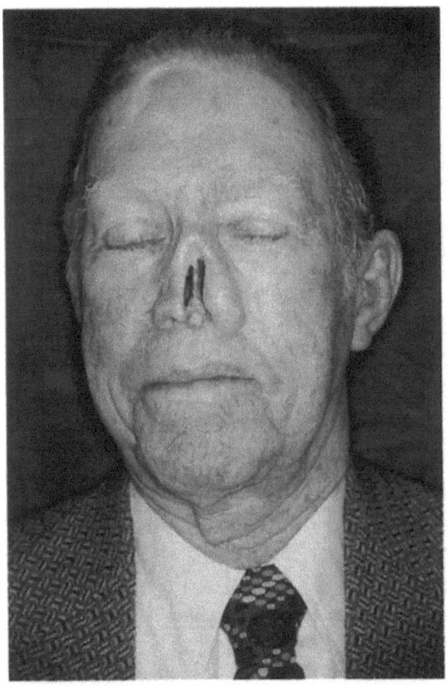

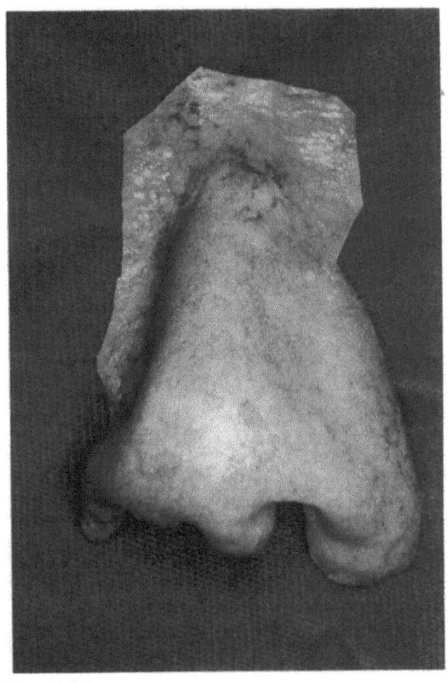

Fig. 7.53 **Fig. 7.54**

Fig. 7.53. Frontal view of patient

Fig. 7.54. Extreme close up of nasal prosthesis showing intrinsic staining and thin margins

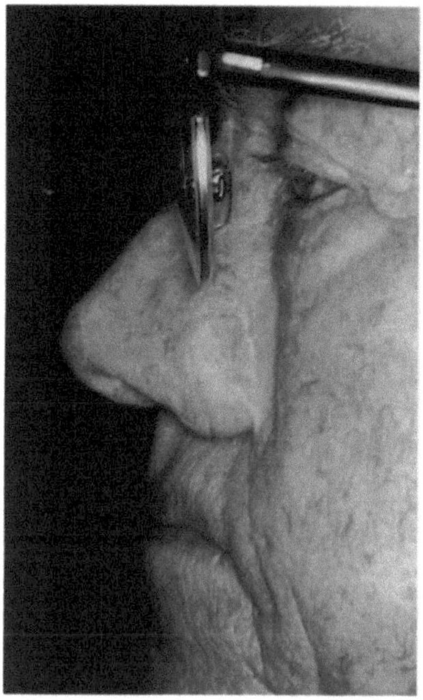

Fig. 7.55

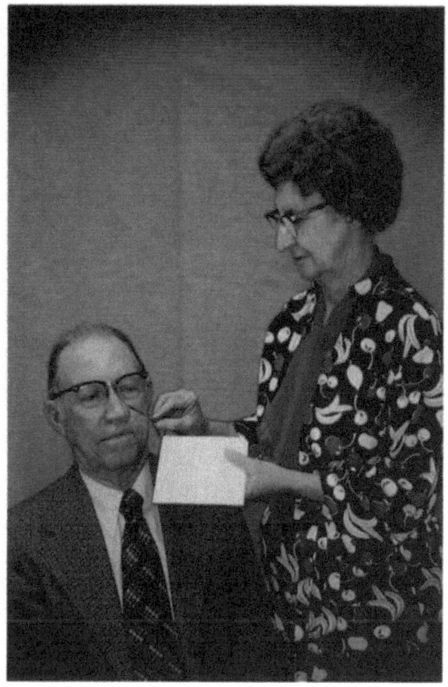

Fig. 7.56

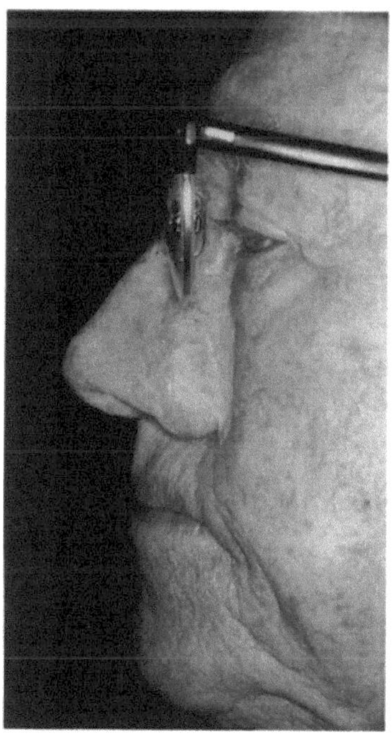

Fig. 7.57

Fig. 7.55. Close up view of prosthesis in place before use of "Margi-Seal"

Fig. 7.56. Wife of patient applying "Margi-Seal" preparation

Fig. 7.57. Close up of margin area after application of "Margi-Seal"

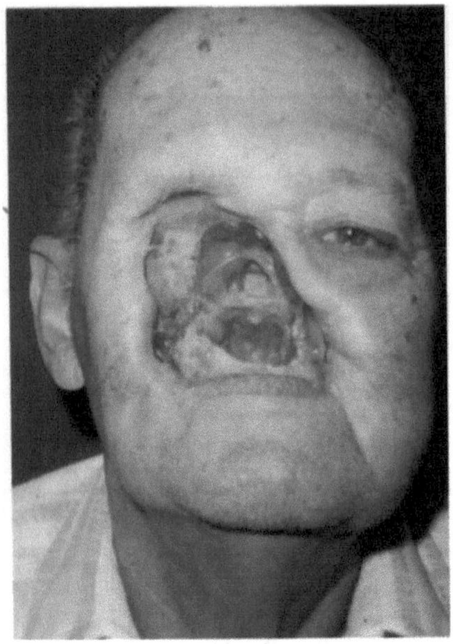

Fig. 7.58

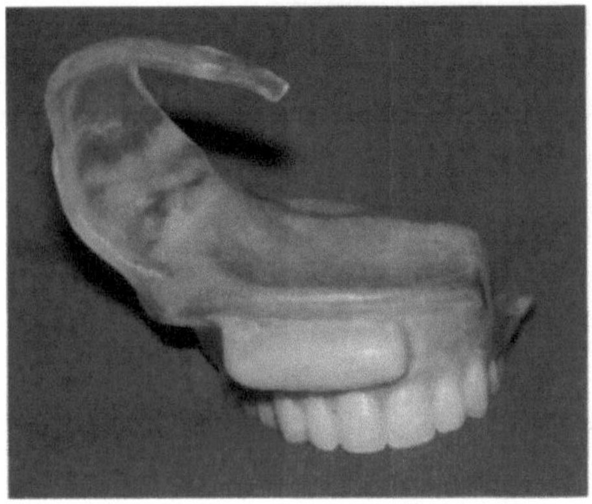

Fig. 7.59

Fig. 7.58. Patient with large palatal and facial defect

Fig. 7.59. Intraoral prosthesis

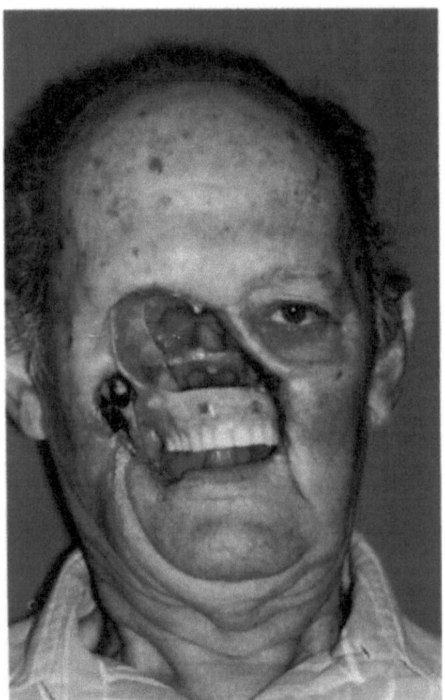

Fig. 7.60

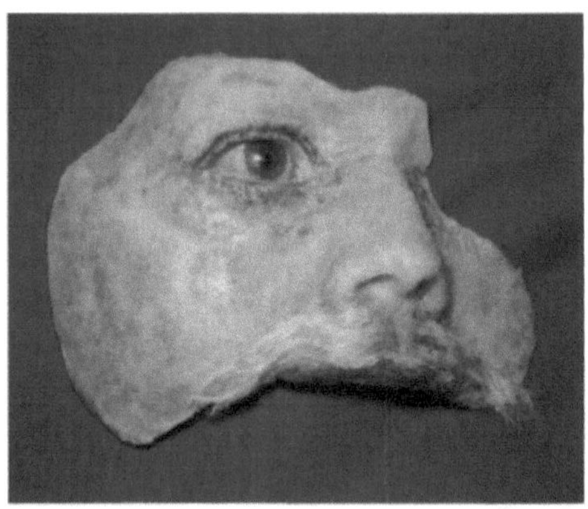

Fig. 7.61

Fig. 7.60. Intraoral prosthesis inserted showing extension to roof of orbit for stabilization

Fig. 7.61. Medical adhesive type A combined with MDX4-4210 facial prosthesis

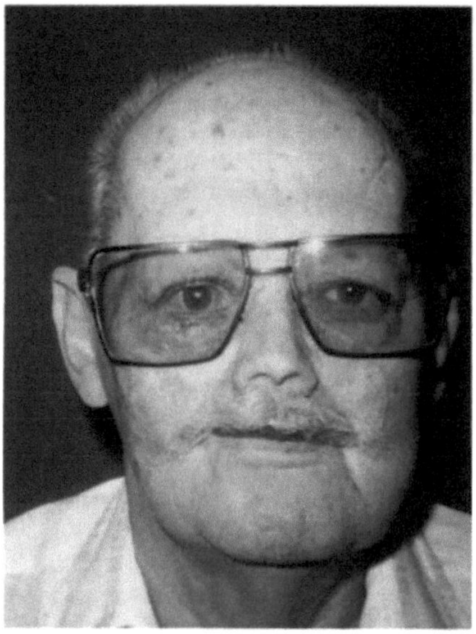

Fig. 7.62. Prosthesis positioned over defect

This type of silicone material offers many advantages over PVC, urethane, and other silicones when used for making facial prosthesis. Some of these are:

- No catalysts or curing agents are required.
- The material is compatible with a wide range of pigments and colorants.
- It can be processed in gypsum molds.
- It is easily modified and recolored.
- It contains no plasticizers which makes the material very stable and long lasting.
- Color stability is much better than PVC or polyurethane.
- Post-cure coloring is simple and long lasting.
- The margins can be easily adapted to the patient by the Margi-Seal technique, which makes the prosthesis indistinguishable from the surrounding skin. These advantages are best demonstrated by Figs. 7.58–7.62.

As the scope of maxillofacial prosthetic programs continually improve and expand to all cancer treatment centers, and well-trained, competent personnel become more readily available to work with the physicians managing the primary care and surgical rehabilitation, the quality of survival of cancer patients will be greatly improved.

References

1. Annual Report of the Department of Dental Oncology, The University of Texas System Cancer Center, M.D. Anderson Hospital and Tumor Institute, 1981
2. Nakamoto, R.Y.: "Use of Immediate Obturators in Maxillary Resections", Project Report, The University of Texas System Cancer Center, M.D. Anderson Hospital and Tumor Institute, 1971

3. Hahn, G.W.: "Vitallium Mesh Mandibular Prosthesis", J. Prosthet. Dent., 14:777–784, 1964
4. Anderson, R.R.: "Complete Dentures for Patients Who Have Had Radiation Therapy for Head and Neck Cancer", Project Report, The University of Texas System Cancer Center, M.D. Anderson Hospital and Tumor Institute, 1970
5. Udagama, A.: "Biocompatibility and Physical Properties of Medical Adhesives Used in Maxillofacial Prosthetics", Thesis, Indiana University, School of Dentistry, Indianapolis, 1975
6. Udagama, A. and Drane, J.B.: "Use of Medical-Grade Methyl Triacetoxy Silane Cross-linked Silicone for Facial Prostheses", J. Prosthet. Dent., 48:86–88, 1982
7. Udagama, A.: "Facial Prosthetic Laboratory and Clinical Procedures". Audio-Visual Tapes, Continuing Education Course, The University of Texas Health Science Center at San Antonio, 1981

Chapter 8. Series of Case Examples

James E. Hamner, III

1. Case No. 1: Squamous Cell Carcinoma

This 53 year-old Indian male presented with an extensive area of homogenous leukoplakia, involving a large portion of his left buccal mucosa (see Fig. 8.1). He was a resident of the State of Kerala in the southern tip of India. His mixed tobacco habit included "pan" (betel quid with tobacco) and "bidi" (a homemade cigar). He had practiced these tobacco habits for many years. The lesion was painless, but he had noticed it inside his mouth.

This individual was followed for three years in our Indian study. Figure 8.2 demonstrates a squamous cell carcinoma arising in the same site as the original leukoplakia. This is a good example of malignant transformation from a white lesion of the oral cavity, since the patient persisted in his tobacco habits, regardless of the advice not to do so. When the cancer was detected, he was immediately referred for treatment. The malignancy was removed by surgery, proved to be moderately well-differentiated on histopathologic examination, and the patient was alive two years post-operatively with no known metastases.

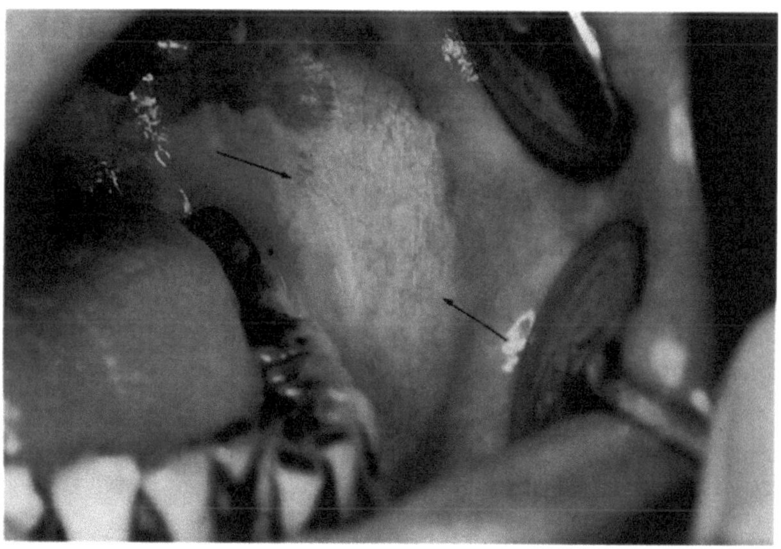

Fig. 8.1. Homogenous leukoplakia (*arrows*), left buccal mucosa, 53 year-old Indian male. (Courtesy of Dr. F.S. Mehta and Dr. D.K. Daftary)

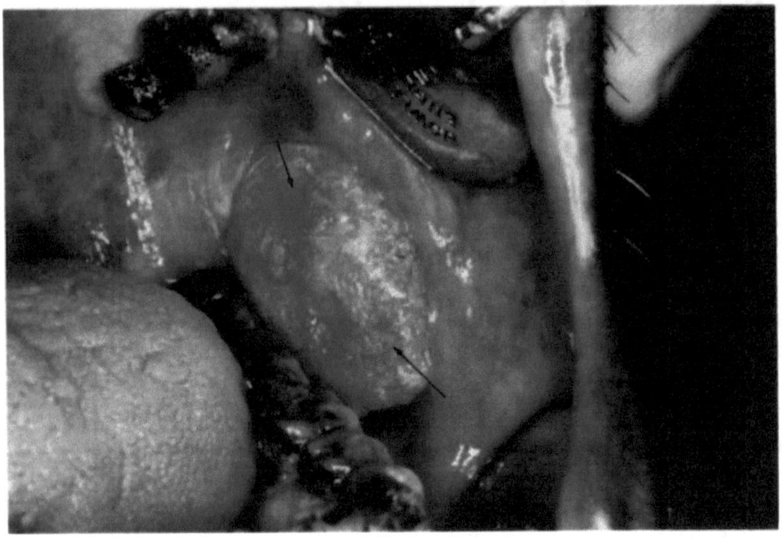

Fig. 8.2. Squamous cell carcinoma (*arrows*), arising from the same leukoplakia site in the above patient, three years later. (Courtesy of Dr. F.S. Mehta and Dr. D.K. Daftary)

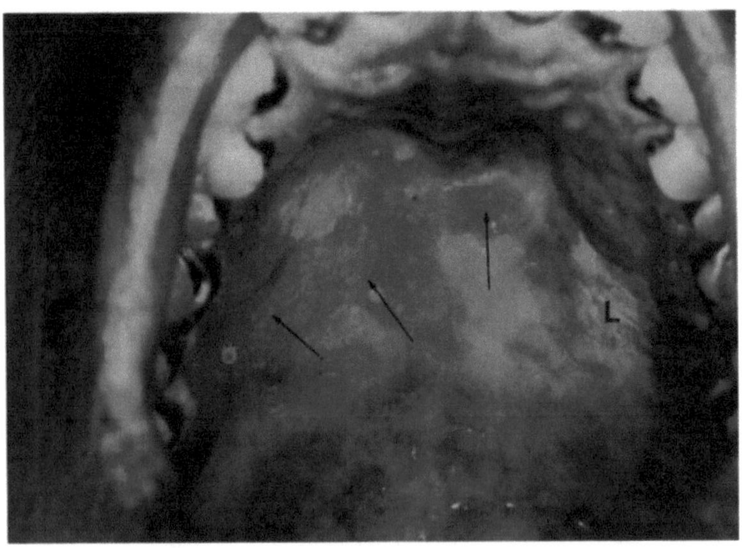

Fig. 8.3. Erythroplakia (*arrows*) and leukoplakia (*L*) occurring together in the hard palate of a 36 year-old Indian female. (Courtesy of Dr. F.S. Mehta and Dr. D.K. Daftary)

2. Case No. 2: Squamous Cell Carcinoma

Figure 8.3 illustrates both erythroplakia and homogenous leukoplakia, occurring simultaneously on the hard palate of a 36 year-old Indian female, who lived along the coastal region of Andhra Pradesh State in India. The erythrop-

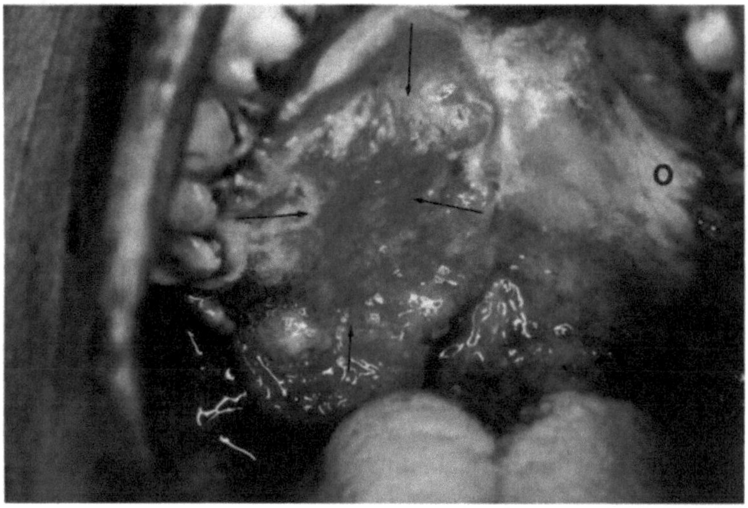

Fig. 8.4. Malignant transformation of erythroplakia to carcinoma (*arrows*); leukoplakia = (o) remained the same, two years later. (Courtesy of Dr. F.S. Mehta and Dr. D.K. Daftary)

lakia lesion was the larger one, extending from the right alveolar ridge to beyond the midline of the palate, with adjacent whitish-pink patches. The main leukoplakia lesion was confined to the left posterior portion of the palate. This woman had a long history of practicing the "chutta" habit – reverse smoking of a homemade cigar.

Two years later the erythroplakia area had progressed to frank carcinoma on the right side of the palate (see Fig. 8.3). The leukoplakia lesion on the left posterior palate appeared clinically to be about the same size and texture as it had been two years previously (compare Fig. 8.4 to Fig. 8.3). This case is an excellent example of the dangerous potential of all erythroplakic lesions in the oral cavity to transform to carcinoma. An original biopsy of the erythroplakia lesion two years earlier revealed marked epithelial atypia, and the patient was advised to discontinue her tobacco habit – to no avail.

The patient was treated by radiation therapy, but died three years later.

3. Case No. 3: Cemento-Ossifying Fibroma

(A) History of Present Illness

A 16 year-old Negro girl was referred to the National Cancer Institute, with a provisional diagnosis of recurrent maxillary tumor. This was her first National Institutes of Health admission. Approximately 5 years before, at the age of 11, the patient became aware of a painless, progressive swelling of the right side of the face. She sought treatment from a private physician, who performed a partial intraoral resection of the maxillary tumor. No further difficulty was experienced until about 2 years later, when the painless swelling recurred in the same area, necessitating a second operation.

The postoperative course progressed well until approximately 6 months prior to the present admission, at which time the painless swelling recurred for the second time. Although the face was moderately swollen about the right cheek region, there was no pain, difficulty in swallowing, impairment of vision, weight loss, or lymphadenopathy. At this time the patient was referred to the National Institutes of Health for further evaluation and treatment.

(B) Physical Examination

A complete physical examination revealed a 16 year-old girl who was essentially normal except for right facial asymmetry with maxillary and palatal swelling caused by a recurrent tumor of unknown etiology. Hematology, urinalysis, and bacteriology findings were within normal limits.

(C) Dental Examination

All the of the teeth were present, with the exception of four impacted third molars and the missing left mandibular first molar. Moderate dental caries were noted. The most striking finding was a large, firm, buccal and palatal expansion of the right maxillary alveolar ridge, extending from the right cuspid to the second molar tooth (Fig. 8.5). The overlying mucosa was slightly erythematous but nonuclerated.

(D) Radiographic Findings

A Panorex radiograph demonstrated a large radiolucent, radiopaque lesion causing extensive destruction of the right maxilla with extension into the hard palate (Fig. 8.6). The lesion had spread through the lower portion of the medial wall of the right maxillary antrum into the right nasal cavity. The entire alreolar ridge was involved with spreading of the teeth roots. The periapical and occlusal dental films indicate a partial loss of the right maxillary premolar roots and the buccal roots of the first molar, probably as a result of surgical trauma during the previous partial resections, since the roots exhibited no histologic evidence of resorption. Chest x-ray films showed no evidence of metastatic lesions.

(E) Hospital Course

Biopsy. Eight days following the patient's admission to the hospital, the right maxillary first and second premolars and the first molar were extracted under local anesthesia. A biopsy specimen was then taken through the periapical region to obtain tumor tissue from deep within the sockets. No excessive bleeding was encountered. Grossly, the tissue was glossy white, could be cut with a

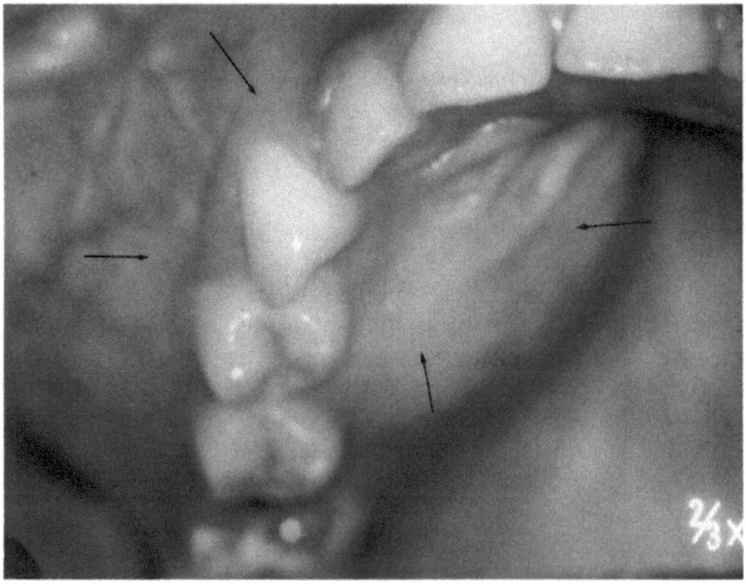

Fig. 8.5. Firm buccal and palatal swelling (*arrows*) from a right maxillary tumor in a 16 year-old Negro female

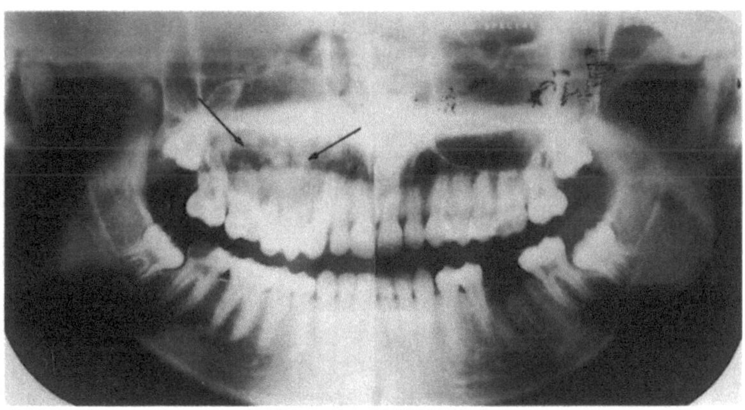

Fig. 8.6. Panorex radiograph revealing a large radiolucent-radiopaque tumor (*arrows*) in the right maxilla and antrum

scapel, and had a "gritty" consistency. Histopathologic study revealed trabeculae of alveolar bone on the periphery of the sections. They polarized with the customary dark and light lines of parallel birefringence indicative of normal mature, lamellar bone. Most of the tissue was composed of fibrous tissue with a marked proliferation of ovoid cells resembling either osteoblasts or cementoblasts. The latter type seemed most likely, since numerous small concentric, basophilic droplets of mineralized tissue were scattered at random among the proliferating cells. These droplets stained red with Masson's trichrome stain, similar to cementum.

The diagnosis indicated a tumor consistent with cementifying fibroma of the right maxilla.

(F) Surgical Procedure

Ten days following the biopsy the patient underwent a right maxillary antrectomy with preliminary tracheostomy under Pentothal and halothane anesthesia. The cheek flap was elevated through a modified Weber-Fergusson incision. The transection was carried just to the right of the midline of the maxilla, along the lateral aspect of the naris on the right, up to the floor of the orbit, which was preserved. Osteotome dissection was similarly carried across the zygoma and posteriorly to free the antrum from the pterygoid plate. Palatal excision was performed after the mucosa of the palate was elevated by sharp dissection and osteotome reflection to the opposite side, leaving the soft palate intact. On removal of the specimen, there was no evidence of the tumor's having been exposed except at the medial aspect of the maxillary transection and along the lateral aspect of the right naris. Therefore, a second specimen, which included the remaining portion of the maxilla over the site of the central incisor tooth as well as the entire lateral wall of the right naris and the turbinates and vomer, was removed. Curettage of the lateral antrum was then performed without difficulty. The ethmoids which had been eroded by the tumor, were explored, but no gross tumor was identified. A 13 mu Brown dermatome graft, taken from the skin of the lateral upper right thigh, was placed into the operative defect, covering the exposed raw bone, skin, and subcutaneous tissue of the cheek. Cornish wool packing and 4-0 plain catgut sutures were used to hold the graft in place. The cheek flap was held back in place with 4-0 plain sutures, and the skin was approximated with 5-0 Dermalon. A dental prosthesis was applied immediately to hold the Cornish wool in place. The endotracheal tube was removed from the tracheostomy site, and a No. 7 tracheostomy tube was inserted. The patient withstood the surgical procedure very well; bleeding was the same as usually encountered in such a procedure, and 500 c.c. of whole blood was used for replacement.

Microscopically, the tumor specimen consisted of connective tissue with numerous plump, ovoid cells producing droplets and globules of cementum randomly interlaced with areas of membranous lamellar bone formation (Fig. 8.7). Van Gieson's stain demonstrated a plentiful amount of collagen throughout the tumor. Under polarized light, the bone that was present polarized in dark and light lines of parallel birefringence, indicative of mature lamellar bone.

The diagnosis was cemento-ossifying fibroma of the right maxilla and maxillary antrum.

(G) Postoperative Course

The postoperative course was without incident except for a brief febrile episode which was believed secondary to a partial collapse of the right lung and right-

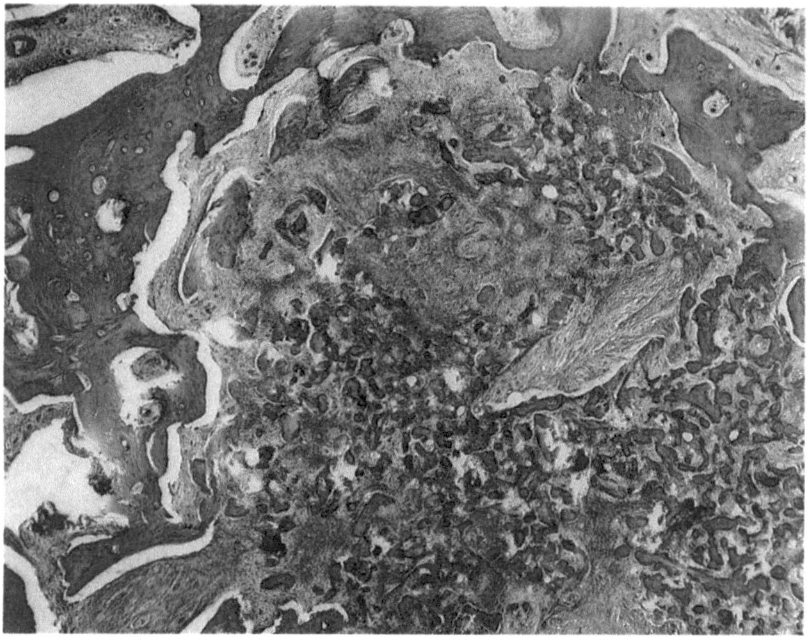

Fig. 8.7. Cemento-ossifying fibroma, right maxilla. H. & E. stain, ×25

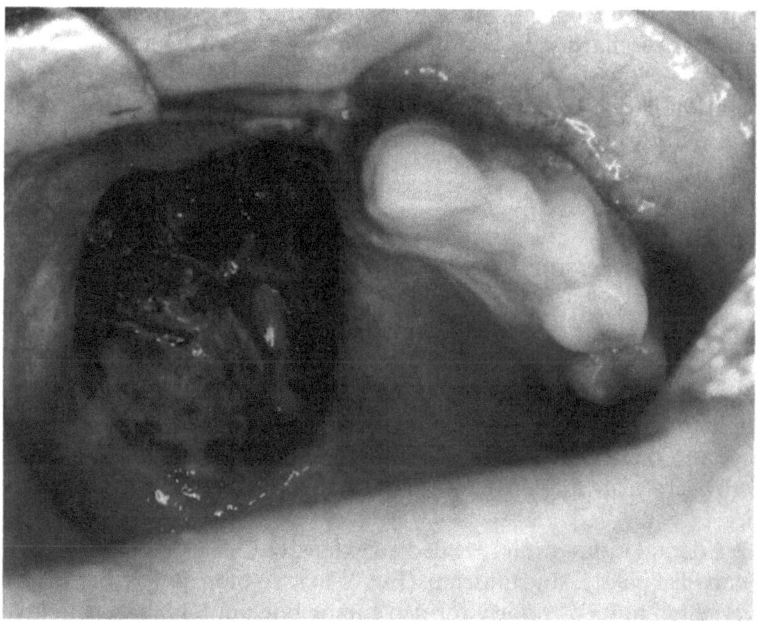

Fig. 8.8. Appearance of the surgical defect one week post-operatively

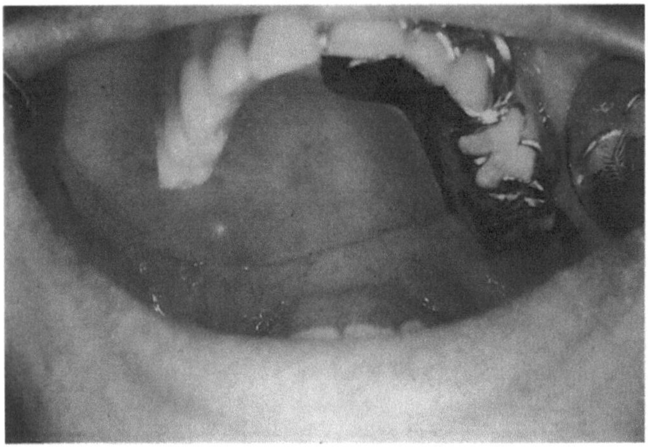

Fig. 8.9. Prosthetic device in place 23 days post-operatively

sided pneumonia. Four days later the patient was afebrile and progressing satisfactorily. One week following the operation the packing was removed, revealing a clean defect with the split-thickness skin graft covering approximately 60% of the surgical defect (Fig. 8.8). Five days afterward, the tracheostomy tube was removed. For the remainder of her hospitalization, the patient's care entailed recurrent debridement of the surgical defect and construction of a partial denture obturator which would enable her to eat without regurgitation of food into the area of the defect (Fig. 8.9). Twenty-three days after the operation the patient was discharged to be followed routinely by the referring physician.

A postoperation check-up 12 months after the surgical procedure revealed a clean surgical defect, no evidence of recurrent tumor, and a continued snug fit of the partial denture obturator.

4. Case No. 4: Osteosarcoma

This 17 year-old Negro male presented with a large swelling of the right maxilla that caused anterior protrusion, extended to the midline of the hard palate (see Fig. 8.10), and antral involvement caused encroachment on the right orbit. His chief complaints were pain and swelling. Only five maxillary anterior incisor teeth remained, and these teeth exhibited ramphant dental caries. The mandibular molar teeth were also missing, and his remaining mandibular teeth were in poor repair.

The panorex dental radiograph revealed an extensive radiopague tumor mass in the right maxilla, palate, and antrum (Fig. 8.11). A biopsy was performed and showed large amounts of poorly formed tumor bone in a highly malignant sarcomatous stroma (Fig. 8.12).

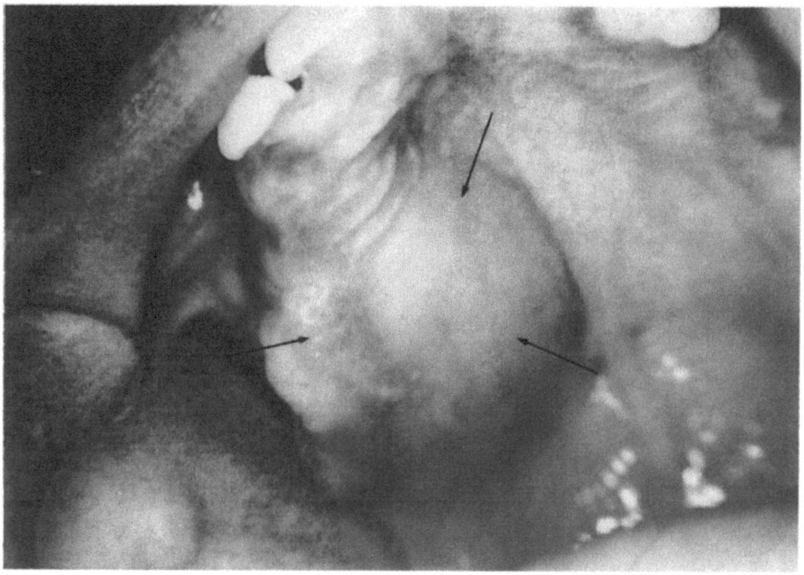

Fig. 8.10. Clinical appearance of a huge, firm right maxillary-antral-palatal tumor (*arrows*) in a 17 year-old Negro male

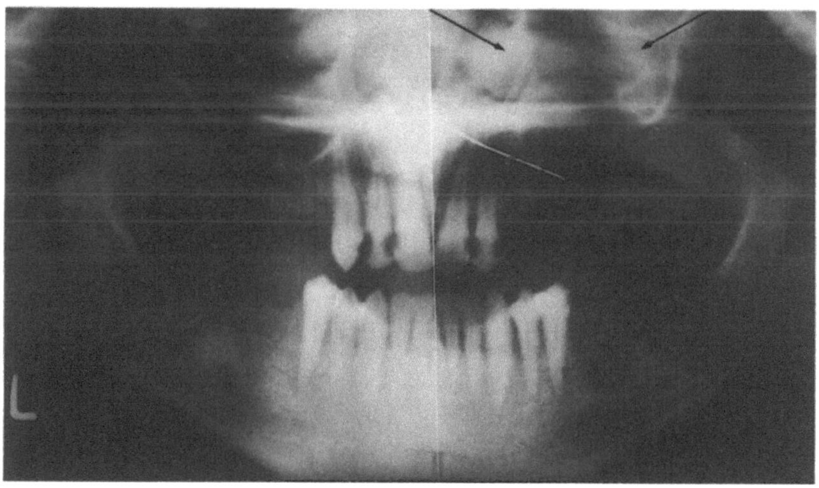

Fig. 8.11. Panorex film of an osteosarcoma (*arrows*) in the right maxilla, antrum, and palate of a 17 year-old Negro male

Because of its rapid onset, the highly malignant histopathologic nature of the tumor, the difficulty of the surgical involvement, and the patient's election of options, it was decided to treat the tumor by radiation therapy. He received 4,900 R to the tumor site with no apparent effect in destroying the osteosarcoma's growth. With this lack of a positive response, the patient went rapidly downhill, and died eight months later. At autopsy, metastatic lesions were noted in the lungs.

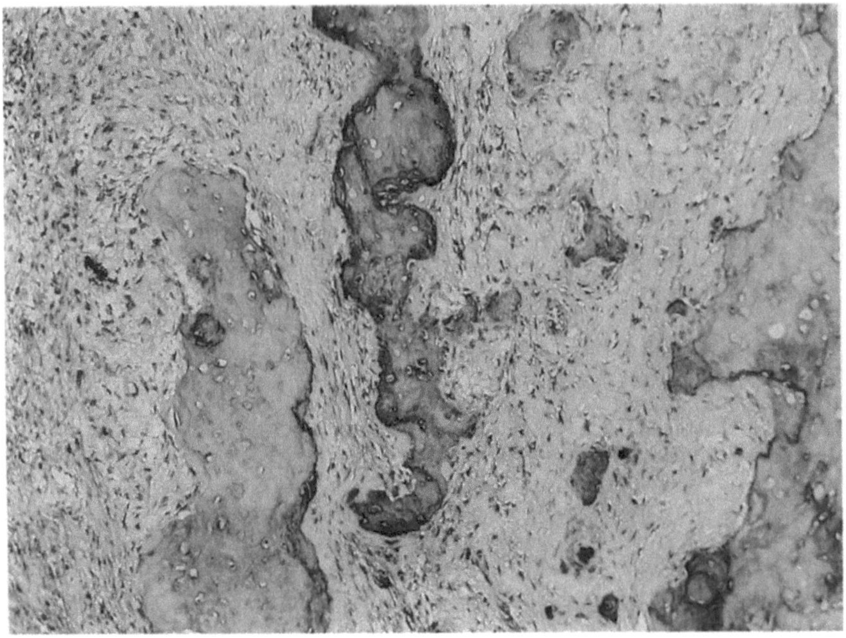

Fig. 8.12. Osteoblastic form of osteosarcoma. H. & E. stain, ×82

5. Case No. 5: Cherubism

(A) Present Illness

This 3 year-old Negro girl was referred to the Clinical Center of the National Institutes of Health in March 1962, with a diagnosis of "familial fibrous dysplasia" of the maxillae and mandible.

(B) Past History

Medical attention was first sought at age 18 months when she presented with a 4-month history of progressive bilateral mandibular swelling. This would place her original onset of symptoms at age 14 months. In September 1960, a mandibular biopsy was interpreted as "fibrous dysplasia"; no therapy was rendered at that time. The disease continued to progress until February 1962, when, at age 3 years, a tracheostomy was performed to relieve her respiratory distress. Upon her first N.I.H. admission her respiratory distress had been relieved by the tracheostomy, but her massive maxillary and mandibular tumor encroachment upon the oral cavity limited oral intake to pureed food. She had had no other operations, illnesses, or known allergies.

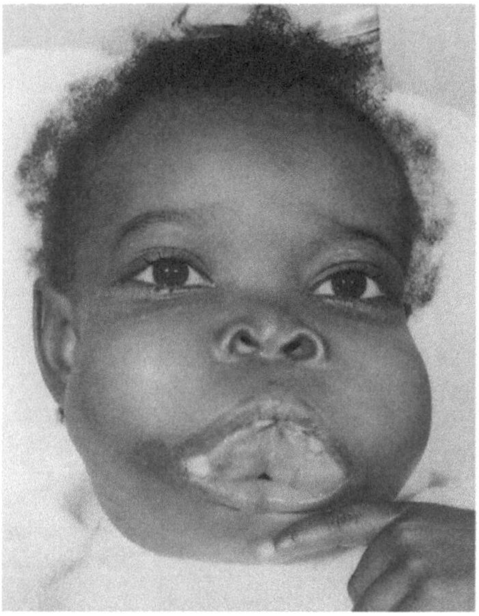

Fig. 8.13

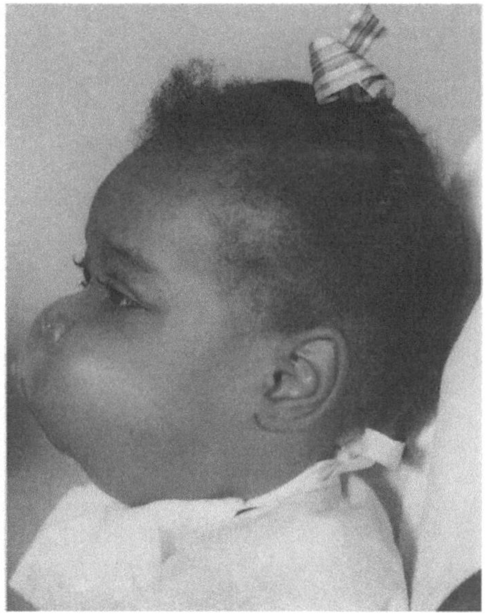

Fig. 8.14

Fig. 8.13. Clinical appearance of severe cherubism in a 3 year-old Negro girl

Fig. 8.14. Side view of the same patient, showing marked protrusion and bulging of the maxillary lesions

(C) Physical Examination

This normally well-developed, alert 3 year-old girl was admitted with subsiding pneumonitis. Any attempt to allow nasal pharyngeal breathing caused acute respiratory distress, and the well-functioning tracheostomy tube was mandatory. The positive physical findings were related entirely to the grossly obvious massive bilateral tumor enlargement of the mandible and maxillae (Figs. 8.13 and 8.14). The intra-oral protrusion of the palate, encroaching upon the floor of the mouth which was essentially obliterated by the mandibular enlargement, made adequate examination of the tongue and pharynx impossible. The maxillary enlargement also extended medially to nearly obliterate the nares. The deciduous dentition had erupted in a haphazard fashion with numerous missing teeth. There was diffuse shotty lymphadenopathy in both necks, but no axillary or inguinal nodes were palpable.

(D) Radiographic Examination

Lateral head radiographs demonstrated numerous multilocular radiolucencies separated by thin, gracile radiopaque septa of bone in both the mandible and maxillae (Fig. 8.15). The jaws were markedly expanded with tumor involvement of both antra as well. The anterior portions of her jaws were affected, in addition

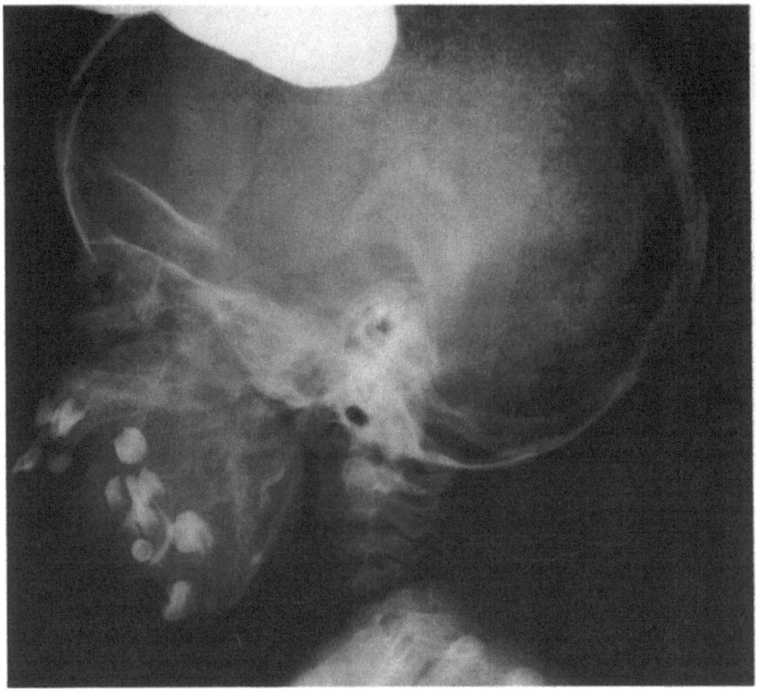

Fig. 8.15. Lateral head view on her admission radiograph with multilocular radiolucencies in the maxillae and mandible, and unerupted teeth appearing to float in radiolucent spaces

to the posterior regions of the mandibular angles, rami, and maxillary tuberosity. Many teeth were obviously missing, or arranged in a distorted manner, appearing to float in the radiolucent spaces. Her chest film and skeletal radiographic survey were negative for any other pathologic lesions.

(E) Laboratory Data

The admission hemogram was normal except for an elevated 13,000 leukocyte count with 38% mature polymorphonuclear neutrophils, 40% lymphocytes, 6% monocytes, and 16% eosinophils. Her hemogram returned to 9,800 leukocytes with 62% polymorphonuclear neutrophils, 30% lymphocytes, 4% monocytes, and 4% eosinophils in the early postoperative course. Urinalysis was unremarkable. Blood chemistries and electrolytes were normal except for an elevated serum alkaline phosphatase of 26 King-Armstrong units (normal for a child in our laboratory is 13–20 King-Armstrong units).

(F) Hospital Course

The decision to proceed with surgery was based on the child's severe respiratory, masticatory, and speech problems. A staged procedure was undertaken, ap-

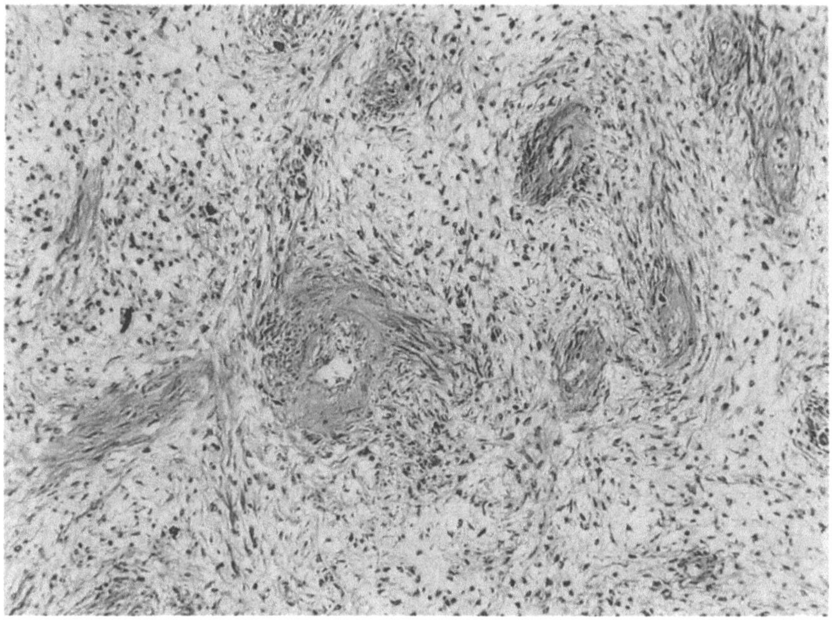

Fig. 8.16. Loose fibribular stroma seen in cherubism lesions. H. & E. stain, ×80

proaching the more symptomatic maxillae first, with the plan of palliative resection and/or curettement of all possible tumor, while attempting to restore facial and palatal contours.

On April 4, 1962, under fluothane and nitrous oxide general anesthesia, she had a bilateral subperiosteal maxillectomy with partial antraectomy. A Weber-Fergusson incision was made bilaterally from the midline of the upper lip and carried paranasally on either side. It was impossible to free the tumor intact from the antra and maxilla due to lack of fibrous encapsulation. Therefore, the center of the tumor was enucleated, and the remaining identifiable tumor tissue was curetted from the large defects. The ethmoid areas were involved with tumor also and were carefully curetted. The tumor was so large that gross cosmetic deformity remained after its removal. An attempt was made to leave periosteum and some fragments of bone in the midline. The large maxillary antral defects were packed with iodoform gauze, and the wound was closed with 4-0 chromic and silk. The palate itself was not incised, as it was possible to scoop tumor off the palate and still leave it intact.

All of the various tumor specimens exhibited a similar microscopic picture of proliferating fibroblasts in a uniform pattern, forming a loose fibrillar stroma (Fig. 8.16). The fibroblasts had an eosinophilic cytoplasm, distinct plump nuclei, and prominent nucleoli. Giant cells were quite plentiful, with a dozen or so nuclei present in many of them. The van Gieson stain demonstrated the distinct, peculiar perivascular cuffing of collagen seen around capillaries in cherubism lesions (Fig. 8.17). A substantial amount of mucopolysaccharide was detected

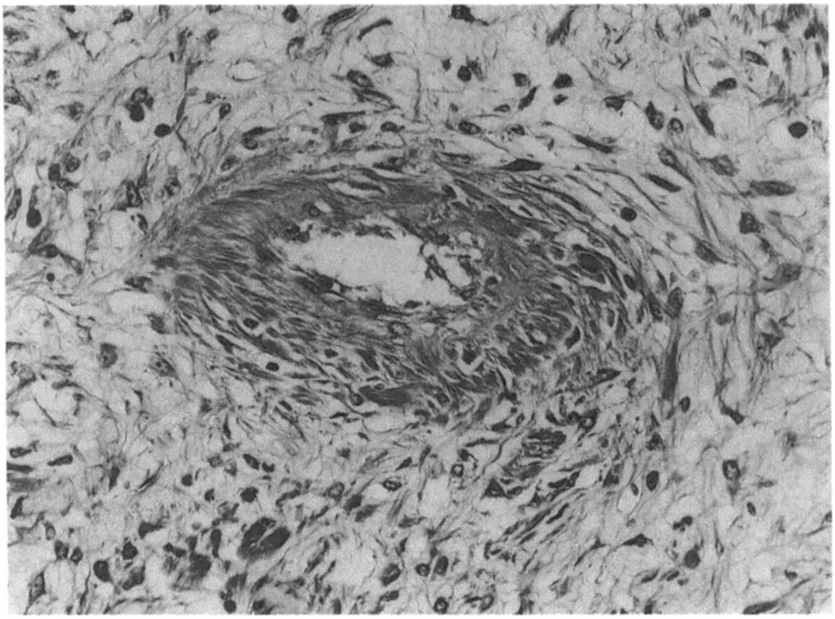

Fig. 8.17. Perivascular cuffing of collagen, characteristic for cherubism. Van Gieson stain, 1250

in the stromal tissue, using the Rinehart and azure blue pH 4.5 staining methods. Bony trabeculae were absent. The histopathologic diagnosis was cherubism.

Postoperatively, the patient fared well. After further evaluation, it was deemed that she would tolerate radical excision of her mandibular tumor lesions. Under similar inhalation general anesthesia on July 16, 1962, she underwent bilateral partial mandibulectomy. Tumor was more apparent and bulky in the patient's left mandible than in the right side. An intact bony septum divided the mandible at the midline preventing direct continuity of tumor from one side of the mandible to the other. Tumor had eroded through the cortex of the mandible anteriorly, superiorly, and inferiorly from the angles to the midline. Some cortex remained on either side of the angles, but tumor tissue extended up into the condylar portions. The bulk of the main tumor was removed as single specimens from each side of the mandible, and the remaining portions were curetted as cleanly as possible. The bony cortex at the angles was deliberately fractured in an attempt to lessen the size of the mandible and give a better cosmetic result. No packing was used, and the wound was closed with interrupted 3-0 plain catgut. A pressure dressing was applied to assist in maintaining the molded realigned contour of the mandible.

The histologic sections were similar to those seen in her maxillary tumor; the diagnosis again was cherubism. The pressure dressing was removed after 2 days, and the sutures were removed on the 6th postoperative day. The child tolerated this surgical procedure well, having a mild recovery period. By late July she was eating by mouth, and her esophageal feeding tube and tracheos-

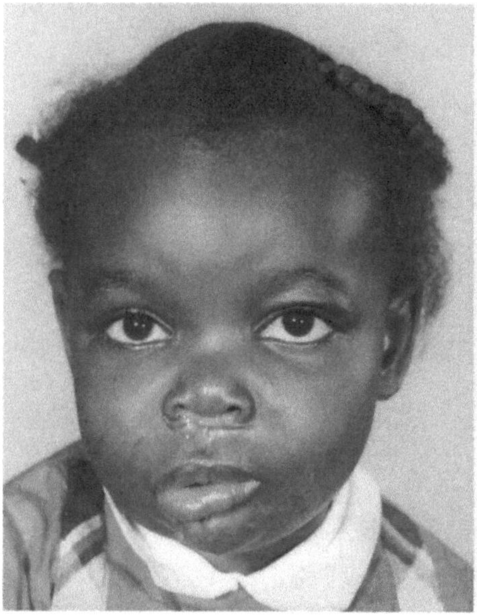

Fig. 8.18

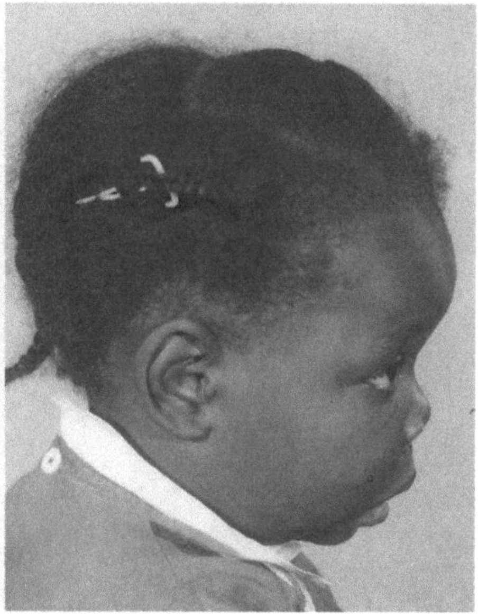

Fig. 8.19

Fig. 8.18. Frontal view, 7 months and 4 months respectively from her maxillary and mandibular surgery. Note the marked improvement

Fig. 8.19. Side view of the same patient for the same time periods postoperatively

tomy tube had removed. On her discharge on August 6, 1962, she was breathing normally and had no difficulty swallowing semisolid foods.

Figures 8.18 and 8.19 show the marked improvement in her clinical appearance 7 months postoperative from her maxillary and 4 months postoperatively from her mandibular surgery.

(G) Readmissions

There were three subsequent readmissions in 1963 and 1964 which revealed a normally developing child with no unusual findings or clinical evidence of tumor regrowth, and with a remarkable cosmetic improvement in her appearance. Mandibular radiographs demonstrated a minimal increase in the radiolucent cherubism lesions; however, one left maxillary radiolucency was noted to encroach upon the orbital region. Because she was eating normally, breathing without difficulty, and learning to articulate, no therapy was felt indicated at this time.

On March 1, 1967, the little girl was readmitted and hospitalized through April 8, 1967. She presented with marked progression of her maxillary lesions (Fig. 8.20). Tumor again displaced an intact palate, partially obliterating the oral cavity and preventing complete closure of her mouth. In addition, scarring contracture prevented approximation of her lips with resultant constant drool-

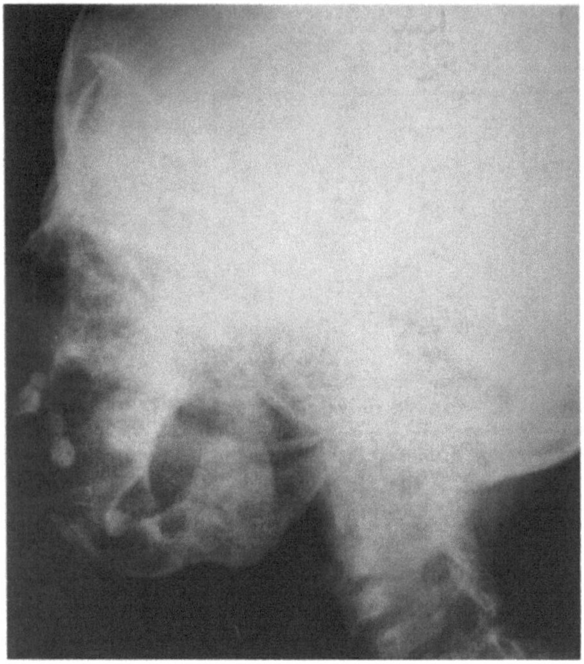

Fig. 8.20. Lateral head film depicting progression of her maxillary lesions in an active growth phase, 5 years after her original surgery

ing. On March 20, 1967, a preoperative tracheostomy was done under general anesthesia, and a recontouring procedure of the maxillae was performed. Fibrous tumor tissue was curetted from the maxillary antra, the nasal cavity, the sphenoids, and the ethmoids. Tumor had extended up to the left orbital floor. The previous upper and lower lip incisions were modified in order to free the lip contracture. The child withstood the surgery extremely well in spite of profuse bleeding from the tumor during its removal, requiring six units of blood. The histopathologic diagnosis was cherubism.

Postoperatively, cosmetic improvement was remarkable with the lips being free and mobile within the limits of the right mandibular nerve paralysis from her original surgery.

Subject Index

Functional Partial Laryngectomy

Conservation Surgery for Carcinoma of the Larynx

Editors: **M.E. Wigand, W. Steiner, P.M. Stell**
1984. 211 figures, 88 tables. Approx. 335 pages.
ISBN 3-540-13175-2

Contents: Introduction into Conservation Surgery for the Larynx. - Basics of Diagnosis and Planning of Therapy. - Vertical Partial Resection of the Larynx. - Horizontal Partial Resection of the Larynx. Surgical Management of the Lymphatic System. - Radiotherapy and Chemotherapy. - Postoperative Course After Vertical and Horizontal Partial Laryngectomy. - Final Synopsis of Conservating Surgery for Carcinoma of the Larynx. - Subject Index.

Internationally recognized laryngologists, pathologists and radiologists from 16 countries have combined their efforts in this book to provide a comprehensive survey of current diagnostic and surgical methods for cancer of the larynx. Their contributions reflect the state of the art in their particular fields and cover such important aspects of the preservation of laryngeal function as

- mass screening for early detection of cancer by means of magnifying and illuminating endoscopy
- the significance of intra - and postoperative histological examinations in surgical management
- new partial laryngectomy techniques based on narrow approaches to the primary tumor or discrete handling of regional lymphatic tissue
- the ise of the CO_2 laser in microsurgical resections
- the treatment of regional metastases based on careful consideration of possible side effects and increased oncological risks for the patient, and
- the adjuvant role of radio- and chemotherapy in the management of laryngeal cancer.

For the young laryngologist this book will serve as a comprehensive guide to the numerous modes of surgical treatment currently available for laryngeal carcinomas; for the experienced surgeon it will provide a fascinating survey of accepted and controversial techniques as performed by distinguished colleagues.

Springer-Verlag
Berlin
Heidelberg
New York
Tokyo

MIX
Papier aus verantwortungsvollen Quellen
Paper from responsible sources
FSC® C105338

If you have any concerns about our products,
you can contact us on
ProductSafety@springernature.com

In case Publisher is established outside the EU,
the EU authorized representative is:
Springer Nature Customer Service Center GmbH
Europaplatz 3, 69115 Heidelberg, Germany

Printed by Libri Plureos GmbH
in Hamburg, Germany